Blueprints

CLINICAL CASES
IN SURGERY

SECOND EDITION

SURGERY

Michelle Li, MD
Attending in General Surgery
California Pacific Medical Center
San Francisco, California

Stephanie C. Lin, MD
Attending in Vascular Surgery
Mills-Peninsula Hospital
Burlingame, California

Aaron B. Caughey, MD, MPP, MPH, PHD (Series Editor)
Assistant Professor in Residence
Department of Obstetrics, Gynecology, and Reproductive Sciences
University of California, San Francisco
San Francisco, California

D0231517

Wolters Kluwer | Lippincott Williams & Wilkins
Health
Philadelphia • Baltimore • New York • London
Buenos Aires • Hong Kong • Sydney • Tokyo

Acquisitions Editor: Nancy Anastasi Duffy
Managing Editor: Stacey L. Sebring
Marketing Manager: Jennifer Kuklinski
Production Editor: Jennifer D.W. Glazer
Designer: Doug Smock
Compositor: International Typesetting and Composition
Printer: R.R. Donnelley & Sons—Crawfordsville

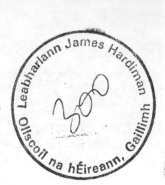

351 West Camden Street
Baltimore, MD 21201

530 Walnut Street
Philadelphia, PA 19106

Printed in the United States of America

First Edition, 2002, Blackwell Science

Library of Congress Cataloging-in-Publication Data

Li, Michelle.
 Blueprints clinical cases in surgery/Michelle Li, Stephanie C. Lin,
Aaron B. Caughey.—2nd ed.
  p. ; cm.—(Blueprints. Clinical cases)
 Includes index.
 ISBN-13: 978-1-4051-0493-7
 ISBN-10: 1-4051-0493-7
 1. Surgery—Case studies. I. Lin, Stephanie C. II. Caughey,
Aaron B. III. Title. IV. Title: Clinical cases in surgery. V. Series.
 [DNLM: 1. Surgical Procedures, Operative—Case Reports.
2. Surgical Procedures, Operative—Problems and Exercises.
3. Perioperative Care—Case Reports. 4. Perioperative Care
—Problems and Exercises. WO 18.2 L693b 2007]
RD34.L44 2007
617—dc22

                              2006026470

The publishers have made every effort to trace the copyright holders for borrowed material. If they have inadvertently overlooked any, they will be pleased to make the necessary arrangements at the first opportunity.

To purchase additional copies of this book, call our customer service department at **(800) 638-3030** or fax orders to **(301) 223-2320**. International customers should call **(301) 223-2300**.

Visit Lippincott Williams & Wilkins on the Internet: http://www.LWW.com. Lippincott Williams & Wilkins customer service representatives are available from 8:30 am to 6:00 pm, EST.

07 08 09 10
3 4 5 6 7 8 9 10

Dedication

To the faculty and residents at the University of California, San Francisco: I still hear and try to live by the tenets of your wisdom, and I feel now more than ever the security of your support and everlasting friendship. To my family and friends: Every day I am grateful for the privilege of being a part of your lives. To the very special people at New York Presbyterian Hospital: I would not be here without you, as coworkers, mentors, and friends, and that is a gift that I can never repay.
Stephanie

With greatest appreciation to my mentors, colleagues, partners, and patients; for continuing to help me learn the art of medicine and the practice of surgery. And with gratitude to my friends and family, who keep it all in perspective.
Michelle

To my family, Aidan, Ashby, and Susan
Aaron

Preface

Blueprints Clinical Cases in Surgery is designed to supplement and enrich the clinical experience of the medical student or subintern rotating through surgery. The cases we have chosen reflect the broad scope of problems encountered in this very diverse field. From elective outpatient evaluations to emergent inpatient consultations and perioperative management considerations, our goal has been to cover those scenarios that are most likely to be encountered on Boards, inservice or shelf examinations, and rounds. As such, the majority of the cases are basic general surgery based; however, a small sampling of the more common urologic, orthopedic, otolaryngologic and neurosurgical problems are presented as well.

Understanding the diagnosis and management of surgical disease requires a firm grasp of the fundamentals of many specialties, including internal medicine, pediatrics, neurology, radiology, pathology, and anesthesia. Therefore, we encourage readers to use their background knowledge in these fields to develop comprehensive diagnostic and therapeutic options in these cases. In particular, it is important to remember that not all "surgical" patients require an operation!

Case Format

The cases are designed to take you through the clinical thought process, beginning with a chief complaint (or consultation request), proceeding through the history, exam, and diagnostic tests, and ending with diagnosis and/or management. The specific case components are described in further detail below.

Title/Chief Complaint (CC/ID): These are common presenting symptoms or signs which are meant to suggest a broad differential diagnosis to begin the thought process.

History of Present Illness (HPI): The HPI is the initial descriptive history as given by the patient and/or elicited by the examiner, and may include a brief review of pertinent systems. At the end of the HPI, the reader should reconsider or refine the differential diagnosis, think about findings that might be anticipated on physical exam, and begin to plan what diagnostic tests (if any) to order. Some of this process has been formalized in the thought questions.

Past History (PMHx/PSHx): The past medical, surgical, social, and family histories, medication lists and allergies are meant to augment the HPI and to put the patient's presenting complaint into context. It is important to consider how baseline medical status will impact the differential diagnosis and eventual treatment plans.

Vital Signs (VS)/Physical Exam (PE): These are critical components of the patient evaluation. The findings in this section will provide information for further narrowing the differential diagnosis, and should be used to confirm or justify the need for specific diagnostic tests. It is important to note that in the interest of space, we have presented only a representative selection of pertinent positives and negatives. If a portion of the history or PE that you are interested in is not discussed, assume it to be normal or noncontributory.

Labs/X-ray: Again, we have included only the pertinent positive and negative findings. Common abbreviations are used, as well as the standard format for the complete blood count and electrolyte panels (see list). We have included images with many of the cases to further enhance the experience of incorporating these visual tools into the diagnostic process.

Thought Questions and Discussion: These open-ended questions are meant to stimulate the thought processes related to diagnosis, pathophysiology, and treatment. These are located throughout each case, often at natural decision points. It is intended that you read these questions and then spend some time reflecting on possible answers, prior to continuing on with the case. The discussion section follows immediately, so try not to read ahead. Consider actually writing the answers down, or if working in a group, discussing the possibilities.

Multiple Choice Questions: These are meant to be in-service or Board-style (shelf-exam) questions, and should be completed at the **conclusion** of each case. These questions and answers provide additional information about the case diagnosis, and address other conditions in the differential that are worth knowing about. In some cases, we have used the multiple choice section to introduce or discuss conditions that are less closely related to the actual case in order to touch on important material not described elsewhere in the book.

In addition to proceeding through the cases in an orderly fashion, we offer a few more suggestions on how to get the most out of these surgical cases:

1. **Approach the cases as you approach your patients.** Read the information carefully, pay attention to details and "key phrases," and think about what you would ask or do next.
2. **Note the obvious as well as the subtle signs of patient discomfort.** Much of the information gathered from the sick patient is nonverbal. Vital signs, language, attitude,

and the way in which a patient sits or moves may all give important clues in evaluating pain, fear, and disability. These signs may often be the most reliable sources of information in the stoic or hypochondriac patient.

3. **Keep the timecourse in mind.** Surgeons encounter emergent, urgent, semi-elective, and elective cases. The relative luxury of working up a stable, asymptomatic patient is obviously different than the combined diagnosis and management of, for instance, a trauma victim. *Patient safety and well-being must always come first.* Any unstable or marginal patient should be regularly subjected to an evaluation of the ABC's (Airway, Breathing, Circulation—almost always a correct management answer on rounds!). Ensuring the integrity of the ABC's will always supercede making a specific diagnosis (e.g. by CT scan). In reality, however, diagnostic evaluation, triage, and management are usually occurring in parallel. Don't forget about the patient while trying to determine the disease.

4. **Think about operations you've seen.** This will enhance your understanding of the case presentations, as it will link the dynamic of the OR to the perioperative process. We have generally stayed away from technical commentary and most operations are not specifically described at the end of the cases. Instead, we have focused primarily on evaluation and diagnosis since it really is the cornerstone of what we do.

5. **Read about topics that you want to know more about.** Standard texts and literature searches can augment your understanding of the many complex diseases described herein.

6. **Remember that surgery, like all of medicine, is a constantly changing field.** Check with the surgeons with whom you are working to find out the latest information on diagnosis and treatment. Recognize that institutional preferences may color their (and your) experience, opinions and treatment algorithms. Understand the rationale for these differences, and ask questions when you need to!.

We hope that you will find these cases to be fun, interesting and informative, and a good complement to your experience on the surgical services. Good luck in your studies!

Michelle LI, MD
Stephanie Lin, MD
Aaron B. Caughey, MD, MPP, MPH, PHD

Contents

Abbreviations/Acronyms

Normal temp= 98 - 99° F

AAA	abdominal aortic aneurysm
ABCs	Airway, Breathing, Circulation
ABG	arterial blood gas
ABI	ankle brachial index
ACTH	adrenocorticotropic hormone
ALT	alanine aminotransferase (same as SGPT)
AO	alert and oriented (i.e., to person, place, time, reason)
appy	appendectomy
ASA	aspirin (acetylsalicylic acid)
ASD	atrial septal defect
AST	aspartate aminotransferase (same as SGOT)
AVSS	afebrile, vital signs stable
BE	barium enema
BP	blood pressure
BM	bowel movement
BPH	benign prostatic hypertrophy
BUN	blood urea nitrogen
CABG	coronary artery bypass grafting
CAD	coronary artery disease
CBC	complete blood count
CBD	common bile duct
CC/ID	chief complaint and identification
CEA	carcinoembryonic antigen
CHF	congestive heart failure
CMT	cervical motion tenderness
CNS	central nervous system
COPD	chronic obstructive pulmonary disease
Cr	creatinine
CRC	colorectal cancer
CRI	chronic renal insufficiency
CT	computed tomography
CTA	clear to auscultation
CXR	chest x-ray
ddx	differential diagnosis
DM	diabetes mellitus
DP	dorsalis pedis (pulse)

DVT	deep venous thrombosis
ECG	electrocardiogram
ED	Emergency Department
EGD	esophagogastroduodenoscopy
EOMI	extraocular movements intact
ERCP	endoscopic retrograde cholangiopancreatography
ESR	erythrocyte sedimentation rate
FFP	fresh frozen plasma
FM	face mask
FNA	fine-needle aspiration
GxPx	gravida x, para x
GER	gastroesophageal reflux
GERD	gastroesophageal reflux disease
GI	gastrointestinal
GIB	gastrointestinal bleed
Hb	hemoglobin
hCG	human chorionic gonadotropin
Hct	hematocrit
HDL	high density lipoprotein (cholesterol)
HEENT	head, eyes, ears, nose, throat
HIV	human immunodeficiency virus
HPI	history of present illness
HR	heart rate
HTN	hypertension
IBD	inflammatory bowel disease
ICU	intensive care unit
IMA	inferior mesenteric artery
INR	International Normalized Ratio
IV	intravenous
IVF	intravenous fluid
JVD	jugular venous distension
KUB	kidneys/ureter/bladder (x-ray)
LA	left atrial
LDH	lactate dehydrogenase
LDL	low density lipoprotein (cholesterol)
LES	lower esophageal sphincter
LFTs	liver function tests
LHRH	luteinizing hormone-releasing hormone
LLQ	left lower quadrant
LMP	last menstrual period
LR	lactated Ringer (solution)
LUQ	left upper quadrant
LV	left ventricular
Lytes	electrolytes

MEN	multiple endocrine neoplasia
MI	myocardial infarction
MRI	magnetic resonance imaging
MVA	motor vehicle accident
MVI	multivitamin
NAD	no apparent distress
NC	nasal cannula
NG	nasogastric
NGT	nasogastric tube
NKDA	no known drug allergies
nl	normal
NPO	nil per os (nothing by mouth)
NS	normal saline (solution)
NSAID	nonsteroidal anti-inflammatory drug
NSVD	normal spontaneous vaginal delivery
NT/ND	nontender/nondistended
OR	Operating Room
PA	posteroanterior
PE	physical examination
PERRLA	pupils equally round and reactive to light and accommodation
PID	pelvic inflammatory disease
Plts	platelets
ppd	packs per day
PRBC	packed red blood cells
PSA	prostate-specific antigen
PT	prothrombin time
PTT	partial thromboplastin time
PUD	peptic ulcer disease
PVD	peripheral vascular disease
pyh	pack year history
RA	right atrial OR room air
RBC	red blood cell
RLQ	right lower quadrant
RQ	respiratory quotient
RR	respiratory rate
RRR	regular rate and rhythm
RUQ	right upper quadrant
RV	right ventricular
SBO	small bowel obstruction
SGOT	serum glutamic-oxaloacetic transaminase
SGPT	serum glutamic-pyruvic transaminase
SIADH	syndrome of inappropriate (secretion of) antidiuretic hormone

SMA	superior mesenteric artery
T&A	tonsillectomy and adenoidectomy
TIA	transient ischemic attack
TIPS	transjugular intrahepatic portosystemic shunt
TM	tympanic membrane
TPN	total parenteral nutrition
TSH	thyroid-stimulating hormone
T_4	thyroxine
TTP	tender to palpation
TURP	transurethral resection of the prostate
UA	urinalysis
UTI	urinary tract infection
VMA	vanillylmandelic acid
VS	vital signs
WBC	white blood cell (count)
WD/WN	well-developed, well-nourished
WNL	within normal limits
XR	x-ray

$$\text{CBC:} \quad \text{WBC} \begin{matrix} \text{Hb} \\ \hline \text{Hct} \end{matrix} \text{Plts} \qquad \text{LYTES:} \begin{array}{c|c|c} \text{Na} & \text{Cl} & \text{BUN} \\ \hline \text{K} & \text{CO}_2 & \text{Cr} \end{array} \text{glc}$$

I

Abdominal Pain

Abdominal Pain with Nausea

CC/ID: Previously healthy 22-year-old woman with abdominal pain, nausea, vomiting, and anorexia.

HPI: Ms. X presents to the Emergency Department (ED) with 18 hours of crampy abdominal pain increasing in intensity over the last few hours, worse in the right lower quadrant (RLQ). Her pain started approximately 2 hours after eating a taco for lunch and was followed by some nausea and three episodes of bilious vomiting that did not relieve her pain. Since lunch, she has had no desire to eat and has only kept down a few sips of tea. No prior episodes of similar pain. Last menstrual period (LMP) was "about 3 weeks ago."

THOUGHT QUESTION

- What do you think are the most likely diagnoses?
- What other information and physical findings will assist in sorting through the differential?

DISCUSSION

In this young healthy woman, acute appendicitis and gynecologic processes such as pelvic inflammatory disease (PID), ovarian torsion, and ectopic pregnancy should probably be high on your list. Other possibilities would include cholecystitis, incarcerated or strangulated hernia, urinary tract infection (UTI)/pyelonephritis, viral syndromes, bowel obstruction, pancreatitis, and mesenteric adenitis. Questions regarding sexual activity, birth control, urinary pain or frequency, bowel habits, hernias (i.e., masses that may be noted to come and go), history of prior surgeries, or risk factors for pancreatitis (e.g., alcohol or other drug use, gallstones) will

3

offer important information that can help to narrow the differential. The physical examination should begin as you are gathering the history, because some findings will be evident before touching the patient. For instance, patients with peritoneal inflammation will often draw their knees up to relax the overlying abdominal wall. In addition, any movement, even slight, can cause abdominal pain. Of course, the abdominal examination itself will allow you to assess for pain, referred pain, tympany (as with obstruction), masses, and evidence of prior surgeries.

CASE CONTINUED

On further questioning, you find that she has been passing stool and gas and has had no symptoms of dysuria or urinary frequency, no notice of groin or belly button bulges, and no vaginal discharge. She has not been sexually active in the past 6 months.

VS: Temp 99.5°F, BP 95/50, HR 100

PE: *Gen:* Thin woman in moderate distress, lying flat on her back, very still, knees drawn up. AO × 3. Bumping into her gurney causes her to wince in pain. *Abdomen:* No scars. Soft, flat with slight fullness and rebound tenderness in the RLQ. No other masses, voluntary guarding. Nontympanitic. There is tenderness to percussion and palpation over McBurney's point*, but deep palpation of the LLQ elicits pain at McBurney's point as well (positive Rovsing's sign). No hernias are found. She has no obturator or psoas signs. *Pelvic:* No discharge. No CMT. No clear adnexal masses, but RLQ tenderness on palpation of the R adnexa. *Rectal:* Nontender, nl tone. No masses. Heme negative.

Labs: WBC 13, with a left shift and an amylase of 150. The remainder of the CBC and LFTs are within normal limits. Urinalysis shows a few red cells and a few white cells but is otherwise clean. Urine pregnancy test is negative.

*Comment: McBurney's point is a point located one-third the distance from the anterior superior iliac spine to the umbilicus (Fig. 1-1). Positive psoas and obturator signs are suggestive of a retrocecal appendix. The former is elicited on passive extension of the hip; the latter on passive internal rotation of the flexed hip. A painful mass on digital rectal examination may also be suggestive of a retrocecal appendix.

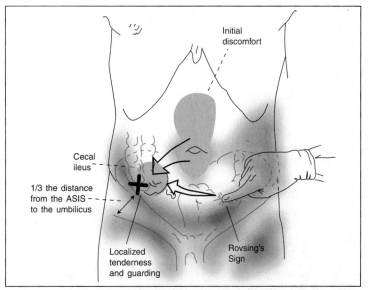

FIGURE 1-1. McBurney's Point (marked by an "X") is located at a point one-third the distance from the right anterior superior iliac spine (ASIS) to the umbilicus, sometimes thought of as approximately 4 cm from the right ASIS. This is the most common site of localized RLQ tenderness in cases of acute appendicitis. Rovsing's sign indicates pain referred to the RLQ upon palpation of the LLQ. (*Illustration by Shawn Girsberger Graphic Design.*)

QUESTIONS

1-1. Given these findings, you suspect the patient has a surgical abdomen. Which of the following is the most common diagnostic study ordered?

    A. Barium enema
    B. Abdominal ultrasound
    C. Computed tomography (CT)
    D. Magnetic resonance imaging (MRI)
    E. Colonoscopy

1-2. The "classic" progression of symptoms in acute appendicitis is

    A. Nausea/vomiting, crampy epigastric pain, RLQ pain.
    B. RLQ pain, crampy epigastric pain, nausea/vomiting.
    C. Crampy epigastric pain, dysuria, nausea/vomiting.
    D. Crampy epigastric pain, nausea/vomiting, RLQ pain.
    E. Nausea/vomiting, constipation, abdominal distension.

1-3. The incidence of retrocecal appendix is
A. <5%.
B. 15% to 20%.
C. 40% to 50%.
D. 65% to 75%.
E. >85%.

1-4. Neoplasms are found in ~0.5% of appendectomies. Which of the following is the most common type?
A. Adenocarcinoma
B. Carcinoid
C. Lymphoma
D. Melanoma
E. Metastatic tumor

ANSWERS

1-1. C. The data in this case are consistent with acute appendicitis. In many centers, the history, physical, and laboratory findings are enough to warrant a trip to the OR for appendectomy. However, because of the potential for other confounding diagnoses, particularly in women or in older patients in whom other pathology is more common (e.g., diverticulitis, cancer), imaging studies may be a useful adjunct.[1] Ultrasound is an excellent tool to evaluate for biliary disease and ovarian pathology and has an 80% sensitivity and 90% specificity for acute appendicitis. The classic findings in acute appendicitis, when seen, are a noncompressible appendix and a "target sign," which is the distended lumen and thickened wall of the appendix seen on end. CT allows for evaluation of most intra-abdominal processes and can be very helpful in the patient with atypical presentations of abdominal pain. Common findings in appendicitis (95% sensitivity, 90% specificity) include thickened appendiceal walls and pericecal or RLQ inflammation and fat stranding. Occasionally, a fecalith may be seen. The appendix may not fill with contrast secondary to pathologic obstruction of the lumenal orifice. Plain films may be ordered as part of a routine abdominal pain workup but are best for evaluation of free air or bowel obstruction and only rarely show a RLQ fecalith suggestive of appendicitis (30% sensitivity, 50% to 80% specificity). In the context of this patient's history and exam, plain x-ray studies would not offer any additional significant useful information.

[1] Sensitivity and specificity are as reported in Surgery: *Basic Science and Clinical Evidence* (2001), Ch. 32.

In this case, it would be justified to go straight to the operating room (OR). A 10% to 20% negative appendectomy rate is commonly accepted because of the significant morbidity and mortality associated with a missed ruptured appendix. Laparoscopy can be used for both diagnosis and treatment, but at this time open appendectomy remains the standard of care.

Observation plays no role in the patient with an acute abdomen. However, in patients in whom the diagnosis is equivocal, serial exams may save an unnecessary trip to the OR. Patients who present early in the course of appendicitis may develop classic signs over the next few hours; other patients may have their symptoms resolve with hydration and time. In the absence of complications (e.g., abscess/peritonitis/sepsis), patients seldom have temperature elevations of >1° above normal.

In a patient who has had a prolonged time course to her symptoms and/or who has had an abscess identified on imaging studies (most commonly in very young or in elderly patients), the treatment is broad-spectrum antibiotics (covering gram-positive, gram-negative, and anaerobic organisms), percutaneous drainage of the defined abscess, and interval (delayed) appendectomy, usually after about 6 weeks.

1-2. D. The "classic" presentation history is one of crampy/vague abdominal pain followed by nausea and/or vomiting, progressing to pain localized to the RLQ. However, this presentation really only occurs in ~50% of cases.

1-3. B. Diagnosis may be somewhat more difficult in patients with a retrocecal appendix, because local inflammation will be less likely to involve the anterior parietal peritoneum. As such, it is important to perform a rectal exam and to look for psoas and obturator signs in patients with a suspicious history.

1-4. B. Carcinoid accounts for most tumors found in the appendix. When tumors are <2 cm in size, appendectomy is considered curative. For larger tumors, right hemicolectomy is recommended.

SUGGESTED ADDITIONAL READING

Hagendorf BA, Clarke JR, Burd RS. The optimal initial management of children with suspected appendicitis: a decision analysis. J Pediatr Surg 2004;39:880–885.

Jones PF. Suspected acute appendicitis: trends in management
    over 30 years. Br J Surg 2001;88:1570–1577.
Kraemer M, Franke C, Ohmann C, et al. Acute Abdominal Pain
    Study Group. Acute appendicitis in late adulthood: incidence,
    presentation, and outcome: Results of a prospective multicenter
    acute abdominal pain study and a review of the literature.
    Langenbecks Arch Surg 2000;385:470–481.
Pinto Leite N, Pereira JM, Cunha R, et al. CT evaluation of
    appendicitis and its complications: imaging techniques and key
    diagnostic findings. AJR Am J Roentgenol 2005;185:406–417.

Abdominal Pain Following Meals

CC/ID: 45-year-old woman with colicky RUQ pain.

HPI: Ms. X presents to urgent care with several hours of crampy, now fairly constant pain in her right upper quadrant. The pain sometimes radiates to her right shoulder blade. She notes that her symptoms began shortly after dinner the previous evening and have gradually worsened. She has been intermittently nauseated but has not had any episodes of emesis. She believes she may be developing a fever. She does have a history of pain in this location, usually after meals, but it has never been this bad and has always been short-lived. She has no appetite.

PMHx: Negative

PSHx: G$_3$P$_3$, perimenopausal; mild HTN, no meds required; no h/o abdominal surgery

VS: Temp 38.1°C, BP 140/85, HR 105

PE: *Gen:* Obese woman in minimal distress, able to move around with some effort. *HEENT:* Mucous membranes slightly dry, eyes anicteric. *Chest:* CTA bilaterally. *Abdomen:* No scars; nondistended; some guarding, but otherwise soft with TTP in the right upper quadrant. No rebound tenderness. Cessation of deep inspiration upon palpation of the right subcostal area (positive Murphy's sign). *Pelvic:* No tenderness, masses, discharge. *Rectal:* nl tone, nontender, no masses, heme negative.

THOUGHT QUESTION

- What is your differential diagnosis at this point? What is the significance of the positive Murphy's sign?

- Would the diagnosis change if the patient was jaundiced or icteric?
- What diagnostic studies would be most helpful to confirm or rule out your suspicions?

DISCUSSION

The differential diagnosis for right upper quadrant (RUQ) pain should include biliary diseases, such as cholelithiasis, cholecystitis, and cholangitis; pneumonia; peptic ulcer disease; acute pancreatitis; appendicitis; renal colic; and gonococcal perihepatitis (Fitz-Hugh-Curtis syndrome). In addition, any woman of child-bearing age should be evaluated for possible ectopic pregnancy. A positive Murphy's sign is suggestive of acute cholecystitis.

Charcot's triad is characterized by biliary colic (RUQ pain), fever (+ /– chills), and jaundice. This trio of findings is significant for acute cholangitis, which can progress to systemic decompensation if not adequately addressed. Patients with cholecystitis may also have some mild jaundice, but as a rule, the findings are less pronounced than with cholangitis.

Lab tests should include a CBC (particularly to examine white cell count) and LFTs. The best imaging modality for examination of the biliary system is ultrasound. Plain XRs will infrequently show calcified stones but may give information regarding obstruction or free air, if these were of concern (not really consistent in this patient's case). CT is excellent for evaluating other organs but is generally less preferable to ultrasound for looking at the gallbladder.

CASE CONTINUED

Labs: WBC 14 with a left shift. Total bilirubin, alkaline phosphatase, and amylase are at the upper limits of normal. Transaminases are WNL. Urinalysis is negative for signs of UTI. Urine pregnancy test is negative.

Imaging: Ultrasound shows stones in a mildly dilated gallbladder. There is gallbladder wall thickening and pericholecystic fluid. The diameter of the CBD is at the upper limit of normal. See Figure 2-1.

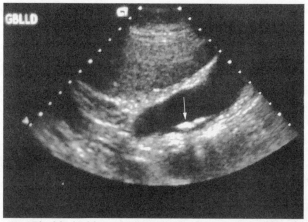

FIGURE 2-1. The black oblong shape extending from the right side of this lateral ultrasound image is the gallbladder. Note the echogenic (bright white) gallstones along the bottom side of the gallbladder sac, which leave shadows distal to the transducer. (*Image provided by Department of Radiology, University of California, San Francisco.*)

The patient likely has acute cholecystitis based on physical, laboratory, and ultrasound findings. She should be admitted for IV fluids and antibiotics. The end point is usually resolution of symptoms and normalization of lab tests. The standard of care in most centers is to perform cholecystectomy before discharge. The former thinking was that patients should recover for a period of 6 weeks and then return for elective cholecystectomy, but a number of patients have recurrent attacks before that time. Furthermore, these patients are at risk for gallstone pancreatitis and its associated morbidity and mortality. The technique of laparoscopic cholecystectomy has facilitated removal of the gallbladder in the acute setting.

 QUESTIONS

2-1. What features make up Reynold's pentad?
   A. Fever, nausea, epigastric pain, anemia, rash.
   B. RUQ pain, jaundice, emesis, headache, tingling.
   C. Jaundice, fever, RUQ/biliary pain, mental status changes, hypotension.
   D. Fever, back pain, icterus, hematemesis, diarrhea.

2-2. What are the classic "F"s of gallstone disease?
  A. Female, fat, fertile, forty.
  B. Female, fifty, fair, fit.
  C. Fellows, forty, fraternal, febrile.
  D. Fellows, fifty, fat, freckled.

2-3. CT is often less preferable to ultrasound for imaging the gallbladder because
  A. Other organs cannot be evaluated.
  B. It is difficult to estimate gallbladder size on CT.
  C. The rib cage interferes with adequate visualization.
  D. Gallstones can be similar in density to bile and are often difficult to see on CT.

2-4. Acalculous cholecystitis:
  A. Is more common than calculous disease.
  B. Typically occurs in otherwise healthy patients.
  C. Usually involves sludge in the gall bladder.
  D. Is the precursor to gangrenous cholecystitis.

ANSWERS

2-1. C. Reynold's pentad includes the findings of Charcot's triad (indicating cholangitis), with the addition of mental status changes and hypotension or shock. These suggest progression to a septic state. In the patient with cholangitis, IV antibiotics are the rule, but failure to improve mandates decompression of the CBD. This may be done in an open fashion, but most centers would proceed with an endoscopic (ERCP) approach. If the patient had a more elevated amylase, elevation in transaminases, and/or findings of CBD obstruction, a diagnosis of acute pancreatitis might be entertained. Treatment is similar to that for acute cholecystitis, usually with cholecystectomy after clinical stabilization and before discharge from the hospital.

2-2. A. Known risk factors for gallstones include female sex, obesity, multiparity, and age >40.

2-3. D. Because gallstones may be difficult to visualize on CT, this modality is usually not an optimal first-line imaging study. However, if the history and exam are equivocal, CT may offer more specific information regarding other intra-abdominal processes.

2-4. C. Acalculous cholecystitis occurs primarily in critically ill patients following trauma, sepsis, or other serious illnesses requiring prolonged intensive care or parenteral nutrition. More rarely, it may be caused by vasculitis, gall bladder torsion, or infection. In these situations, gall bladder motility and emptying is impaired and may lead to dehydration of the bile.

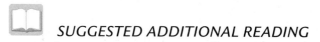

SUGGESTED ADDITIONAL READING

Abou-Saif A, Al-Kawas FH. Complications of gallstone disease: Mirizzi syndrome, cholecystocholedochal fistula, and gallstone ileus. Am J Gastroenterol 2002;97:249–254.

Bhattacharya D, Ammori BJ. Contemporary minimally invasive approaches to the management of acute cholecystitis: a review and appraisal. Surg Laparosc Endosc Percutan Tech 2005;15:1–8.

Lillemoe KD. Surgical treatment of biliary tract infections. Am Surg 2000;66:138–144.

Yusoff IF, Barkun JS, Barkun AN. Diagnosis and management of cholecystitis and cholangitis. Gastroenterol Clin North Am 2003;32:1145–1168.

Lower Abdominal Pain

CC/ID: 72-year-old man with lower abdominal pain and diarrhea.

HPI: Mr. X presents with a 3- to 4-day h/o crampy left greater than right lower abdominal pain and occasional blood-spotted loose stools. He has a h/o intermittent blood in his stool but has always attributed this to his hemorrhoids. He has had no recent changes in his food intake—he tends to eat a "balanced" diet but states that in the past his doctors have told him he should eat more fiber. He has had no nausea or vomiting but believes he has had some fevers. Per his history, colonoscopy done ~5 years ago showed some "pits," but no other findings that he can remember.

PMHx: HTN, CAD, former smoker (35 pyh), BPH

PSHx: Open cholecystectomy, some sort of "look around" in his abdomen during the war, TURP

Meds: "Blood pressure medicine," aspirin, MVI, "something else for my heart"

VS: Temp 38.5°C, BP 130/85, HR 65

PE: *Gen:* AO × 3, pleasant elderly man in moderate distress. *HEENT:* Anicteric, mucous membranes dry. *Chest:* Scattered wheezes throughout. *CV:* RRR, S_4 gallop, no murmurs or rubs. *Abdomen:* Well-healed midline and R subcostal scars; normal active bowel sounds; soft, nondistended, with TTP in the LLQ >RLQ and a questionable fullness in the LLQ; no guarding or rebound; no hernias. *Rectal:* Easily reducible, noninflamed prolapsing internal hemorrhoid, heme neg.

THOUGHT QUESTION

- Why is this patient febrile? What effect may his medications have on his clinical presentation?
- To what may the patient be referring in regards to his last colonoscopy?

DISCUSSION

You would expect that an infection or other inflammatory process is causing this patient's fever. However, in the elderly population, it is common for patients not to be able to mount a significant febrile response—this should be considered when examining the patient's vital signs. In addition, many cardioactive medications can cause bradycardia and/or hypotension, which may confound the picture. Febrile patients are generally tachycardic, suggesting that this patient may be on a beta-blocker or calcium channel blocker. Such considerations will have an impact on management in the older patient.

"Pits" or "pockets" or "pouches" are among the terms that patients remember in trying to describe diverticula. He could also be referring to ulcers or other manifestations of IBD. A thorough history can help to sort out these possibilities.

CASE CONTINUED

Labs: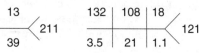

Imaging: *Abdominal series:* No dilated loops of bowel, no free air, no stones. *CT:* Diverticula throughout the distal colon. 2 × 2 cm enhancing fluid collection adjacent to the sigmoid colon. See Figure 3-1.

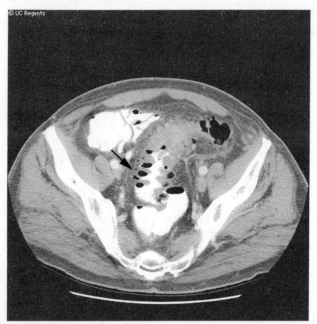

FIGURE 3-1. In this CT of the pelvis, diverticula are seen as small black (air-filled) spaces adjacent to the (rectal) contrast. Note that as you follow the contrast anteriorly, the lumen narrows and stranding, inflammation, and free air are seen. (*Image provided by Department of Radiology, University of California, San Francisco.*)

You diagnose the patient with acute diverticulitis with localized abscess and start him on a course of broad-spectrum antibiotics. There is usually no need to operate for acute sequelae of diverticula in the absence of frank peritonitis or persistent bleeding. Some recommend prophylactic sigmoidectomy when the acute infection has passed, whereas others reserve surgery until at least a second episode has occurred. If there is a large or well-organized fluid collection, percutaneous drainage may be advisable.

 QUESTIONS

3-1. Diverticulitis differs from diverticulosis in that
   A. Diverticulitis refers to disease of the left colon, whereas diverticulosis is of the right colon.

B. Diverticulitis occurs in the elderly, whereas diverticulosis occurs in the young.
C. Diverticulitis describes an inflammatory process, often associated with perforation, whereas diverticulosis describes an anatomic condition, sometimes associated with bleeding.
D. Diverticulitis is a surgical emergency, diverticulosis is not.

3-2. Colonoscopy is contraindicated in this scenario because
A. There is nothing to biopsy.
B. Insufflation can exacerbate a perforation.
C. Pus will be tracked proximally.
D. Sedation should be avoided in these patients.

3-3. A negative colonoscopy screen for cancer generally means that the next screen should be in
A. 6 to 18 months
B. 2 to 3 years
C. 3 to 5 years
D. 7 to 10 years

3-4. A potential complication of diverticulitis is
A. Stricture
B. Inflammatory bowel disease
C. Short gut syndrome
D. Hemorrhoids

ANSWERS

3-1. C. *Diverticulosis* refers to the presence of diverticula, which are outpouchings of the colon wall. *Diverticulitis* refers to inflammation of a diverticulum or diverticula. Diverticula that become inflamed tend to be more common on the left and those that bleed tend to be more common on the right. However, either process can occur in either location and in any age group. Neither condition absolutely mandates surgical intervention; this decision should be based on the patient's clinical condition and response to nonoperative management.

3-2. B. Insufflation can cause or exacerbate a perforation and is generally contraindicated in this situation.

3-3. D. Although the exact recommendations change frequently, most health care providers would agree that a 3- to 5-year interval between sigmoidoscopy or 7 to 10 years between colonoscopy is appropriate, given negative findings on the initial study and no other risk factors or signs (e.g., family history, blood in stool).

3-4. A. Complications of diverticulitis include stricture, perforation, and fistula (to bladder, skin, vagina, or other bowel).

SUGGESTED ADDITIONAL READING

Buckley O, Geoghegan T, O'Riordain DS, et al. Computed tomography in the imaging of colonic diverticulitis. Clin Radiol 2004 Nov;59:977–983.

Chung CC, Tsang WW, Kwok SY, et al. Laparoscopy and its current role in the management of colorectal disease. Colorectal Dis 2003;5:528–543.

Stollman N, Raskin JB. Diverticular disease of the colon. Lancet 2004;363:631–639.

Whetsone D, Hazey J, Pofahl WE 2nd, et al. Current management of diverticulitis. Curr Surg 2004;61:361–365.

Acute Epigastric Pain

CC/ID: 31-year-old man with acute-onset epigastric pain.

HPI: Mr. X presents with severe unrelenting pain felt just above his umbilicus. The pain is sharp and nonradiating. He specifically remembers being on his way to a client meeting when the pain began and has not felt relief since. He has never had a history of similar pain. He denies any nausea, vomiting, fever, chills, or sweats and had been eating normally until the onset of symptoms. He takes an occasional antacid for "heartburn" or "stomach cramps" but did not get any relief from doing so in this instance.

PMHx: Negative

PSHx: Tonsillectomy in childhood.

SHx: Smokes ~1 ppd.

VS: Temp 37.9°C, BP 110/70, HR 110

PE: *Gen:* Fit young man in moderate distress. *Chest:* Clear, without rales or signs of consolidation. *Abdomen:* Min. distended, no scars, quiet, firm, slightly tympanitic; diffuse TTP. *Genitals:* No scrotal swelling, redness, or TTP. *Rectal:* nl tone, no masses, heme negative.

THOUGHT QUESTION

- What is the differential diagnosis in this young man with acute onset of pain?
- Is there any significance to his h/o "heartburn"?
- What is the role of acid hypersecretion in peptic ulcer disease (PUD)?
- What studies do you want to order?

DISCUSSION

The acuity of symptoms in this patient suggests an abrupt event such as perforation or torsion. As in this case, patients can remember very specifically the time at which symptoms began. Perforation can occur in the stomach, duodenum, gallbladder, appendix, or other hollow viscus. Torsion can occur in any segment of non-fixed bowel or in the ovaries or testicles.

The patient's h/o smoking puts him at risk for PUD. Other risk factors associated with PUD are use of NSAIDs, alcohol, and steroids. In addition, his symptoms suggestive of reflux disease may indicate that he is an acid hypersecreter and specifically at risk for duodenal ulcer. Conversely, patients with gastric ulcer have a defect in mucosal defense and generally have normal or below average acid secretion. As a result, acid-reducing medications (histamine receptor blockers and proton pump inhibitors) tend to be more effective in patients with duodenal ulcer. Regardless, the ddx in this patient should still include other common causes of abdominal pain, such as appendicitis, cholecystitis, nephrolithiasis, and UTI. Lab tests, including WBC, chemistry panel, LFTs, and urinalysis, can help to support or exclude some of these other inflammatory processes.

CASE CONTINUED

Labs: CBC, chemistry panel, LFTs, and UA are ordered and return with normal values.

Imaging: *Abdominal series:* Shows a normal bowel gas pattern with no distended loops or air-fluid levels. A thin rim of air is seen between the diaphragm and the liver in the upper right abdomen. See Figure 4-1.

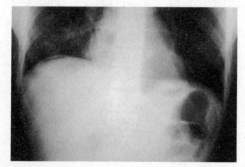

FIGURE 4-1.
This is an upright plain XR in which free air is seen as a thin sliver between the right hemidiaphragm and the (solid non–air-bearing) liver. It is not specific for a particular source of air. (*Image provided by Department of Radiology, University of California, San Francisco.*)

Given the specific acute history, physical examination, laboratory findings, and evidence of free air, you decide that the patient most likely has a perforated ulcer. He subsequently undergoes an uncomplicated upper midline laparotomy with identification of a perforated duodenal ulcer and repair of the defect with an omental (Graham) patch.

In patients with a prior ulcer history, a definitive antiulcer operation is often recommended at the same time as the perforation repair, provided there is little peritonitis. Patients without an ulcer history may undergo patch repair alone, but longitudinal studies suggest that recurrence rates may be high. Surgical options from least to most morbid include highly selective (parietal cell) vagotomy, truncal vagotomy with pyloroplasty, and vagotomy and antrectomy with Billroth (I or II) reconstruction. Because highly selective vagotomy carries a low morbidity and has the benefit of not requiring an accompanying gastric-emptying procedure (innervation to the antrum and pylorus is spared), it would be a good option in this patient with duodenal disease. However, not all centers are experienced in this technique, thus necessitating one of the other procedures. Vagotomy with pyloroplasty is probably the most commonly performed in this scenario. Billroth reconstructions are most appropriate for obstructing or pyloric ulcers but carry significant morbidity and may not be feasible in the acute setting. It is important to note that any procedure that preserves any amount of vagal innervation or any capacity for antral gastrin production may lead to an incomplete cure; not surprisingly then, historical recurrence rates for highly selective vagotomy are 5% to 20%; for vagotomy with pyloroplasty, 10% to 15%; and for vagotomy and antrectomy, <2%.

QUESTIONS

4-1. Bleeding peptic ulcers are usually anatomically associated with

A. The posterior duodenum, with erosion into the gastroduodenal artery.

B. The greater curvature of the stomach, with erosion into the gastroepiploic artery.

C. The anterior antrum, with bleeding from the omentum.

D. The pylorus, with erosion into the pancreatic vessels.

4-2. Gastric outlet obstruction in PUD results from
A. Blood clots pooling in the antrum.
B. Overwhelming ileus.
C. Poor digestion and breakdown of large food particles.
D. Edema and scarring leading to narrowing of the gastric outlet.

4-3. The patient position in which free air is best visualized on plain XRs is
A. Supine.
B. Right lateral decubitus.
C. Upright.
D. Trendelenburg.

4-4. Zollinger-Ellison syndrome is associated with severe peptic ulcers secondary to excessive elaboration of
A. Gastrin.
B. Somatostatin.
C. Histamine.
D. Chloride.

ANSWERS

4-1. A. Although bleeding may come from any source along the rich collateral blood supply of the stomach and duodenum, the most common association is with posterior ulcers eroding into the gastroduodenal artery.

4-2. D. Narrowing of the gastric outlet results from the inflammatory processes of PUD. Medical treatment may be attempted, but surgical intervention is usually necessary. Gastric outlet obstruction may also result from malignancy, which can be diagnosed on endoscopic exam.

4-3. C. Upright CXR is useful to evaluate for free air in the abdomen. Alternatively, in the patient who is unable to sit upright, a *left* lateral decubitus film (i.e., left side down) can be used to demonstrate free air between the liver and lateral abdominal wall.

4-4. A. A gastrin-secreting tumor or "gastrinoma" is the principal culprit in Zollinger-Ellison syndrome. Patients have elevated serum gastrin levels and severe PUD. These tumors are often associated with the pancreas but can occur anywhere within the "gastrinoma triangle," which is defined by the junction of the cystic duct and the common bile duct, the junction of the second and third portions of the duodenum, and the junction of the neck and the body of the pancreas.

SUGGESTED ADDITIONAL READING

Behrman SW. Management of complicated peptic ulcer disease. Arch Surg 2005;140:201–208.

Boey J, Choi SK, Poon A, et al. Risk stratification in perforated duodenal ulcers: A prospective validation of predictive factors. Ann Surg 1987;205:22–26.

Jamieson GG. Current status of indications for surgery in peptic ulcer disease. World J Surg 2000;24:256–258.

Zittel TT, Jehle EC, Becker HD. Surgical management of peptic ulcer disease today—indication, technique and outcome. Langenbecks Arch Surg 2000;385:84–96.

Abdominal Pain in a Drinker

CC: Abdominal pain, nausea, and vomiting × 1 day.

HPI: Mr. X is a 56-year-old man who presents to the emergency department with a 1-day hx of sharp epigastric pain that radiates to the back. He is nauseated and has been unable to keep anything down since having bacon and eggs the previous morning. He denies any hx of aspirin or NSAID use and has no previous hx of peptic ulcer disease.

PMHx: Negative

PSHx: Appendectomy as a child

Meds: None

All: NKDA

SHx: Drinks 1 to 3 pints of tequila a day, smokes 2 ppd, tried speed "once or twice" in the past.

VS: Temp 38.2°C, BP 125/60, HR 120, RR 22, O_2 sat 95% on RA

PE: *Gen:* WD/WN man, lying on the gurney with knees drawn up, AO × 4. *HEENT:* PERRL, EOMI, anicteric. *Lungs:* CTA bilaterally, no crackles or wheezes. *CV:* RRR, no murmurs/rubs/gallop. *Abdomen:* Soft, slightly distended, very TTP in epigastrium with focal rebound tenderness, no referred pain, well-healed RLQ scar. *Rectal:* nl tone, heme neg, no masses.

THOUGHT QUESTION

- What is in your differential at this point? What studies would you like to obtain first?

DISCUSSION

The differential diagnosis with this presentation is very broad. Although appendicitis is unlikely because the patient has had his appendix removed, it is still possible to have acute inflammation of the appendiceal stump. The differential also includes bowel obstruction, perforated viscus, peptic ulcer disease, Mallory-Weiss tear, pancreatitis, cholecystitis, and acute MI. Distinguishing among these should begin with blood work, an ECG, and a three-way abdominal XR series (i.e., KUB, upright abdomen, and CXR), which is useful as an initial screening study to rule out free air and bowel obstruction.

CASE CONTINUED

Labs: WBC 15; Hct 49; Plts 248; BUN 28; Cr 1.3; Lytes nl; glucose 198; Ca 7.6; Mg 1.8; Phos 2.4; AST 80; ALT 42; AlkP 98; Tbili 1.0; amylase 789. UA: Negative.

Imaging: *ECG:* No ischemic changes. *XR:* No free air or air-fluid levels, sentinel loop in LUQ.

THOUGHT QUESTION

■ How do these results affect your differential diagnosis?

DISCUSSION

These objective findings make a perforated viscus, cholecystitis, and MI less likely. Hyperamylasemia is consistent with pancreatitis, but it is important to remember there are other sources of amylase in the body (e.g., salivary glands, fallopian tubes, small bowel), and local disturbances of these organs (e.g., salivary tumor, salpingitis, SBO) can lead to elevations in the amylase level. A *lipase* level, which is more specific for the pancreas, can be helpful in confirming the source of hyperamylasemia. The hemoconcentration and slightly elevated BUN and creatinine are consistent with intravascular volume depletion, which occurs in pancreatitis as a result of regional retroperitoneal inflammation, systemic microvascular injury (e.g., thrombosis, increased permeability, etc.), and resultant "third-spacing" of fluid. The LFTs are consistent with alcoholic hepatitis (i.e. a 2:1 AST:ALT ratio) but not with obstructive biliary disease. On *plain films,* classic (but not specific) findings for pancreatitis include diffuse ileus or a sentinel loop (e.g., single, dilated, air-filled loop of small bowel in the region of inflammation). *CT* may show pancreatic inflammation or necrosis.

CASE CONTINUED

Lipase and LDH levels added on the initial labs return with values of 503 and 246, respectively. ABG shows a mild mixed respiratory and metabolic alkalosis. Based on the patient's presentation, history of alcohol abuse, and the above findings, you diagnose the patient with acute alcohol-induced pancreatitis. He is admitted, put on bowel rest (NPO), and begun on aggressive IV fluid hydration.

QUESTIONS

5-1. How many of Ranson's admission criteria does this patient meet?
- A. 0
- B. 1
- C. 2
- D. 3
- E. 4

5-2. Which of the following is a rare cause of pancreatitis?
- A. Gallstones
- B. Alcohol use
- C. MRCP
- D. Coxsackie B virus
- E. Diabetes

5-3. Acute pancreatitis
- A. rarely leads to respiratory distress.
- B. has a high mortality rate when associated with necrosis and infection.
- C. may cause gastric perforation.
- D. is preceded by pseudocyst formation by at least six weeks.
- E. has an incidence of 10% to 20%

5-4. Standard management of acute pancreatitis includes
  A. Emergent ERCP.
  B. Antibiotics.
  C. Fresh frozen plasma infusion.
  D. Pancreatic debridement and drainage.
  E. Careful hemodynamic monitoring.

ANSWERS

5-1. B. This patient meets only one of Ranson's early criteria. A patient who has three of the criteria at the stated times has a 15% to 30% mortality; this mortality rate increases with the increasing number of criteria met. It is important to remember that amylase and lipase levels are *not* included in Ranson's criteria and do not have predictive value. See Table 5-1.

TABLE 5-1 Ranson's Criteria for Acute Pancreatitis

Early (within 24 hrs)	Late (>48 hrs)
Age >55 years	Hct drop of 10%
WBC >16	Pao_2 <60
AST >250	Total calcium <8
Glucose >200	Base deficit >4
LDH >350	BUN increase of >5
	Fluid sequestration of >6 L

5-2. D. In the United States, alcohol use is the most common cause of pancreatitis, whereas in other industrialized countries, gallstone pancreatitis is more common. Gallstones cause pancreatitis when a stone passing through the common bile duct blocks the pancreatic duct. These two etiologies account for >90% of all cases of acute pancreatitis. This variation in etiologies also affects the patient profile, because gallstone-induced disease more commonly involves women and younger patients, whereas alcohol-induced disease tends to involve older men. More rare causes of pancreatitis include hypercalcemia; hyperlipidemia; familial, idiopathic (e.g., after ERCP) or structural anomalies (e.g., obstructing tumor, pancreas divisum); scorpion bite; infection; pregnancy; and many different drugs (e.g., steroids, diuretics, warfarin, and azathioprine). Diabetes can be a rare complication of pancreatitis but is not a cause.

5-3. B. The presentation of acute pancreatitis varies from mild to fulminant, but pulmonary dysfunction occurs in two-thirds of patients. Retroperitoneal hemorrhage, often associated with necrosis, can result in hypotension and blue discoloration of the flanks (*Grey-Turner* sign), umbilicus (*Cullen* sign), and inguinal ligament (*Fox* sign). Other complications include sepsis, shock, multiple-system organ failure, pseudocyst, and abscess. As a result of such complications, acute pancreatitis (which has an incidence of only 0.14% to 1.3%) has a significant mortality rate of 6% to 20%. *Necrotizing pancreatitis* occurs in 5% to 10% of cases with an increased mortality of >50%. Such severe disease is often heralded by jaundice and hypotension. *Pseudocysts* usually present with persistent pain or ileus after an acute episode of pancreatitis. Most occur in the head of the pancreas, and management can be either by observation or drainage (open, percutaneous, endoscopic, or laparoscopic), depending on its size and symptoms. See Figure 5-1.

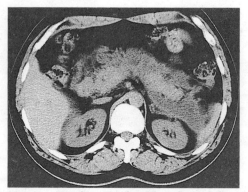

FIGURE **5-1.** Acute pancreatitis: CT showing inflammatory exudates surrounding the pancreas. (*Used with permission from Patel PR. Lecture Notes on Radiology. Oxford: Blackwell Science, Ltd., 1998:136.*)

5-4. E. Aggressive IV fluid resuscitation is the most important initial treatment to avoid hypovolemia and inadequate end-organ perfusion. Close monitoring (including Foley catheter for urine output, frequent ABGs or continuous O_2 saturation, and arterial and/or central venous pressure monitors) is essential. Serial laboratory tests are also necessary to follow and correct any metabolic disturbances. Antibiotics are not indicated for uncomplicated acute pancreatitis but are reserved for infected necrosis, sepsis, or failure to improve with supportive care alone. Surgical debridement and drainage (open or closed) is recommended only for infected necrosis. ERCP, cholecystectomy, and other surgical procedures for ductal obstruction are performed in the setting of gallstone pancreatitis.

SUGGESTED ADDITIONAL READING

Bell RH Jr. Current surgical management of chronic pancreatitis. J Gastrointest Surg 2005;9:144–154.

Clancy TE, Benoit EP, Ashley SW. Current management of acute pancreatitis. J Gastrointest Surg 2005;9:440–452.

Nathens AB, Curtis JR, Beale RJ, et al. Management of the critically ill patient with severe acute pancreatitis. Crit Care Med 2004;32:2524–2536.

Tenner S. Initial management of acute pancreatitis: critical issues during the first 72 hours. Am J Gastroenterol 2004;99:2489–2494.

Werner J, Feuerbach S, Uhl W, et al. Management of acute pancreatitis: from surgery to interventional intensive care. Gut 2005;54:426–436.

Abdominal Pain with Distension

CC/ID: 37-year-old woman with a 2-day h/o abdominal pain, distension, and vomiting.

HPI: Ms. X presents to the ED with gradually worsening symptoms. She had eaten dinner two nights before without difficulty but later that evening had several episodes of bilious emesis. She tried drinking some fluids this morning, but again threw up and has had no appetite since. She c/o diffuse abdominal discomfort and bloating that comes and goes and is somewhat crampy in nature. Her last bowel movement was the morning before last. She is unsure if she is passing flatus. She reports an episode of similar pain about a year or two ago, but it resolved in a few hours.

PMHx: None

PSHx: Appy 15 years ago; nevus on back removed 5 years ago

Meds: None

VS: Temp 37.7°C, BP 110/70, HR 100

PE: *Gen:* Mod distress, moving relatively easily. *HEENT:* Mucous membranes dry. *Chest:* Clear bilaterally. *Abdomen:* Well-healed RLQ scar; moderately distended with occasional high-pitched rumblings on auscultation; tympany on percussion; diffuse TTP without guarding or rebound; no discrete masses or hernias. *Rectal:* No masses, normal tone, no stool in the vault; heme neg.

THOUGHT QUESTION

- What is the likely source of this otherwise healthy patient's symptoms?

■ How will you support this diagnosis?

■ What additional findings will affect your management decisions?

DISCUSSION

The patient has a history and findings suggestive of bowel obstruction. Any patient presenting with abdominal distension, nausea, and vomiting, and with even a remote h/o prior abdominal surgery should have this in his or her differential. She could also have other causes of discomfort, including any inflammatory process (e.g., cholecystitis) with associated ileus. Radiographic findings can sometimes suggest functional ileus versus mechanical obstruction. This is more true of CTs than of plain films, as the former can often demonstrate a specific site of obstruction, at which there is a transition point between proximal bowel dilatation and distal bowel decompression. However, plain XRs are usually sufficient to diagnose SBO. The patient's overall clinical picture and imaging studies will guide management; the commonly described rule of thumb is to "never let the sun set on a (complete) bowel obstruction."

CASE CONTINUED

You place an NGT to help the patient decompress her stomach, give her 2 L of crystalloid, and order labs that show a metabolic (contraction) alkalosis, consistent with her h/o vomiting. Her WBC count is mildly elevated at 11,000. An abdominal series is performed. There is no free air, but supine and upright films reveal dilated loops of bowel with multiple air-fluid levels. There is a small amount of stool seen in the descending colon and a paucity of air in the rectum. See Figure 6-1.

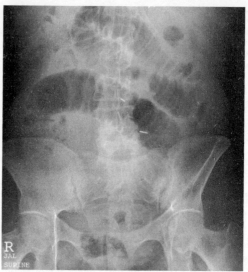

FIGURE 6-1. In this KUB (abdominal plain film), a single dilated loop is seen crossing transversely across the mid-portion of the image. Note the paucity of air in the rectum (pelvis). This pattern is suggestive of bowel obstruction, and additional upright images might be expected to show air-fluid levels. (*Image provided by Department of Radiology, University of California, San Francisco.*)

THOUGHT QUESTION

- The patient is hemodynamically stable and nonacidotic. How do you wish to proceed? What if she were acidotic or hemodynamically unstable? If her abdominal pain was worsening or localizing? If she suddenly passed gas and/or was hungry?

DISCUSSION

Passage of air or stool, or air in the rectum on XR (before digital examination), suggests a partial or early complete bowel obstruction. Many of these patients can be managed expectantly, with resolution of symptoms occurring with hydration and GI decompression (via NGT to low continuous wall suction). A deteriorating clinical picture (i.e., worsening or localizing abdominal pain, increasing abdominal distension, acidosis, hypotension) or further findings of complete bowel obstruction (i.e., complete absence of flatus or stool, massive dilation of proximal bowel) mandate surgical intervention, as irreversible bowel ischemia and/or perforation and sepsis can result. Serial exams and x-rays may be helpful in guiding these decisions. In addition, a partial bowel obstruction that does not resolve after a trial of expectant management may require surgical intervention as well. Improvement and possible spontaneous resolution of a partial obstruction is often heralded by return of flatus and appetite.

QUESTIONS

6-1. The number one cause of SBO in the developed world is
A. Hernias.
B. Adhesions.
C. Cancer.
D. Large food particles.

6-2. Closed loop obstruction occurs when bowel
A. Inflow is compromised.
B. Outflow is compromised.
C. Inflow and outflow are compromised.
D. Walls collapse upon themselves.

6-3. An internal hernia may result from
A. The bowel twisting on its vascular pedicle.
B. An inguinal defect.
C. An iatrogenic mesenteric defect.
D. The bowel telescoping on itself.

6-4. A postoperative patient on narcotics has not had a BM in 4 days. You might expect to find on XR
A. A single massively dilated loop of bowel with air-fluid levels.
B. Diffuse air in the bowel without air-fluid levels.
C. Air in the biliary tract.
D. No air in the abdomen.

ANSWERS

6-1. B. The most common cause of SBO in industrialized countries is adhesions, usually postoperative. Hernias are the next most common. Cancer is often a factor in large bowel obstruction.

6-2. C. In closed loop obstruction, both inflow and outflow of bowel contents are compromised. Examples of this include volvulus and appendiceal fecalith. This type of obstruction rarely resolves spontaneously.

6-3. C. Internal hernias may occur through any iatrogenic or congenital space in the abdomen, including such openings as mesenteric defects or the foramen of Winslow. Bowel twisting on itself is a volvulus. Herniation through an inguinal defect is, by definition, an external hernia. Bowel telescoping on itself is an intussusception. Any of these processes may cause a bowel obstruction.

6-4. B. Functional ileus usually results in a diffuse pattern of mildly dilated bowel without massive distension or significant air-fluid levels. However, ileus in the immediate postoperative period is common and seldom requires radiographic evaluation or surgical intervention.

SUGGESTED ADDITIONAL READING

Choi HK, Chu KW, Law WL. Therapeutic value of gastrografin in adhesive small bowel obstruction after unsuccessful conservative treatment: a prospective randomized trial. Ann Surg 2002;236:1-6.

Fleshner PR, Siegman MG, Slater GI, et al. A prospective, randomized trial of short versus long tubes in adhesive small-bowel obstruction. Am J Surg 1995;170:366-370.

Maglinte DD, Heitkamp DE, Howard TJ, et al. Current concepts in imaging of small bowel obstruction. Radiol Clin North Am 2003;41:263-283, vi.

Abdominal Pain with Diarrhea

CC: Intermittent bloody diarrhea and abdominal pain for several years.

HPI: Mr. X is a 31-year-old man who reports intermittent episodes of diarrhea and abdominal pain for the past several years. The diarrhea is occasionally streaked with blood. The episodes generally last for a few days and then seem to go away spontaneously. The most recent episode 1 month ago was his worst yet, with severe diffuse abdominal pain and cramping after eating a few raw carrots. He also had a fever. He has lost about 15 pounds since these episodes began.

PMHx: PUD, arthritis

PSHx: None

Meds: Pepcid, ASA prn

All: NKDA

SHx: Nonsmoker, occasional beer on weekends, no illicit drugs

FHx: No known family members with "bowel problems," no family cancers

THOUGHT QUESTION

- What is in your differential diagnosis?
- What studies should you perform to narrow the differential?

DISCUSSION

The differential for intermittent abdominal pain and diarrhea is broad. It includes appendicitis, diverticulitis, inflammatory bowel disease, infection (bacterial, protozoal, and fungal), and ischemic colitis. Other possibilities are sprue, lymphoma, sarcoidosis, radiation enteritis, and irritable bowel syndrome. You could begin with basic lab tests (CBC, electrolytes) and stool cultures and, provided the patient is not acutely ill, proceed to a sigmoidoscopy or colonoscopy. Barium enema may also be an option in patients who are nontoxic. If the patient is acutely ill, you should consider a CT of the abdomen and pelvis.

CASE CONTINUED

VS: Temp 37.8 °C, BP 123/56, HR 67, RR 12

PE: *Gen:* WD/WN man in no acute distress, somewhat pale appearing, AO × 4. *HEENT:* PERRL, EOMI, conjunctiva injected, mucous membranes pale pink, aphthous ulcer on lower lip. *Lungs:* CTA bilaterally. *CV:* RRR, no murmurs. *Abdomen:* Soft, slightly distended and tympanitic, mildly tender to palpation over the RLQ, bowel sounds hyperactive. *Rectal:* nl tone, brown stool, trace heme positive, ulcerated skin tag at 8 o'clock. *Ext:* clubbing, no edema or cyanosis.

Labs: 10 $>$―$<$ 188   lytes and LFTs WNL; albumin 2.8; stool
         38
cultures negative.

Imaging: *Colonoscopy:* Rectum with "cobble-stoned" mucosa, rest of colon normal except cecum, which shows several 2-cm deep linear ulcers; biopsies are taken of these areas.

THOUGHT QUESTION

- What do you expect to see upon microscopic examination of the biopsies? What are some other clinical features that might be seen in this disease?

DISCUSSION

In light of this patient's anemia, ulcerated lesions of the mouth and anus, conjunctivitis, and history of arthritis, you might predict that this patient will have Crohn's colitis. On biopsy, you would therefore expect to see inflammatory cells near the crypts, with granulomas and possibly crypt abscesses. The submucosa may be edematous with lymphoid aggregates and fistulous tracts. Serositis may also be present. Crohn's colitis can involve all layers of the intestinal wall and is often discontinuous or segmental, whereas ulcerative colitis generally involves only the mucosa and is contiguous beginning at the rectum (perianal involvement is rare). Crypt abscesses and pseudopolyps are common in ulcerative colitis, whereas granulomas are rare.

Crohn's colitis is a chronic inflammatory disorder of the intestinal tract. It most often involves the terminal ileum and proximal colon, but any part of the gastrointestinal tract (from mouth to anus) is susceptible. In fact, extraintestinal manifestations (i.e., eyes, skin, joints, and liver) are also common. Crohn's disease involves abscess, ulcer, and fistula formation, followed by fibrosis and stricturing. The bowel wall is edematous with "creeping fat." The symptomatic triad of abdominal pain, diarrhea, and weight loss usually presents in young adulthood and often remains undiagnosed for several years.

QUESTIONS

7-1. Medical management of Crohn's colitis relies primarily on
A. Anti-peristaltic agents.
B. Total parenteral nutrition.
C. Immunosuppressive agents.
D. Sulindac.

7-2. Rectovaginal fistula complicating Crohn's colitis
A. Requires emergent proctectomy.
B. Can often be treated medically with steroids and metronidazole.
C. Is a successful application for fibrin glue injection.
D. Are easier to treat than those following obstetrical trauma.

7-3. Surgical resection of Crohn's colitis
  A. Is curative.
  B. Is contraindicated for complications of the disease.
  C. Is indicated for failed medical therapy.
  D. Involves resection of as much bowel as possible.

7-4. Complications of inflammatory bowel disease
  A. are not necessarily confined to the gastrointestinal tract
  B. always require surgical intervention
  C. never require extensive colon resection
  D. should always be managed with total proctocolectomy

ANSWERS

7-1. C. Inhibition of peristalsis can lead to ileus and toxic dilatation, particularly during acute flares. Therefore, antispasmodics and opiates may be used to decrease hypermotility and diarrhea, respectively, but they are used with extreme caution in patients with inflammatory bowel disease. TPN is sometimes used with bowel rest during an acute episode. Immunosuppressive and anti-inflammatory drugs have been the mainstay of medical therapy, with recent advances involving immunotherapy (e.g., infliximab).

7-2. B. Rectovaginal fistula is uncommon, but it has been reported following obstetrical trauma as well as associated with Crohn's colitis. Fibrin glue injection is an option for treatment, but most fistulae respond to antibiotic therapy (metronidazole) and anti-inflammatory medication. Proctectomy may be required for refractory and complex rectal disease.

7-3. C. Because of a very high recurrence rate, surgical resection is palliative only and is reserved primarily for complications of Crohn's disease or for cases where medical therapy has failed. Resection is limited to as little involved bowel as necessary. Lysis of adhesions is also usually required. Strictures are treated with stricturoplasty rather than resection whenever possible. Resection may be indicated when there are high-grade dysplastic changes unassociated with inflammation in regions of long-standing colitis, which are at high risk for malignant degeneration. As with Crohn's disease, surgical resection for ulcerative colitis is indicated for complications (i.e., bleeding), refractory disease, and dysplastic changes. Unlike Crohn's, resection in ulcerative colitis can be curative when the entire colon and rectum are removed.

7-4. A. Sixty percent of patients with primary sclerosing cholangitis have inflammatory bowel disease, and 30% of patients with primary sclerosing cholangitis develop cholangiocarcinoma. Fistulas in Crohn's disease can involve any adjacent structure (i.e., other bowel loops, skin, bladder, urethra, vagina, rectum). Small bowel obstruction can occur, particularly after ingestion of high fiber foods. These episodes can usually be managed expectantly. Toxic megacolon and free perforation are rare but serious complications of both Crohn's and ulcerative colitis. The reasonable surgical treatment of toxic megacolon is total colectomy with ileostomy; this can be performed expeditiously and without excessive dissection in the pelvis, allowing for proctectomy in the future when the patient is more stable. Other complications of ulcerative colitis include hemorrhage and obstruction, usually due to a rectal stricture.

SUGGESTED ADDITIONAL READING

Baert F, Vermeire S, Noman M, et al. Management of ulcerative colitis and Crohn's disease. Acta Clin Belg 2004;59:304–314.

Froehlich F, Juillerat P, Mottet C, et al. Obstructive fibrostenotic Crohn's disease. Digestion 2005;71:29–30.

Loftus EV Jr. Management of extraintestinal manifestations and other complications of inflammatory bowel disease. Curr Gastroenterol Rep 2004;6:506–513.

McNamara DA, Brophy S, Hyland JM. Perianal Crohn's disease and infliximab therapy. Surgeon 2004;2:258–263.

Michetti P, Juillerat P, Mottet C, et al. Therapy of mild to moderate luminal Crohn's disease. Digestion 2005;71:13–18.

Epigastric Pain with Early Satiety

CC: Abdominal pain for several months.

HPI: Mr. X is a 46-year-old Japanese man who recently moved to the United States. Since arriving here several months ago, he has noted intermittent sharp epigastric pain that seems to be relieved by eating. He has also tried Maalox with some relief of symptoms. He has had a few episodes of vomiting (nonbloody), but his appetite otherwise seems normal. Despite this, he still has lost 10 pounds in the last few months. Upon further questioning, the patient describes several months of what sounds like early satiety with eating. He denies any change in his bowel movements and has not noted any dark or bloody stools.

PMHx: None

PSHx: None

Meds: None

All: NKDA

SHx: Occasional sake, 1 ppd cigarettes for 30 years, no IV drug use

FHx: Maternal aunt had "stomach problems."

VS: Afebrile, BP 124/69, HR 78

PE: *Gen:* Thin man, no acute distress. *HEENT:* Unremarkable, no *Virchow's node. CV:* RRR. *Lungs:* CTA bilaterally. *Abdomen:* Soft, NT/ND, fullness in epigastrium, no hepatosplenomegaly, no Sister Mary Joseph's node. *Ext:* Warm, well-perfused. *Rectal:* Guaiac positive, brown stool; no masses.

Labs: 7 > 38 < 210; lytes and LFTs WNL; *Helicobacter pylori* Ab pending

THOUGHT QUESTION

■ What is the recommended management for this patient?

DISCUSSION

In a patient with epigastric pain and heme-positive stools, active peptic ulcer disease is a concern. With the added findings of weight loss, possible abdominal mass, and early satiety, malignancy rises on the differential. Both of these can be evaluated using upper endoscopy or barium swallow. On endoscopy, an early cancer may appear as a simple shallow ulcer, a small polyp, or a flat plaque. More advanced cancers tend to appear raised and ulcerated with irregular borders. Only biopsy can distinguish between a malignant ulcer and a benign one. Endoscopic ultrasound can show disruption of the gastric wall layers by tumor. With barium swallow, pathology may appear as an ulceration, gastric mass, loss of mucosal detail, or a distorted gastric silhouette. *CT* is useful to assess for infiltration of the gastric wall, ulceration, and metastases.

CASE CONTINUED

The patient undergoes an esophagogastroduodenoscopy (EGD). He is found to have a shallow ulcer in the fundus. Biopsies are taken and reveal adenocarcinoma. Ultrasound performed during endoscopy reveals infiltration of the mucosa and submucosa anteriorly, but it is unable to assess the nodal status. CT shows no hepatic or other distant metastases.

THOUGHT QUESTION

■ What are the management options for this patient?

DISCUSSION

Gastric cancers tend to spread intramurally via lymphatics and metastasize hematogenously or via direct extension to adjacent organs. Because of the vast capillary and lymphatic network within the gastric wall, even gastric cancers detected early have a 15% chance of nodal metastasis. The natural history of gastric carcinoma is one of obstruction and hemorrhage; therefore, resection and/or reconstruction is indicated in all cases (even if cure is not possible) unless there is evidence of diffuse metastatic disease or other contraindications to surgery. Surgical resection is the only hope for cure. Controversy exists regarding the utility (survival benefit versus operative morbidity) of extended perigastric lymphadenectomy and routine splenectomy or partial pancreatectomy. Chemotherapy has limited use, and improved survival rates have not been shown. Palliation can be surgical, endoscopic (e.g., fulguration, stenting), or with radiation. Mean survival in palliative cases is less than 6 to 9 months. Overall 5-year survival is 50% to 70% for stage I disease; this drops to 30% to 40% for stage II; and only 10% to 20% for stage III.

CASE CONTINUED

The patient undergoes an uncomplicated total gastrectomy with Roux-en-Y esophagojejunostomy. Postoperatively, he complains of heartburn, bloating, malabsorptive diarrhea, and continued weight loss. You decide that his symptoms are likely related to the loss of the gastric reservoir. Therefore, you have a nasointestinal feeding tube placed under fluoroscopic guidance to be used for slow, continuous nutritional supplementation while the patient adapts to his new gastrointestinal (GI) anatomy.

QUESTIONS

8-1. One of the most well-established risk factors for gastric cancer is
   A. Pernicious anemia.
   B. *Helicobacter pylori*.
   C. Hyperplastic polyps.
   D. Dietary fats.

8-2. Gastrointestinal stromal tumors
  A. Are common GI tract neoplasma.
  B. Are differentiated as benign or malignant based on tumor size and a number of mitotic figures.
  C. Can be treated with simple enucleation.
  D. Are associated with frequent distant metastases on presentation.

8-3. Resection for gastric lymphoma
  A. Minimizes the risk of hemorrhage and perforation with chemotherapy.
  B. Is curative for >75% of invasive tumors.
  C. Is less morbid than gastrectomy for carcinoma.
  D. Requires extensive lymphadenectomy.

8-4. Linitis plastica is
  A. Diffuse tumor infiltration of the stomach.
  B. Diffuse desmoplastic reaction to the cancer.
  C. A good prognostic sign.
  D. Seen in most cases.

ANSWERS

8-1. A. The median age of patients with gastric cancer is 65 years, and almost two-thirds of patients are male. Hyperplastic polyps occur in <1% of the population but account for 70% to 80% of all gastric polyps. Atypia is rare and is considered not premalignant. On the other hand, *adenomatous polyps* have a risk of carcinoma of 10% to 20%. Chronic atrophic gastritis is often associated with intestinal metaplasia and mucosal dysplasia, both of which are frequently found in mucosa adjacent to a carcinoma. The chronic gastritis found with pernicious anemia is characterized by fundic mucosal atrophy, loss of parietal and chief cells, hypochlorhydria, and hypergastrinemia. There is a two- to threefold increase in gastric cancer in patients with pernicious anemia. Gastric cancer is more common in Japan and China than in the United States and is believed to be related to environmental carcinogens in the diet. *Helicobacter pylori* infection may be associated with development of gastric cancer, but the evidence is not definitive. There may be a slightly increased risk of carcinoma in the gastric remnant after gastric resection (particularly Billroth II), but only at more than 25 years after initial surgery.

8-2. B. Altered tumor growth factor expression and chromosomal abnormalities are also frequent in these tumors.

8-3. A. Gross bleeding is uncommon with gastric lymphoma, but occult bleeding and anemia are present in 50% of patients. More than half of gastrointestinal lymphomas occur in the stomach, the most common site of extranodal lymphoma. Gastrectomy allows accurate histologic identification, local cure, and prevention of future hemorrhage or perforation related to deeply infiltrating tumor. However, chemoradiotherapy alone is also an option. In contrast to adenocarcinoma, positive margins do not predict local recurrence if postoperative radiation therapy to the gastric bed is performed. In fact, survival is primarily related to disease stage at time of diagnosis.

8-4. B. Linitis plastica is rare (10%) in gastric carcinoma cases. It results from gastric induration secondary to a diffuse desmoplastic reaction to the tumor. Linitis predicts a poor prognosis.

ADDITIONAL SUGGESTED READING

Aviles A, Nambo MJ, Neri N, et al. The role of surgery in primary gastric lymphoma: results of a controlled clinical trial. Ann Surg 2004;240:44–50.

Cuschieri A, Weeden S, Fielding J, et al. Patient survival after D1 and D2 resections for gastric cancer: long-term results of the MRC randomized surgical trial. Surgical Co-operative Group. Br J Cancer 1999;79:1522–1530.

Degiuli M, Sasako M, Calgaro M, et al. Italian Gastric Cancer Study Group. Morbidity and mortality after D1 and D2 gastrectomy for cancer: interim analysis of the Italian Gastric Cancer Study Group (IGCSG) randomised surgical trial. Eur J Surg Oncol 2004;30:303–308.

MacDonald JS, Smalley SR, Benedetti J, et al. Chemoradiotherapy after surgery compared with surgery alone for adenocarcinoma of the stomach or gastroesophageal junction. N Engl J Med. 2001 (6);345:725–730.

Maeta M, Yamashiro H, Saito H, et al. A prospective pilot study of extended (D3) and superextended para-aortic lymphadenectomy (D4) in patients with T3 or T4 gastric cancer managed by total gastrectomy. Surgery 1999;125:325–331.

Wils J. Treatment of gastric cancer. Curr Opin Oncol 1998; 10:357–361.

Abdominal Cramping with Bloody Stools

CC/ID: 18-month-old boy with a 1-day h/o intermittent, sudden, severe, colicky abdominal pain associated with runny reddish stools.

HPI: Ms. X is an otherwise healthy toddler who has become progressively fussy over the last day. His mother tells you that she believes his belly is the source of his discomfort, but he himself is unable to clearly state what is bothering him. She goes on to tell you in this same period she has noticed his stools have become loose and dark reddish in color. He has had no recent change in his diet, but she believes his appetite over the day is a little decreased. He vomited once this morning, before coming to your office.

THOUGHT QUESTION

- What is the differential diagnosis for abdominal pain in this age group?
- What features or characteristics of this pain will aid your diagnosis?
- What do you think of the description of his stool?

DISCUSSION

The differential diagnosis of abdominal pain in a toddler includes acute appendicitis, Meckel's diverticulitis or ulcer, intussusception, and gastroenteritis. Appendicitis in a child can be difficult to diagnose by history, because the patient is frequently unable to describe the exact site or onset of symptoms. However, the pain is generally persistent, gradually worsens to the point of perforation, abates, and then returns as peritonitis ensues. Intussusception is marked by episodic, colicky pain lasting for a few minutes, interspersed with periods of comfort and relative normalization. The pain of gastroenteritis is nonspecific but may mimic any of the above. Both appendicitis and gastroenteritis are usually accompanied by fever.

The quality of the stool suggests the presence of blood. This may be associated with infectious causes, although frankly reddish stool is uncommon in that circumstance. More often, the description of blood mixed with mucus ("currant jelly stool") is suggestive of intussusception and is the result of vascular compromise, ischemia, and ultimately mucosal injury and necrosis of the involved bowel.

CASE CONTINUED

Further questioning reveals that the child has in fact seemed "normal," although perhaps a bit lethargic in the periods when he is not crying in pain. The "episodes" last for a few minutes and occur one to three times an hour. As you are speaking with the mother, the child begins to scream. Telling you this is what she means, she tries to comfort her son, but for several minutes he is inconsolable. As he is placed on the examining table, you note that he draws his knees up to his chest.

VS: Afebrile, BP 100/65, HR 130

PE: *Gen:* WD/WN toddler, agitated, but becoming quieter. *Chest:* Clear. *Abdomen:* Soft, with a palpable sausage-like mass in the right upper quadrant/flank; no tympany.

Labs: CBC and chemistry panel are within normal limits.

THOUGHT QUESTION

■ Are there any other tests you would like to order?

DISCUSSION

The constellation of history and physical findings is highly suspicious for intussusception. Ultrasound (US) can often identify this pathology (seen as a mass with 2 lumens, making a "bull's-eye"). However, the test of choice is a BE, which is both diagnostic and, in 60% to 90% of cases, therapeutic. In the event of an irreducible intussusception or an uncertain reduction, surgery is indicated. Most frequently, this entails simple open reduction of the intussusceptum (the invaginated or internal proximal part) from the intussuscipiens (the receiving distal part). However, if manual decompression is not possible or if viability is in question, bowel resection may be necessary. Recurrence occurs in ~5% of patients after either intervention. In this instance, repeat BE may resolve the problem. Mortality is rare.

QUESTIONS

9-1. Which of the following regarding intussusception is true?
A. 1:2 male-female predominance.
B. Incidence is 10/1000 population.
C. 90% occur in patients >2 years of age.
D. The ileocecal valve is commonly involved.

9-2. The classic triad of abdominal ("sausage-like") mass, pain, and currant jelly stools is noted in what percent of children presenting with intussusception?
A. <10
B. 30 to 35
C. 60 to 70
D. >90

9-3. The imaging test of choice for a suspected Meckel's diverticulum is
A. Angiography.
B. CT.
C. MRI.
D. Nuclear medicine scan.

9-4. Meckel's diverticulum is associated with the "rule of 2s." Which of the following is one of the rules?
A. incidence in the population is 2%.
B. Located 2 inches from the ileocecal valve.
C. Often diagnosed in twins.
D. less than 2 cm long.

ANSWERS

9-1. D. Ninety percent of cases occur *before* the age of 2 years. The cause in young children is idiopathic and generally involves the ileocecal valve. It was previously thought that hypertrophic Peyer's patches were the lead point for intussusception, but it is now believed that the lymphoid hyperplasia is the result rather than the cause of the ischemic insult. In older children, ~10% are caused by a Meckel's diverticulum. Polyps, gastrointestinal duplications, hemangiomas, and tumors are all causes of intussusception in older children.

9-2. B. Only about one-third of patients with intussusception will clearly have all three of the "classic" findings.

9-3. D. A ^{99m}technetium-pertechnate scan is the imaging modality of choice, although false results may occur with enteric duplications.

9-4. A. A Meckel's diverticulum is typically found approximately 2 *feet* from the ileocecal valve and is usually about 2 *inches* long. It occurs in about 2% of the population and is most commonly seen in children younger than 2 years.

ADDITIONAL SUGGESTED READING

DiFiore JW. Intussusception. Semin Pediatr Surg 1999;8:214–220.
Hadidi AT, El Shal N. Childhood intussusception: a comparative study of nonsurgical management. J Pediatr Surg 1999;34: 304–307.
Lin SL, Kong MS, Houng DS. Decreasing early recurrence rate of acute intussusception by the use of dexamethasone. Eur J Pediatr 2000;159:551–552.
Sorantin E, Lindbichler F. Management of intussusception. Eur Radiol 2004;14 Suppl 4:L146–154.
Yalamarthi S, Smith RC. Adult intussusception: case reports and review of literature. Postgrad Med J 2005;81:174–177.

Chronic Abdominal Pain

CC: Chronic abdominal pain for the past year.

HPI: Ms. X is a 53-year-old woman with a h/o DM, HTN, and hyperlipidemia. She has developed a "fear of eating" over the past year because she reproducibly gets steady diffuse abdominal pain and diarrhea 30 minutes after every meal. The pain usually lasts 2 to 3 hours and is unrelieved by antacids, vomiting, or belching. The pain initially occurred only after eating solids, but now occurs with all oral intake. She has lost nearly 40 lbs during this time.

PMHx: As above

PSHx: No abdominal operations

Meds: Glyburide, HCTZ, Zocor

All: NKDA

SHx: 60 pack-year smoker, currently 1/2 ppd; past heavy drinker, no illicit drugs

THOUGHT QUESTION

- What should you consider in your differential and how will you proceed with your workup?

DISCUSSION

The differential should start with common disorders such as pancreatitis, cholecystitis, partial small bowel obstruction, and malignancy. This patient does have a history of prior alcohol use but no known cholelithiasis and no previous abdominal operations. In addition to postoperative adhesions, other causes of small bowel obstruction include internal hernias, intussusception, and malignancy. All should be ruled out by laboratory, radiographic, and

49

possibly endoscopic evaluation. At that point, one can entertain the more rare entity of mesenteric ischemia, particularly in a patient with multiple risk factors for atherosclerosis and unexplained significant weight loss.

CASE CONTINUED

VS: Afebrile, BP 142/57, HR 86, weight 108 lbs, height 5'6"

PE: *Gen:* Well-developed, thin woman, no acute distress. *Abdomen:* Scaphoid, soft, mildly TTP in the periumbilical region, faint bruit heard in the epigastrium, normoactive bowel sounds. *Ext:* Soft tissue wasting in hands and calves; no edema or cyanosis, 1+ distal pulses. *Rectal:* nl tone, brown stool, trace heme positive.

Labs: WBC 8; Hct 36; Plts 300; Na 142; K 4.7; BUN 30; Cr 1.5; LFTs WNL; amylase 108; Cl 108; CO_2 24.

Imaging: *KUB:* No air-fluid levels, free air, or dilated loops of bowel. *CT with IV/PO contrast:* Liver, pancreas, and spleen normal appearing; gallbladder thin-walled, no pericholecystic fluid; difficult to visualize celiac and SMA trunks, IMA normal; small and large bowel unremarkable; no masses; no pneumatosis intestinalis or portal venous air.

THOUGHT QUESTION

- What are the possible causes of/risk factors for chronic mesenteric ischemia?
- What are the imaging modalities used to make this diagnosis?

DISCUSSION

Chronic mesenteric ischemia is almost exclusively a result of atherosclerosis but occurs more frequently in women than men for unclear reasons. Because of the rich collateralization of the bowel vasculature, chronic intestinal ischemia generally requires the involvement of at least two of the three visceral vessels (i.e. celiac, SMA, IMA) with >50% stenosis. Other causes include fibromuscular dysplasia, arteritis, neurofibromatosis, and median arcuate ligament syndrome (external compression of the celiac artery). Gastric ulcers sometimes develop as a manifestation of chronic ischemia. Average time from symptom onset to diagnosis is 9 months. Patients with chronic mesenteric ischemia are at high risk for acute intestinal infarction.

As with all vascular disorders, duplex ultrasonography is an excellent first-line study, especially in these typically thin patients. Flow velocity patterns are used to assess for stenoses. Computed tomography (CT) is useful to help rule out other causes of abdominal pain and, in the acute setting, to better visualize signs of bowel ischemia (pneumatosis, portal venous air, bowel wall edema, or infarction). Arteriography should be performed to confirm the diagnosis, to treat focal lesions (angioplasty, stenting, or thrombolysis), and to define the anatomy for revascularization.

? QUESTIONS

10-1. Which of the following is true about bowel perfusion?
   A. In the small bowel after a meal, blood flow increases within 20 minutes, peaks at 30 to 60 minutes, and remains elevated for 90 to 100 minutes.
   B. In the colon after a meal, blood flow increases within 2 hours and remains elevated for 4 hours.
   C. Blood flow through all three visceral arteries is required to adequately perfuse the small and large bowel.
   D. Ischemia progresses transmurally starting from the serosa to the mucosa.

10-2. Nonocclusive mesenteric ischemia
   A. Is caused by severe vasodilation of the visceral arteries.
   B. Results from shower emboli from a diseased aorta.
   C. May be treated with papaverine infusion into the SMA even if there is evidence of bowel infarction.
   D. May be associated with digitalis and cocaine use.

10-3. Mesenteric venous thrombosis
   A. Involves some form of hypercoagulable state.
   B. Occurs acutely.
   C. Can be treated only with bowel resection.
   D. Accounts for 30% of patients with acute intestinal ischemia.

10-4. Which of the following is characteristic of early acute mesenteric ischemia?
   A. Coagulopathy.
   B. Constipation.
   C. Elevated lactate.
   D. Vomiting.

ANSWERS

10-1. A. The colon does not increase its blood flow in response to normal foodstuffs, but flow does increase in the inferior mesenteric artery in response to lactulose. Gradual occlusion of any of the visceral vessels or acute occlusion of either the celiac or inferior mesenteric artery may be tolerated by virtue of collateralization, but acute occlusion of the SMA alone is generally sufficient to produce ischemia and infarction.

10-2. D. Nonocclusive mesenteric ischemia is responsible for 20% of cases of acute mesenteric ischemia and is caused by severe *vasoconstriction* of the visceral arteries. It generally occurs in low cardiac output situations and with the use of vasopressors. Acute mesenteric ischemia is often caused by atheroembolism from cardiac or aortic sources, but those would be considered examples of occlusive disease. Papaverine infusion into the SMA is a therapeutic option, provided there is no evidence of infarction. In the setting of bowel infarction, immediate operative intervention is indicated.

10-3. A. As long as there is no sign of bowel infarction, mesenteric venous thrombosis is treated with long-term anticoagulation. However, a low threshold for exploration and even "second-look" exploration is important given the high morbidity and mortality associated with necrotic bowel. Bowel infarction is generally associated with thrombosis of the smaller venous tributaries rather than the large ones, because obstruction of a large vein (i.e., superior mesenteric vein) can be compensated via the interconnections with the portal venous system.

10-4. D. Acute mesenteric ischemia is most often a result of cardiac embolism to the SMA, generally from atrial fibrillation, MI, or dilated cardiomyopathy. More than one-third of patients with acute SMA embolism have had a previous peripheral arterial embolism. Acute embolic mesenteric ischemia presents with abrupt abdominal pain and gastrointestinal tract emptying (i.e., diarrhea, vomiting). Delay in diagnosis contributes to significant mortality (>50%).

The diagnosis of acute mesenteric ischemia requires a high index of suspicion, because there are often no specific physical findings and no reliable diagnostic lab tests. Lactate levels may be elevated, but this is usually a very late finding that occurs when infarction is already present. Bloody stool may be reported, and the patient's pain is often out of proportion to the physical exam (i.e., significant abdominal tenderness with a soft nondistended abdomen).

ADDITIONAL SUGGESTED READING

Burns BJ, Brandt LJ. Intestinal ischemia. Gastroenterol Clin North Am 2003;32:1127–1143.

Chang JB, Stein TA. Mesenteric ischemia: acute and chronic. Ann Vasc Surg 2003;17:323–328.

Cleveland TJ, Nawaz S, Gaines PA. Mesenteric arterial ischaemia: diagnosis and therapeutic options. Vasc Med 2002;7:311–321.

Schoots IG, Koffeman GI, Legemate DA, et al. Systematic review of survival after acute mesenteric ischaemia according to disease aetiology. Br J Surg 2004;91:17–27.

Tendler DA. Acute intestinal ischemia and infarction. Semin Gastrointest Dis 2003;14:66–76.

Abdominal Pain in the Immunocompromised Patient

CC/ID: 36 year-old man with acute-onset abdominal pain, nausea, and vomiting

HPI: The patient is an HIV-positive (CD4 count 400, viral load undetectable) man with a 36-hour history of abdominal pain. The pain is somewhat diffuse, but seems to be worse in the RLQ. He has intermittent fevers and occasional sweats. He reports that he often has diarrhea several times a day, but states that that is common because of his medications. His last bowel movement was the day before last. His appetite is diminished.

THOUGHT QUESTION

- How does this patient's HIV status affect your evaluation?
- Would it make a difference in your thinking if his CD4 count were 1000? 100?

DISCUSSION

Strictly speaking, an HIV-positive patient should undergo the same careful evaluation and workup as any other patient. However, it is important to remember that patients with immune dysfunction (including patients on chemotherapy) will be at increased risk for certain opportunistic infections that do not affect immunocompetent individuals. These may lead to abdominal pain that is due to nonoperative causes, such as splenomegaly, hepatomegaly, pancreatitis, and enterocolitis/typhlitis.

CASE CONTINUED

You obtain further history that he has had episodes of similar discomfort in recent weeks, but that they were previously self-limited. He has lost a few pounds in the last month, but hasn't thought much of it.

PMH: as per HPI. No history of AIDS-defining illnesses. Asthma in childhood

PSH: Cervical lymph node biopsy about 2 years ago

MEDs: Highly active anti-retroviral therapy (HAART)

SH/H: Denies tobacco or alcohol use. He is a recovered IVDA, now clean and sober for a little over two years.

 THOUGHT QUESTION

 ■ How will you proceed with your examination?
 ■ What do you expect to find?

 DISCUSSION

Obviously, a focused exam will be centered on the abdomen. In a patient who usually has loose stools, the absence of bowel activity is worrisome for a possible bowel obstruction or ileus. These may be specifically related to immune-compromise (e.g., cytomegalovirus [CMV colitis, with or without perforation], CMV cholecystitis, lymphoma), or to the usual causes in a "virgin" abdomen (hernia, tumor). Therefore, your exam should include a thorough inspection for hernia (inguinal/umbilical/ventral) and lymphadenopathy (including cervical, supraclavicular, axillary, and inguinal node basins).

 CASE CONTINUED

Exam: Afebrile. HR 105 BP 100/60

Gen: Thin man in moderate discomfort. *Lymph nodes:* Shotty nodes in all basins without dominant nodules. *Abdomen:* Slightly distended but soft, with some tympany; diffusely TTP, most prominent in the RLQ. No rebound, slight guarding. Questionable fullness in the RLQ. No scars or hernias. *Rectal:* heme negative

Labs:

$$145 \mid 98 \mid 22$$

$$8 >\text{--------}< 110 \qquad \text{---------------------}< 101$$

$$35 \qquad\qquad 3.2 \mid 32 \mid 1.0$$

LFTs, amylase, urinalysis WNL

THOUGHT QUESTION

- Given that the patient is afebrile and has a normal white blood cell count, how do you wish to proceed? Any additional tests or imaging studies?

DISCUSSION

It is important to remember that immunocompromised patients may not be able to mount a fever or rise in WBC, which makes the absolute value of these markers difficult to interpret in a possible surgical abdomen. In addition, a blunted inflammatory response may contribute to a relatively benign exam, even in the face of an intra-abdominal catastrophe.

The patient has a contraction alkalosis that is consistent with his history of emesis. His exam is suggestive of a bowel obstruction, with a possible evolving process in the RLQ (e.g., volvulus, intus-susception, ischemia). Although it would not be wrong to place an NGT and to obtain an abdominal XR series (to rule out free air, look for air-fluid levels, check for dilated bowel, etc.), the extended differential diagnosis in these patients is such that abdominal CT will offer the highest yield.

CASE CONTINUED

Abdominal CT shows a complete SBO with a transition point in the RLQ. There appears to be an associated mass, but it is difficult to discern because of nearby stranding. At exploration, a small bowel tumor is found. Pathology ultimately returns with lymphoma.

QUESTIONS

11-1. For the patient above, appropriate intraoperative management will include:

A. Closure of the abdomen, with referral for radiation and chemotherapy.

B. Partial small bowel and mesentery resection of the affected segment.

C. Total small bowel resection.

D. Placement of a feeding gastrostomy or jejunostomy.

E. Ileostomy.

11-2. Lymphoma is not usually considered to be a surgical disease. Under which of the following conditions would chemotherapy be the appropriate first-line management?

A. When the diagnosis is unclear or cell-typing is not available.

B. Hemodynamically significant bleeding.

C. Perforated viscus.

D. Weight loss and pain.

E. When there are no signs of extra-abdominal lympadenopathy.

11-3. What is the most common malignant neoplasm of the small bowel?

A. Adenocarcinoma.

B. Leiomyoma.

C. Carcinoid.

D. Lymphoma.

E. Sarcoma.

11-4. Postoperative infection risk with which of the following organisms is the same in HIV-infected as it is in non-HIV-infected patients?

A. *Staphylococcus aureus?*

B. Cytomegalovirus.

C. *Pneumocystis carinii.*

D. *Streptococcus pneumoniae.*

E. *Mycobacterium avium* (MAC).

ANSWERS

11-1. B. Treatment of primary small-bowel lymphoma is mainly surgical. The patient in question should undergo complete resection of the tumor, which will include partial small bowel resection and a wedge of mesentery. For patients with positive margins, adjuvant therapy is recommended. The survival for completely resected intestinal lymphoma is about 50%.

11-2. D. The role of the surgeon in lymphoma is usually limited to biopsy of a single peripheral lymph node to establish a tissue diagnosis. Abdominal surgery is rarely required except in the absence of peripheral lymphadenopathy, where it may be necessary to obtain intra-abdominal tissue for diagnosis or assessment of the spleen for decision-making regarding radiation versus chemotherapy. As with any patient, when hemodynamically significant bleeding, obstruction, or perforation occurs, laparotomy is indicated.

11-3. A. The most common malignant neoplasm of the small bowel is adenocarcinoma, followed by carcinoid, lymphoma, and sarcoma. Leiomyoma is the most common benign neoplasm of the small bowel.

11-4. A. Opportunistic infections in patients with a depressed immune status may be the result of pathogens such as *Pneumocystis carinii*, toxoplasmosis, cryptococcus, cytomegalovirus (CMV), herpes viruses, cryptosporidium, *Mycobacterium avium* (MAC), or tuberculosis. *Streptococcus pneumoniae* is the most common bacterial pathogen causing pneumonia in patients with HIV. Immune response to *Staphylococcus* sp. infection does not require cell-mediated immunity, and is not more common in HIV-infected patients.

ADDITIONAL SUGGESTED READING

Hodin RA and Matthews JB. Small Intestine, in Norton JA, Bollinger RR, Chang AE, Lowry SF, Mulvihill SJ, Pass HI, Thompson RW. (eds): Surgery: Basic Science and Clinical Evidence. New York: Springer-Verlag, 2001: 617–646.

Lefor AT, Phillips EH. Spleen, in Norton JA, Bollinger RR, Chang AE, Lowry SF, Mulvihill SJ, Pass HI, Thompson RW. (eds): Surgery: Basic Science and Clinical Evidence. New York: Springer-Verlag, 2001:763–785.

Lipsett PA. Hepatitis C and HIV Infection, in Cameron JL (ed): Current Surgical Therapy, 8th ed. Philadelphia: Mosby, 2004:1129–1135.

II

Other GI Tract Symptoms

Heartburn

CC/ID: 40-year-old woman with "severe heartburn" occurring two to three times per week.

HPI: The patient presents with a several year h/o "heartburn" for which she has tried multiple different over-the-counter remedies, including Maalox, Mylanta, Tums, Pepcid, Axid, and Zantac. More recently, she had been prescribed omeprazole in progressively escalating doses, and is now taking the maximum dose with some improvement in symptoms. She is frustrated because these medications do not offer her as much relief as they once did. Furthermore, if she forgets to take her medications, she is likely to get a bitter taste in her mouth, especially when she lies down to sleep. She denies any hoarseness, chest pain, difficulty swallowing, cough, or other respiratory problems.

PMHx: Fibromyalgia

PSHx: Rhinoplasty 10 years ago

Meds: As above; birth control pills

VS: AVSS

PE: *Gen:* Pleasant, no distress. *HEENT:* Anicteric, mucous membranes moist; no halitosis. *Neck:* No lymphadenopathy. *Chest:* Clear bilaterally. *Abdomen:* Soft, obese, nontender, nondistended, no masses, no scars.

THOUGHT QUESTION

- What is gastroesophageal reflux disease (GERD)? What are its causes?
- What are your options for further evaluating this patient?

DISCUSSION

GER is defined as abnormal reflux of gastric contents into the esophagus. This occurs secondary to failure of the antireflux barrier and may be caused by decreased lower esophageal sphincter (LES) tone, delayed gastric emptying, dysfunctional esophageal motility with loss of peristalsis, increased intra-abdominal pressure due to obesity or large meals, or iatrogenic injury to the LES.

Forty to fifty percent of Americans experience monthly symptoms of heartburn, and 10% experience these symptoms daily. Consequently, it is not really cost effective to endoscope all patients with classic symptoms in order to document esophagitis. Instead, empiric treatment (often with proton pump inhibitors or other antacids) is frequently attempted first. In this patient who has failed such therapy, further (invasive) evaluation is certainly warranted to confirm the clinical diagnosis and to validate the treatment strategy.

In a patient with typical symptoms, endoscopic findings of esophageal erosions or ulcers are fairly specific for GER. Esophageal biopsy can verify esophagitis. If endoscopy is normal (which may happen if a patient has been treated with antacid medications), then 24-hour pH probe monitoring can confirm the diagnosis. Esophageal manometry necessarily accompanies this procedure, because identification/localization of the LES is required for proper probe placement. It also gives information about esophageal motility. Barium swallow is generally used in patients with signs or symptoms of stricture, dysphagia, paraesophageal hernia, or other anatomic abnormalities.

CASE CONTINUED

You perform an EGD and find the salmon-colored appearance of columnar-lined epithelium in the distal esophagus. This area is biopsied and confirms intestinal metaplasia. There are no signs of ulceration or stricture. The gastric and duodenal portions of the exam are normal. Manometry reveals normal motility with adequate peristaltic pressures (i.e., you expect reliable esophageal clearance). pH probe monitoring confirms the diagnosis of reflux. With these findings, you schedule the patient for a laparoscopic Nissen (360-degree) fundoplication.

THOUGHT QUESTION

- What is the significance of the EGD findings? What are these changes called?
- What impact will this have on your long-term management plans?

DISCUSSION

The condition in which the tubular esophagus becomes lined with metaplastic columnar epithelium (rather than the normal squamous epithelium) is called *Barrett's* esophagus and is found in 7% to 10% of patients with GER. It is significant because it represents an increased risk for adenocarcinoma, estimated to be 0.2–2.0% per annum, or 30–60 times that of the general population. Treatment is still with acid-reducing medications and antireflux surgery, though regression of the changes is inconsistent. Regardless, patients with Barrett's are advised to undergo regular surveillance endoscopy to identify progressive metaplastic changes or progression to dysplasia. A finding of high-grade dysplasia has been grounds for recommending esophagectomy, on the grounds that there is a high likelihood of occult cancer or inevitable progression to cancer in that setting. Though recent epidemiological studies are challenging this recommendation, it remains the current standard of treatment.

QUESTIONS

12-1. LES dysfunction is the most common cause of GER. Which of the following is a DeMeester component of a competent LES?
- A. Resting LES pressure <6 mm Hg.
- B. Resting LES length <2 cm.
- C. Length of the intra-abdominal LES >1 cm.
- D. Gastric venting (belching).
- E. Therapeutic response to antacids.

12-2. Medical therapy is the first-line management for GER, with esophagitis healing in >90% of cases with intensive therapy. However, the percentage of patients in whom symptoms will recur after withdrawal of medication is

A. 20%.
B. 40%.
C. 60%.
D. 80%.
E. 100%.

12-3. Recommended lifestyle changes for treatment of GER includes

A. Eating within 2 hours of sleep.
B. Eating small meals.
C. Taking muscle relaxants.
D. Drinking more coffee.
E. Increasing alcohol consumption.

12-4. A patient is informed that his EGD for reflux symptoms demonstrates the presence of a hiatal hernia. In response to his request for information about his condition, you tell him that:

A. Sliding (type I) hernias have a peritoneal sac, but rarely progress to incarceration.
B. Peraesophageal (type II) hernias are the most common, and do not require repair.
C. There is no true peritoneal sac in paraesophageal (type II) hernias, so they do not incarcerate.
D. Type III hernias are a combination of types I and II, and should be managed operatively.
E. Hiatal hernias do not need to be addressed until reflux symptoms are under control.

ANSWERS

12-1. C. Resting LES pressure >6 mm Hg, length >2cm, and intra-abdominal length >1 cm are all thought to be important components of LES competence. The DeMeester score attempts to grade reflux severity using these measures. Belching or gastric venting is a normal means of relieving transient episodes of reflux and response to antacids predicts symptom relief following an antireflux procedure. Neither describes LES competence.

12-2. D. Because medical management does not address the mechanical etiology of GER, symptoms will recur in more than

80% of cases within 1 year of drug withdrawal. In some patients, avoiding the prospect of life-long antacid treatment is an indication for surgical intervention.

12-3. B. Minimizing gastric distension by avoiding overeating or eating small meals is a frequently recommended dietary change. Patients should avoid eating within 2 hours of sleep because of postural-related symptoms; additionally, elevating the head of the bed may be helpful. Patients should be counseled to avoid substances that decrease LES pressure, including coffee, nicotine, alcohol, and fatty foods. They are also recommended to avoid anticholinergics, muscle relaxants, and tranquilizers.

12-4. D. Type I hiatal hernias do not have a true hernia (peritoneal) sac; type II do. Sliding hiatal hernias are generally not treated. However, because of the risk of bleeding, incarceration, or strangulation with paraesophageal hernias, patients with type II and III hiatal hernias should be referred for operative repair.

ADDITIONAL SUGGESTED READING

Cappell MS. Clinical presentation, diagnosis, and management of gastroesophageal reflux disease. Med Clin North Am 2005;89:243–291.

Jackson CC, DeMeester SR. Surgical therapy for Barrett's esophagus. Thorac Surg Clin 2005;15:429–436.

Shaheen NJ. Advances in Barrett's esophagus and esophageal adenocarcinoma. Gastroenterology 2005;128:1554–1566.

CASE 13

Difficulty Swallowing

CC/ID: 70-year-old man with difficulty swallowing.

HPI: The patient presents to your clinic with a 2- to 3-month h/o increasing difficulty swallowing (solids > liquids). He points to his mid-sternum, stating that it feels as though "things get stuck here." He infrequently feels a need to vomit, but believes that he is eating less, accounting for his ~10 pound weight loss in the last couple of months. He feels maybe a little more tired than usual and has been coughing more, although he notes that he has had a chronic cough related to his years of smoking. He has had no fevers, chills, or sweats.

PMHx: Arthritis, glucose insufficiency, asthma, mild CHF

PSHx: Skin cancer removal, cholecystectomy ~30 years ago

Meds: MVI

SHx: 60 pyh, now smoking ~1/2 ppd; nightly "cocktail"; no illicit drugs

THOUGHT QUESTION

- What will you look for on physical exam?
- What would be the significance of halitosis?
- Does a h/o GERD affect your differential?
- Is there significance to the worsening cough?
- What studies will you order and why?

DISCUSSION

It may be difficult to find any obvious physical signs on exam if intrathoracic pathology is suspected. Patients with a malignancy may show signs of weight loss or wasting if their disease is advanced. Malignant lesions may show spread to cervical or sup-raclavicular lymph node groups, but may also be undetectable by physical examination in the mediastinal, celiac, or gastric regions. Foul-smelling emesis or halitosis suggests obstruction with bacterial degradation of retained food particles. Reflux is nonspecific, but patients may have related findings of Schatzki's ring, achalasia, or Barrett's metaplasia, which is associated with an increased risk of cancer. Coughing is commonly seen when reflux or obstruction causes aspiration and bronchospasm.

A number of studies are integral to the evaluation of esophageal pathology, and most are used in concert to obtain the most complete information. Disorders of motility, such as achalasia, diffuse esophageal spasm, and nutcracker esophagus, are best studied using esophageal manometry. A definitive diagnosis of reflux requires a 24-hour pH probe study, with placement of the probe determined by the location of the lower esophageal sphincter (LES), which is defined on manometry. Esophagogram, using barium or, in cases of suspected perforation, a water-soluble contrast agent, is best for defining esophageal anatomy, deviation (e.g., when the esophagus is displaced by a mass), and perforation. EGD is an important tool for evaluating internal lesions and for obtaining biopsies for tissue diagnosis. Computed tomography (CT) is less useful in evaluating primary esophageal pathology than it is in evaluating local lymph nodes and involvement of other nearby structures. This patient sounds as though he may have a partially obstructing lesion, which could be delineated on esophagogram. If a mass is seen or suggested, EGD would be helpful in obtaining a specimen for diagnosis.

CASE CONTINUED

PE: *Gen:* Thin but fairly vigorous appearing elderly man. *HEENT:* Oropharynx clear; no cervical or clavicular lymphadenopathy. *Chest:* Diffuse wheezes bilaterally. *Cor:* RRR, S_4 gallop. *Abdomen:* Soft, scaphoid, nontender. *Rectal:* heme negative.

You proceed with a barium esophagogram, which shows an irregular filling defect in the middle one-third of the esophagus. An EGD is performed and biopsies are taken.

THOUGHT QUESTION

■ What kinds of tumors occur in the esophagus? What are the most common types of esophageal cancer?

■ Would a smooth filling defect on barium swallow change your differential?

DISCUSSION

Esophageal tumors can be benign (<1%) or malignant. Leiomyoma is the most common benign tumor, but other benign masses include cysts, polyps, lipomas, and hemangiomas. Historically, most esophageal cancers have been of squamous cell, rather than adeno-matous origin. However, adenocarcinoma now accounts for more than half of all new cases diagnosed. Typically, adenocarcinomas occur in the distal one-third of the esophagus, whereas squamous cell cancer occurs in equal proportions throughout its length. Malignant tumors may appear as smooth or irregular defects on esophagogram, but smooth defects tend to be more suggestive of a benign process.

QUESTIONS

13-1. Biopsy returns with adenocarcinoma, and further tests (CT scan, endoscopic ultrasound [EUS], bronchoscopy) reveal no evidence of nodal extension. Appropriate surgical management in a patient with a potentially curable lesion must include
    A. Total or subtotal esophagectomy.
    B. Removal of the tumor only, with primary restoration of GI tract continuity.
    C. Thoracotomy for adequate mediastinal dissection.
    D. Bowel interposition grafting.
    E. Resection of at least 1/2 of the stomach.

13-2. Blood supply to the esophagus includes the
    A. Superior thyroid arteries.
    B. Left pulmonary artery.
    C. Right pulmonary artery.
    D. Right gastric artery.
    E. Splenic artery.

13-3. Barrett's esophagus
   A. Eventually occurs in all patients with reflux disease.
   B. Occurs when columnar epithelium becomes squamous.
   C. Occurs when squamous epithelium becomes columnar.
   D. Increases the risk of squamous carcinoma of the esophagus.
   E. Never progresses >1 cm from the gastroesophageal junction.

13-4. Achalasia is marked by
   A. Absence of peristalsis and failure of the LES to relax with swallowing.
   B. Hyperactive peristalsis and an obstructing lesion at the LES.
   C. Normal peristalsis and a hypertensive LES.
   D. Pathognomonic esophagogram findings.
   E. Requirement for EGD to confirm the diagnosis.

ANSWERS

13-1. A. Total or subtotal esophagectomy is critical if there is any hope for cure, although 5-year survival for resectable esophageal cancers still remains at an abysmal 5% to 20%. Because lymphatics run longitudinally, micrometastatic spread can occur over the entire length of the esophagus even in the presence of a localized lesion. Limited resections are generally reserved only for palliative purposes. Bowel interposition grafting may be used if the stomach cannot be adequately mobilized for a pull-up, but is not mandatory. Esophagectomy can be acceptably accomplished via abdominal and cervical incisions (transhiatal approach), without an absolute requirement for thoracotomy (transthoracic approach).

13-2. A. The superior and inferior thyroid arteries supply the cervical esophagus; bronchial and esophageal arteries supply the mid/thoracic esophagus; and the left gastric and phrenic arteries supply the distal/abdominal esophagus.

13-3. C. Barrett's esophagus occurs in 7% to 10% of patients with GERD and is marked by the metaplastic change of squamous to columnar epithelium in the distal esophagus. Ten percent of patients with Barrett's changes will go on to develop *adeno*carcinoma.

13-4. A. Achalasia is a manometric diagnosis, with failure of relaxation of the LES with swallowing and a lack of peristalsis.

The "classic" esophagogram finding in achalasia is the "bird's beak" deformity, a tapering seen at the LES. However, this finding is not specific or pathognomonic.

ADDITIONAL SUGGESTED READING

Chu KM, Law SY, Fok M, et al. A prospective randomized comparison of transhiatal and transthoracic resection for lower-third esophageal carcinoma. Am J Surg 1997;174:320–324.

Visbal AL, Allen MS, Miller DL, et al. Ivor Lewis esophagogastrectomy for esophageal cancer. Ann Thorac Surg 2001;71:1803–1808.

Wang KK, Wongkeesong M, Buttar NS. American Gastroenterological Association technical review on the role of the gastroenterologist in the management of esophageal carcinoma. Gastroenterology 2005;128:1471–1505.

Weber WA, Ott K. Imaging of esophageal and gastric cancer. Semin Oncol 2004;31:530–541.

Painless Jaundice

CC: Yellow eyes for 1 month.

HPI The patient is a 67-year-old man who is brought in by his family because they believe his eyes look yellow. The man had not noticed anything out of the ordinary, but his wife thinks that his eyes have been a little "less white" for about a month. They are not sure about specific weight loss, but his clothes seem to fit much more loosely now than they had previously. He denies anorexia, nausea, or vomiting. He reports occasional epigastric pain that radiates to his back, but he has attributed this to heartburn. He denies dark urine, light stools, or pruritus. There have been no unusual changes in his bowel habits (diarrhea, constipation, or melena).

PMHx: GERD

PSHx: None

Meds: Maalox prn

All: NKDA

SHx: No tobacco or alcohol use, no illicit drug use

FHx: No known cancers

VS: Afebrile, vital signs normal, weight 71 kg, height 5'11"

PE: *Gen:* WD/WN thin man in no acute distress, skin slightly jaundiced. *HEENT:* PERRL, EOMI, sclera moderately icteric. *Abdomen:* Soft, NT/ND; firm 3- to 4-cm mass felt in RUQ, nonmobile, round, nontender. *Rectal:* nl tone, heme neg, no masses. *Neuro:* grossly nonfocal, AO × 4.

THOUGHT QUESTION

- What is your differential diagnosis?
- What tests will assist in making the diagnosis?

DISCUSSION

The differential diagnosis for jaundice includes prehepatic (hemolysis), hepatic (hepatitis, cirrhosis), and posthepatic/ obstructive (choledocholithiasis, cholangitis, biliary stricture, choledochal cyst, neoplasm) causes. Laboratory tests including liver function tests (transaminases, total and direct bilirubin, alkaline phosphatase) will help to narrow the diagnosis.

Although this patient does not yet have other signs or symptoms suggestive of obstructive hyperbilirubinemia (dark urine, light stools), his presentation (age, weight loss, jaundice, +/-epigastric pain, and a palpable RUQ mass) is most concerning for cancer of the pancreas, ampulla of Vater, or bile ducts. Biliary ductal anatomy is best evaluated with ultrasound. If there is no evidence of dilated common or intrahepatic ducts, then a mechanical (mass) obstruction is unlikely and other diagnoses should be entertained. If dilated ducts and gallstones are present but no mass is obvious, then ERCP will help to document choledocholithiasis and to rule out a malignancy. If dilated ducts but no gallstones are seen, or if there is evidence of a mass, then a computed tomography (CT) is indicated to identify and characterize the obstruction. The palpable mass in the RUQ is not usually the tumor itself, but rather the distended gallbladder. A *Courvoisier gallbladder* (or Courvoisier's sign) is an enlarged, nontender gallbladder associated with jaundice, and is a sign of pancreatic cancer with bile duct obstruction and bile accumulation. It is appreciated in 20% to 25% of patients with painless jaundice.

CASE CONTINUED

Labs: CBC and lytes WNL; AST 218; ALT 185; AlkP 518; Tbili 11.5; Dbili 9.8; albumin 2.7; amylase 184; PT 16.2; PTT 23.5; INR 1.6; serum (tumor marker) CA 19-9 mildly elevated.

Imaging: *Ultrasound:* No gallstones seen, gallbladder distended but without signs of inflammation; dilated intra- and extra-hepatic bile ducts; echogenic mass in the head of the pancreas; pancreas otherwise normal in appearance. *CT:* 4-cm mass in the head of the pancreas, without evidence of liver metastases or portal lymphadenopathy; tumor abuts the portal vein but does not appear to invade it.

THOUGHT QUESTION

■ What are your treatment options at this point?

DISCUSSION

The patient has a pancreatic head mass which is cancer until proven otherwise. ERCP can be performed to better delineate ductal anatomy and to obtain cytologic brushings, but is unlikely to change the primary recommendation, which is surgical. Surgical resection (pancreatico-duodenectomy, or Whipple procedure) is the only potentially curative therapy for a pancreatic head or periampullary tumor. This patient's apparent reasonable functional status and lack of radiographic evidence of metastatic disease make him a potential operative candidate. Chemotherapy and radiation may improve results slightly, but 5-year survival after operation is still poor. Most resectable pancreatic tumors are found in the head of the pancreas, because jaundice prompts evaluation and diagnosis earlier than tumors of the body or tail. If unresectable disease is found, either preoperatively or at the time of surgery, biliary bypass and/or gastroenterostomy can be performed to prevent progression of biliary and duodenal obstruction, respectively. Endoscopic decompression of the bile duct with stenting can be performed if the patient is deemed unfit for surgery or if the disease is advanced and survival is expected to be less than 3 months. However, biliary sepsis and recurrent jaundice are common.

QUESTIONS

14-1. A possible risk factor for pancreatic cancer is
A. *H. Pylori* infection.
B. Aflatoxins.
C. Chronic pancreatitis.
D. Multiparity.
E. Blood type A.

14-2. Most pancreatic carcinomas
A. Originate from ductal epithelial cells.
B. Invade the duodenum at the time of presentation.
C. Are found in the body and tail.
D. Remain localized to the pancreas.
E. Spread hematogenously.

14-3. Which of the following oncogenes is believed to be involved in the pathogenesis of pancreatic cancer?
A. *myc*
B. *her*-2
C. DCC
D. K-*ras*
E. *p53*

14-4. A mass might be difficult to visualize on CT scan when
A. It is of different intensity that the surrounding parenchyma.
B. It is surrounded by fat.
C. It is displacing nearby structures.
D. It is calcified.
E. It is <1–2 cm in size.

ANSWERS

14-1. C. Chronic pancreatitis is a risk factor for pancreatic cancer. Other factors that may be associated are cigarette smoking, family history, high dietary fat, and cholecystectomy (in women). Aflatoxins are a risk factor for hepatocellular carcinoma. *H. pylori* infection and blood type A are risk factors associated with gastric cancer.

14-2. A. Pancreatic ductal tumors involve glandular formation within a dense fibrous matrix. Most patients have evidence of a chronic obstructive pancreatitis. Sixty to seventy percent of pancreatic adenocarcinomas are found in the head of the pancreas, whereas 15% are in the body, 10% in the tail, and 5% to 15% are diffuse. Duodenal invasion is present at the time of diagnosis in only 25% of patients, but symptoms (nausea and vomiting) eventually develop in one-third. Extension beyond the pancreas is typical, with early local invasion of nearby structures (i.e., bile duct, liver, retroperitoneum, visceral and portal vessels, stomach, left adrenal). Tumors (of any type) found at the confluence of the extrahepatic ducts are called *Klatskin tumors*. Lymphatic spread usually precedes hematogenous spread.

14-3. D. *myc* is associated with Burkitt lymphoma, *her*-2 with breast cancer, DCC (deleted in colon cancer) with colon cancer. *p53* is associated with retinoblastoma and a number of other non-pancreatic neoplasms.

14-4. E. CT may not reveal tumors that are <2 cm in size. In the case of pancreatic tumors, a diagnosis can instead be made based on ERCP findings of pancreatic or biliary ductal dilation or with endoscopy and endoscopic ultrasound. The other choices are all features that actually enhance CT visualization. See Figures 14-1 and 14-2.

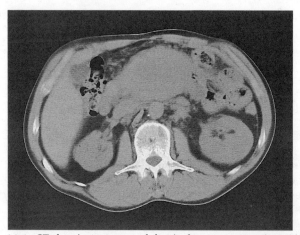

FIGURE 14-1. CT showing an upper abdominal mass: pancreatic carcinoma. (*Used with permission from Patel PR. Lecture Notes on Radiology. Oxford: Blackwell Science, Ltd., 1998:140.*)

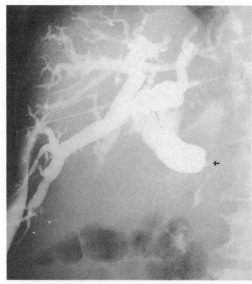

FIGURE 14-2. Transhepatic cholangiogram: tight stricture from pancreatic carcinoma (arrow) causing severe biliary obstruction. (*Used with permission from Patel PR. Lecture Notes on Radiology. Oxford: Blackwell Science, Ltd., 1998:132.*)

ADDITIONAL SUGGESTED READING

Ahmad NA, Lewis JD, Ginsberg GG, et al. Long term survival after pancreatic resection for pancreatic adenocarcinoma. Am J Gastroenterol 2001;96:2609–2615.

Billingsly KG, Hur K, Henderson WG, et al. Outcome after pancreaticoduodenectomy for periampullary cancer: an analysis from the Veterans Affairs National Surgical Quality Improvement Program. J Gastrointest Surg 2003;7:484–491.

Neoptolemos JP, Dunn JA, Stocken DD, et al. European Study Group for Pancreatic Cancer (ESPAC): adjuvant chemoradiotherapy and chemotherapy in respectable pancreatic cancer: a randomized controlled trial. Lancet 2001;358:1576–1585.

Jaundice and Confusion

CC: Jaundice and confusion for 1 day.

HPI: The patient is a 42-year-old woman who is brought in by her family because of increasing confusion for the past day. She also seems to have developed a yellowish hue to her skin. They report that she was fine 2 days ago when the family had gone for a hike in the woods. She is otherwise healthy, without recent anorexia or weight loss. In fact, she eats only organic vegetables and even found some mushrooms on the hike that she made into a quiche for dinner that evening. Her husband and children opted for pizza. She has no recent travel history and has never had a blood transfusion. She is not pregnant and has no known family history of liver disease. She has had no nausea, vomiting, fever, or chills, and has no hx of hepatitis or gallstones.

PMHx: Depression (but no hx of suicide attempts)

PSHx: Appendectomy

Meds: Prozac

SHx: Glass of wine with dinner nightly, no cigarettes or IV drug use, no high risk sexual activity or tattoos

VS: Temp 38.6°C, HR 88, BP 93/45, RR 18, O_2 sat 97% on 2 L NC

PE: *Gen:* WD/WN woman, jaundiced, resting quietly. *Neuro:* Arousable but oriented to self only, moves all extremities, withdraws to pain, no asterixis. *HEENT:* Sclera icteric, PERRL, EOMI, no *fetor hepaticus. Lungs:* CTA bilaterally, no crackles or wheezes. *CV:* RRR, no murmurs. *Abdomen:* Soft, NT/ND, no palpable liver enlargement. *Ext:* No cyanosis or edema.

Labs: WBC 6; Hct 40; Plts 298; PT 54; INR 5.4; PTT 102; lytes WNL; AST 1614; ALT 1823; Alk Phos 314; Tbili 16.2; acetaminophen level <10; hepatitis titers pending.

THOUGHT QUESTION

- What is happening in this patient? What are the possible causes?
- What would be the significance of findings of asterixis or fetor hepaticus?
- What are the principles of management in this setting?

DISCUSSION

Hepatic failure is caused by hepatocyte necrosis. Fulminant hepatic failure is defined by the onset of acute hepatic encephalopathy within 8 weeks of the onset of symptomatic hepatocellular disease in a previously healthy person. Acute hepatitis causes 20% of cases of acute liver failure (10% each hepatitis A and hepatitis B). Acetaminophen overdose accounts for another 20%; cryptogenic (15%) and idiopathic drug reaction (12%) are other causes. More rare causes of acute liver failure include Budd-Chiari syndrome, acute fatty liver of pregnancy, Wilson's disease, heat stroke, and *Amanita phalloides* ingestion. Only about 2000 cases of acute hepatic failure occur in the United States each year, with a mortality of up to 80%. Morbidity and mortality is primarily determined by the course of encephalopathy. This patient likely ingested a toxic dose of the *Amanita phalloides* mushroom, which grows in the wild. She has no other risk factors (e.g., IV drug use, alcoholism, acetaminophen use).

Asterixis and fetor hepaticus are signs that may be seen in hepatic failure. Asterixis is a clinical sign indicating a loss of posture, and is usually manifest by a bilateral flapping tremor at the wrist, metacarpophalangeal, and hip joints. It may also be seen in tongue, foot, and any skeletal muscle. To test for asterixis, extend the patient's arms, spread the fingers, dorsiflex the wrist, and observe for the abnormal "flapping" tremor at the wrist. *Fetor hepaticus* is a musty-sweet breath odor, sometimes described as reminiscent of garlic or urine. It is thought to perhaps be due to the exhalation of mercaptans.

Management of acute liver failure requires aggressive invasive monitoring pulmonary artery catheter, arterial line, Foley catheter, nasogastric tube [NG tube] and treatment. This should include measures to protect against and treat cerebral edema (e.g., intracranial pressure monitor, mannitol), and to maintain a cerebral perfusion pressure >60 mm Hg. The patient may need to be intubated for severe mental status changes or pulmonary failure. Lactulose is given to bind and lessen the amount of free ammonia, which can exacerbate encephalopathy. Judicious treatment of coagulopathy, prevention of sepsis (with prophylactic antibiotics), and prevention or treatment of hypoglycemia are all essential parts of the management algorithm. *N*-acetylcysteine (Mucomyst) is used specifically to treat acetaminophen ingestion.

 ## CASE CONTINUED

The patient rapidly deteriorates and requires intubation for airway protection. Her urine output begins to fall with a concomitant rise in her BUN and creatinine levels. She begins to bleed from her IV sites and is started on a fresh frozen plasma (FFP) drip. She is listed as status 1 for liver transplant.

THOUGHT QUESTION

- What are the indications for liver transplant?

DISCUSSION

The clinical sequelae of liver failure that signal the need for transplantation include intractable ascites, frequent episodes of spontaneous bacterial peritonitis or sepsis, bleeding varices, encephalopathy, coagulopathy, and hepatorenal or hepatopulmonary syndromes. The disease states for which transplant is commonly indicated in adults include hepatitis C (with or without hepatocellular carcinoma), alcoholic liver disease, primary biliary cirrhosis, and cryptogenic disease. In children, biliary atresia and metabolic disorders are two common reasons for transplantation. With the development of split-liver and living-donor grafts, pediatric liver transplantation is now being performed with greater frequency and with reasonable success.

QUESTIONS

15-1. In patients with portal hypertension
  A. Varices develop in fewer than 25% of patients.
  B. The Child classification predicts operative mortality.
  C. Spontaneous bacterial peritonitis usually involves anaerobic microbes.
  D. Caput medusa describes a large umbilical hernia.
  E. All patients who develop varices will eventually experience a GI bleed.

15-2. Transjugular intrahepatic portosystemic shunt (TIPS)
  A. Is used to treat refractory ascites or variceal bleeding.
  B. Is a durable solution for treatment of portal hypertension.
  C. Completely decompresses the portal system.
  D. Leads to neural excitation and hallucinations.
  E. Reduces portal pressure by about 30%.

15-3. Which immunosuppressive agent binds cyclophilin, blocking early T-cell activation and inhibiting macrophage production of IL-1?
  A. Tacrolimus.
  B. Antithymocyte globulin.
  C. Azathioprine.
  D. Cyclosporine.
  E. Glucocorticoids.

15-4. Hepatocellular carcinoma
  A. Is always preceded pathologically by hepatic adenoma.
  B. Is preceded pathologically by focal nodular hyperplasia (FNH).
  C. Is associated with primary metastases to the brain.
  D. Can produce hypertension and diarrhea.
  E. Can be followed with the tumor marker CA 19-9.

ANSWERS

15-1. B. Although two-thirds of patients with portal hypertension develop varices, only two-thirds of those patients will experience a significant variceal bleed. Variceal hemorrhage rarely occurs when the portal pressure gradient (portal minus hepatic venous pressure) is <12 mm Hg. Caput medusa is formed by distended periumbilical venous collaterals that are filled by a recanalized umbilical vein. They may be seen as prominent periumbilical vessels. The development of umbilical and other abdominal wall hernias (e.g., inguinal) is enhanced by the ascites and muscle wasting typical of patients with advanced liver disease. Spontaneous bacterial peritonitis most frequently involves *E. coli*, pneumococci, and streptococci.

The Child-Turcotte classification was originally devised to predict operative mortality and long-term survival in liver failure patients after construction of a portosystemic shunt (Table 15-1). Child's class A patients are believed to be good risk (90% survival at 1 year), whereas class C patients are very poor risk (50% survival at 1 year) for operation. Class B patients are intermediate (66% survival). This classification is now used to estimate hepatic reserve and prognosis in other clinical settings as well.

TABLE 15-1 Child-Turcotte Classification

Class	A	B	C
Bilirubin (mg/dL)	<2	2–3	>3
Albumin (g/dL)	>3.5	3–3.5	<3
Ascites	None	Treatable	Refractory
Encephalopathy	None	Minimal	Severe
Nutrition	Normal	Fair	Poor

15-2. A. A TIPS procedure generally reduces portal pressures by more than 50% by diverting a significant volume of blood from the liver. Patients with hepatic encephalopathy post-TIPS present with mental confusion and even obtundation. This results from decreased hepatic extraction and metabolism of (and therefore increased central exposure to) the neuroactive substances that cause neural *inhibition*. Encephalopathy and hepatic insufficiency occur in 20% to 30% of patients after TIPS.

Patency of the TIPS is followed with serial color duplex ultrasonography. Shunt stenosis and occlusion is approximately 60% at 1 year. Therefore, TIPS is not a good choice for long-term (>2 years) management of nontransplant candidates, but it may be adequate for elderly and high-risk patients who are not candidates for an open operative portosystemic shunt.

15-3. D. Tacrolimus binds to FK binding protein and blocks expression of interleukin-2 receptors on stimulated T cells. Glucocorticoids inhibit interleukin-1 and interleukin-6 synthesis, along with many other T-cell and macrophage functions. Antithymocyte globulin acts by complement-dependent lysis and opsonization. Via inhibition of the cyclophylin enzyme, cyclosporin blocks transcription of early T-cell activation genes (interleukin-2, interleukin-3, interleukin-4, and interferon-γ) and inhibits macrophage production of interleukin-1.

15-4. D. Hepatocellular adenomas histologically lack bile duct architecture and have a very low rate of malignant degeneration. They are more common in women who have used oral contraceptives. There is a significant risk of rupture and intraperitoneal hemorrhage, particularly with pregnancy. Focal nodular hyperplasia (FNH) is usually asymptomatic and rarely bleeds. Large lesions are associated with a central stellate scar. Histologically, focal nodular hyperplasia shows normal-appearing hepatocytes, bile ducts, and Kupffer cells. It is also a benign lesion with no risk of malignant degeneration. Hepatocellular carcinoma is associated with hepatitis infection, cirrhosis, and aflatoxin B1. Paraneoplastic syndromes associated with hepatocellular carcinoma include erythrocytosis, hypercalcemia, hypertension (from angiotensin production), and diarrhea (from vasoactive intestinal peptide or gastrin production). Levels of serum alpha-fetoprotein correlate with tumor size (not CA 19-9, a pancreatic and ovarian tumor marker). Hepatocellular carcinoma has a tendency for local and vascular invasion and metastasizes primarily to the lung. Of note, the most common liver tumor is a metastatic tumor from another site.

ADDITIONAL SUGGESTED READING

Blei AT, Cordoba J; Practice Parameters Committee of the
    American College of Gastroenterology. Hepatic encephalopathy.
    Am J Gastroenterol 2001:96;1968–1976.
Wiesner R, Edwards E, Freeman R, et al. United Network for
    Organ Sharing Liver Disease Severity Score Committee. Model
    for end-stage liver disease (MELD) and allocation of donor
    livers. Gastroenterology 2003;124:91–96.

CASE **16**

Vomiting Blood

CC/ID: 50-year-old man vomiting blood.

HPI: 911 was called after the patient was found by a friend to be very confused and spitting up blood. He is a known alcoholic who has been seen previously in your hospital for assorted injuries sustained while inebriated. You are uncertain of the duration or magnitude of his symptoms, because he is unable to give you much history. As far as you can tell from his records, he has no other significant medical comorbidities and is not on any medications.

THOUGHT QUESTION

- What are your priorities upon the arrival of this patient?
- Are there any services that should be called or notified?
- What are the possible etiologies of this patient's symptoms? Which are the most likely given his drinking hx?

DISCUSSION

Any patient with an acute GI Bleed requires aggressive resuscitation management as guided by the "ABCs": airway, breathing, circulation. While the patient's airway and breathing are secured, two large-bore IVs should be placed (14 or 16 gauge), IV fluids started, and blood made available. A nasogastric tube should be placed and lavaged until clear. Failure of gastric aspirate to clear suggests an ongoing bleed. A Foley catheter to monitor urine output during the resuscitation can assist in assessment of fluid status. It is usually advisable to notify the GI service, because upper endoscopy will be required for diagnosis and/or treatment when the patient is hemodynamically stable.

The patient's alcohol history suggests that his bleed will be related to varices (from cirrhosis with portal hypertension) or possibly to retching (Mallory-Weiss tear). However, ulcer disease and malignancy cannot be ruled out. Other toxicology screening may be warranted. Regardless, focus should first be on resuscitation and stabilization, then diagnosis and management.

CASE CONTINUED

IV access is obtained and intravenous fluids are begun. NG aspirate clears after 800 mL of lavasate. Your evaluation continues.

VS: (after 2 L of LR) Temp 36°C, BP 105/70, HR 105

PE: *Gen:* Dysarthric, AO × 2 (to person, place), confused, smelling of alcohol. *HEENT:* Plethoric, anicteric, PERRLA. *Chest:* Spider angiomata, gynecomastia; otherwise CTA. *Abdomen:* Distended but soft and nontender; fluid wave; nodular liver edge palpable 2 to 3 cm below the costal margin.

Labs:

```
        9                    131 | 96 | 41      Tbili 2.0        PT 16.1 (INR 1.5)
  8 >------< 211          ----+----+----<       AST/ALT 155/73   PTT 37
       27                  4.5 | 20 | 1.3       AP 151
```

The patient is brought to the ICU for observation. Shortly after arrival, he becomes more tachycardic and his NG again begins to drain frank blood. He receives 2 U PRBCs and is started on a vasopressin drip to help constrict his splanchnic circulation. As he stabilizes, an EGD is performed and a significant bleeding esophageal varix is identified and cauterized. He is started on a beta-blocker.

Comment: Another option for endoscopic control of bleeding varices is band ligation. It has been shown in some series to be superior to sclerotherapy because of a slightly lower risk of treatment-related complications. The efficacy of controlling active hemorrhage is approximately equivalent. Beta-blocker therapy can help to decrease portal pressure and may help to decrease the risk of first bleed or re-bleed.

QUESTIONS

16-1. If endoscopic treatment fails, other options to control bleeding include
   A. Gastrectomy.
   B. NGT to high continuous suction.
   C. Transjugular intrahepatic portosystemic shunt (TIPS).
   D. Esophagectomy.
   E. Emergent liver transplant

16-2. Coffee ground emesis is suggestive of
   A. A recent history of coffee ingestion.
   B. Blood clotting defects.
   C. Stagnant blood that has oxidized.
   D. Perforation.
   E. Biliary obstruction

16-3. The five clinical components of the Child's criteria are
   A. Transaminases, coags, hematocrit, mental status, macroglossia.
   B. Fever, ascites, jaundice, hypotension, brittle nails.
   C. Transaminases, ascites, oliguria, anemia, gallstones.
   D. Ascites, encephalopathy, muscle wasting, albumin level, bilirubin level.
   E. Fever, RUQ pain, jaundice, hypotension, mental status changes.

16-4. Bleeding from Mallory-Weiss tears generally
   A. Is pathognomonic of cancer.
   B. Requires massive transfusion.
   C. Only occurs in end-stage cirrhosis.
   D. Mandates surgical resection of the offending lesion.
   E. Resolves without intervention.

ANSWERS

16-1. C. Esophagectomy, gastrectomy, liver transplant, and high NG tube suction are not reasonable management interventions. Other options for bleeding control following failure of endoscopic therapy include balloon tamponade (Minnesota tube or Senstaken-Blakemore tube), TIPS, or open portosystemic shunt. TIPS and portosystemic shunt are procedures meant to decompress the portal system by directing blood flow to the systemic circulation.

TIPS continues to become more common with experience and good comparative study trials. Open portosystemic shunt is done in select centers, but remains uncommonly performed in the emergent situation.

16-2. C. "Coffee grounds" usually suggests older blood that has been oxidized, but does not exclude the presence of an ongoing bleed. It is analogous to melena (as opposed to hematochezia) in lower GIB.

16-3. D. The Child's classification is an assessment of hepatic reserve and is used to assess operative risk (see Case 15, Table 15-1). The clinical findings are indicators of hepatic synthesis, hepatic filtering capacity, and nutritional status. (Muscle wasting is a clinical surrogate for nutritional status.) Transaminases are not an indicator. Choice "E" is Reynold's pentad, and is associated with severe ascending cholangitis.

16-4. E. Bleeding from Mallory-Weiss tears is rarely severe and is usually self-limited in duration. The lesions can be diagnosed endoscopically as a tear at the gastroesophageal junction, and if they have not already stopped bleeding by the time of this exam, can be cauterized or injected.

ADDITIONAL SUGGESTED READING

Banares R, Albillos A, Rincon D, et al. Endoscopic treatment versus endoscopic plus pharmacologic treatment for acute variceal bleeding: a meta-analysis. Hepatology 2002;35:609–615.

Singh P, Pooran N, Indaram A, et al. Combined ligation and sclerotherapy versus ligation alone for secondary prophylaxis of esophageal variceal bleeding: a meta-analysis. Am J Gastroenterol 2002;97:623–629.

CASE **17**

Bleeding per Rectum

CC/ID: 65-year-old man with bright red blood per rectum.

HPI: The patient presents to the VA clinic for a "checkup." On interview, he tells you that his wife made him come in after he mentioned to her that the toilet water was tinged pink following a bowel movement. His stools have otherwise been unremarkable. He is unsure if this has happened much before, because he usually flushes without looking. He is a little lightheaded but has no other complaints. His weight and appetite are unchanged. Colonoscopy 3 1/2 years ago was reportedly normal.

PMHx: HTN, PVD, CAD, DM, hypercholesterolemia; 1 ppd smoker for >40 years

PSHx: Appendectomy, R shoulder surgery

Meds: Simvastatin, glyburide, lisinopril, aspirin, Viagra

VS: Temp 36.5°C, BP 135/80, HR 90

PE: *Gen:* AO × 3, comfortable, NAD. *Chest:* Clear bilaterally. *Abdomen:* normal active bowel sounds, soft, nontender/nondistended; no masses. *Rectal:* Soft stool and gross dark red blood in vault; normal tone; no masses; no obvious hemorrhoids. *Ext:* Warm and well perfused with strong bilateral femoral pulses.

THOUGHT QUESTION

- What is the significance of the dark red blood on examination? How does this correlate with his toilet water?
- What are the most common sources of lower GIB and how are these diagnosed?
- Does his medical/surgical history offer any potential clues to his diagnosis?

DISCUSSION

Dark blood is suggestive of blood that is not fresh, such as that which has traveled for some distance or which has been slow in transit. Because it only takes a few drops of blood to change the color of toilet water, it is seldom helpful to use this finding as a reliable measure of blood loss.

Upper GIB is the most common cause of lower GIB, and for this reason workup should include evaluation of upper GI sources. In this older patient, colorectal cancer and diverticular disease should be high on the differential. Mesenteric ischemia is a possibility, given his medical history and known vascular disease (including CAD). Other considerations would include angiodysplasia, inflammatory bowel disease, or hemorrhoids. Aortoenteric fistula, which is an uncommon but potentially devastating process, should be considered in any patient who has undergone aortic surgery and who presents with any GIB. Serial hematocrits can help to estimate volume loss. Upper and lower endoscopy, angiography, and scintigraphy will assist with the diagnosis.

CASE CONTINUED

You do a rigid sigmoidoscopy in your office and are unable to identify a bleeding source in the anus, rectum, or distal sigmoid colon. While you are doing the examination, a runny clot of blood enters your visual field. You send the patient to the ED, where IVs are started and a hemoglobin returns at 9. A CBC drawn 8 months ago for an infectious workup showed a hemoglobin of 13.5 at that time. NG lavage is clear and bilious. You worry that the patient has an active bleed and arrange to have him admitted to the hospital. An angiogram is performed and a bleeding source is localized to the RLQ and embolized. The patient stabilizes his hematocrit and you arrange for him to have a colonoscopy performed.

QUESTIONS

17-1. In the face of active bleeding, which of the following tests is most *sensitive* for localizing the bleeding source?
A. Angiography.
B. Technetium-labeled RBC scintigraphy.
C. Endoscopy.
D. CT scan.
E. MRI.

17-2. Frankly bloody diarrhea (hematochezia) might be expected in
A. Perforated peptic ulcer.
B. Resolving variceal bleed.
C. Gastritis.
D. Radiation colitis.
E. Anal warts

17-3. A clear bilious nasogastric aspirate suggests
A. The NGT is in the esophagus
B. You have cannulated the bile duct with your NGT.
C. The patient has a cholecystoduodenal fistula.
D. The patient is hyperbilirubinemic.
E. There is a low likelihood that bleeding is proximal to the ligament of Treitz.

17-4. The percent of people with diverticular disease who will ever have a significant episode of bleeding is
A. <1%.
B. 15%.
C. 30%.
D. 50%.
E. >75%

ANSWERS

17-1. B. Tagged cell scans are the most sensitive, with the ability to detect a bleed of ~0.1 mL/min. Angiography requires a fairly brisk bleed of >0.5 mL/min in order to detect a contrast "blush." CT and MRI are infrequently able to precisely identify a gastrointestinal bleeding site. In the face of ongoing hemorrhage, endoscopy can be difficult because the presence of intraluminal blood impairs the ability to adequately visualize the bowel wall.

17-2. D. Inflammatory bowel disease, infection (particularly of the toxin-forming variety), and radiation damage can all present with bloody diarrhea. It is unlikely for a proximal GI tract source to present with gross bleeding from below, although it is possible if the bleeding is very brisk (in which case soft melenic stools or even hematochezia may be seen). Perforated peptic ulcers generally present with symptoms related to peritoneal (free) air and infrequently result in significant bleeding. Anal warts rarely result in large volume bleeds. History is key in evaluating the possibilities.

17-3. E. In evaluating a GIB, an NG aspirate and lavage that returns with clear bilious fluid is a normal finding and indicates that the bleeding source is likely *distal* to the ligament of Treitz. An NG lavage that returns without bile does not exclude a duodenal source. Bloody aspirate, then, implies a proximal source (upper GIB), located in the esophagus, stomach, or duodenum. In this instance, EGD is usually the next step.

17-4. B. Only 15% of patients with diverticulosis will experience a significant bleed from them.

ADDITIONAL SUGGESTED READING

Bounds BC, Friedman LS. Lower gastrointestinal bleeding. Gastroenterol Clin North Am 2003;32:1107–1125.

Cappell MS, Friedel D. The role of sigmoidoscopy and colonoscopy in the diagnosis and management of lower gastrointestinal disorders: endoscopic findings, therapy, and complications. Med Clin North Am 2002;86:1253–1288.

Funaki B. Endovascular intervention for the treatment of acute arterial gastrointestinal hemorrhage. Gastroenterol Clin North Am 2002;31:701–713.

Terdiman JP. Colonoscopic management of lower gastrointestinal hemorrhage. Curr Gastroenterol Rep 2001;3:425–432.

CASE **18**

Guaiac-Positive Stool

CC/ID: 61-year-old man with guaiac-positive stool on routine examination.

HPI: The patient is in his usual state of good health when he presents for his annual physical exam. He has just moved into the area, and this is your first encounter with him. He has no complaints, exercises regularly (runs four times a week), eats well, and has maintained his same weight for "more than 20 years." You perform a complete physical examination that is unremarkable except for the finding of a positive stool hemoccult test.

THOUGHT QUESTION

- What are potential causes of heme-positive stool?
- What additional directed questions will you ask?
- What diagnostic maneuvers would be appropriate at this time?

DISCUSSION

Heme-positive stool may be the result of any bleeding along the GI tract; it is therefore important to consider both upper and lower GI sources. Upper GI sources would include peptic ulcer disease, esophageal varices, gastritis, and others. Lower GI sources would include hemorrhoids, diverticula, colorectal cancer (CRC), and inflammatory bowel disease (IBD). Infectious and traumatic causes may also lead to blood in the stool.

In many cases, directed questions can narrow the differential. A history of ulcer disease, GERD, or alcoholism/cirrhosis may suggest an upper GI source. IBD is generally diagnosed earlier in life. Bright red blood per rectum, blood streaking with stool, and/or prolonged sitting are often

91

seen with hemorrhoids. A family history of cancer or a change in the quality or caliber of stools may be a sign of CRC. In this older patient, it will also be useful to know if and when he last had a screening sigmoidoscopy or colonoscopy.

Regardless of the particulars, any patient over the age of 50 is at risk for CRC, and this should be excluded even if other etiologies seem likely. Double contrast barium enema is a reasonable initial study, because it can delineate colon anatomy and masses >0.5 cm; however, the sensitivity of detecting cancer is only 85% as compared with 95% for colonoscopy. Moreover, a diagnosis can only be made with tissue sampling. Therefore, it is generally recommended that patients with heme-positive stools undergo endoscopy to evaluate for masses and to possibly biopsy any lesions. An anoscopic exam or sigmoidoscopy can often be performed in the office, but this does not replace a complete study. CT colonography (virtual colonoscopy) is less sensitive than colonoscopy, and is not at this time recommended as a standard screening test.

CASE CONTINUED

On further questioning, you learn that the patient does have a distant history of hemorrhoids, but they have not bothered him in years. His stools are soft and regular. He has had no fever, chills, sweats, or diarrhea. His last physician had him undergo what sounds like a flexible sigmoidoscopy ~6 years ago, when he turned 55. He tells you that they removed a couple of polyps, which were all "normal." He has no other significant medical or surgical history. He takes no medications except for multivitamins. His grandfather died of colon cancer.

PE/Labs: You perform an anoscopic examination and find small, noninflamed, internal hemorrhoids. CBC and liver function tests are within normal limits.

Studies: Colonoscopy reveals several small pedunculated polyps scattered throughout the transverse and descending colon, as well as a somewhat larger 3- to 4-cm mass at the hepatic flexure. Pathology on the polyps returns with tubular adenoma. Pathology on the mass returns with adenocarcinoma.

THOUGHT QUESTION

- What will you do or recommend next?

DISCUSSION

Staging may be important at this juncture, but is not critical. The primary objective is oncologic resection of the tumor, since it is possible to obtain staging information at the time of operation. However, CT can help to evaluate the extent of the disease and the presence of metastases, which may alter the surgical plan. This is perhaps more true in tumors of the distal colon and rectum. CT findings in those cases may indicate whether there is a need for adjuvant or neoadjuvant chemoradiation therapy. Regardless of spread, surgical resection is almost always indicated, as many colorectal tumors will go on to bleed or obstruct. In addition, adjuvant therapies are more likely to be beneficial when the primary tumor has been removed. Information about particular tumor characteristics or depth of invasion may be difficult to assess on endoscopic biopsy alone, so other treatment decisions will ultimately be based on analysis of the surgical specimen.

CASE CONTINUED

CT shows no evidence of metastases, with disease apparently confined to the area of the hepatic flexure. The patient is scheduled for surgery.

QUESTIONS

18-1. What is an appropriate operation for this patient?
   A. Right hemicolectomy.
   B. Transverse colectomy.
   C. Low anterior resection.
   D. Abdominoperineal resection.
   E. Total colectomy.

18-2. Which of the following is a risk factor for colorectal cancer?
- A. Low fat diet.
- B. High fiber diet.
- C. IBD.
- D. Hemorrhoids.
- E. Diverticulosis.

18-3. Regarding the Dukes' classification,
- A. It is graded A through D.
- B. It is graded I through IV.
- C. It is defined by tumor size.
- D. It is defined by tumor cell differentiation.
- E. It is only applied to rectal cancers.

18-4. The most common site of colorectal metastases is to
- A. Lung.
- B. Liver.
- C. Spleen.
- D. Stomach.
- E. Brain.

ANSWERS

18-1. A. Right hemicolectomy alone suggests segmental removal of the colon as supplied by the ileocolic, right colic, and possibly the right branch of the middle colic arteries, and is generally appropriate for tumors of the cecum and ascending colon. (Oncologic resections for bowel are performed to the root of the mesentery along the vascular supply, because this is the same route by which the lymphatics drain.) Extended right colectomy implies removal of the colon extending to the area supplied by the middle colic artery as well; this is more likely to offer an adequate margin for the patient in this case. Transverse colectomy is less frequently performed and is unlikely to provide an adequate proximal margin in this patient. Low anterior resection is for distal sigmoid or proximal rectal lesions. Abdominoperineal resection suggests a very low (rectal) lesion, requiring permanent colostomy and closure (oversewing) of the anal opening. Total colectomy is not required.

Laparoscopic techniques for resection are becoming more commonly performed in the surgical treatment of colon cancer. Although there were initial worries about an increase in tumor recurrence, the most complete study to date suggests that this is not the case. It seems likely that this approach will become the standard of care.

18-2. C. Other risk factors include age, obesity, physical inactivity, alcohol, smoking, a positive family history of colon cancer (in a first-degree relative), and familial polyp syndromes (Gardner's, familial polyposis coli). Low fat, high fiber diets are thought to be protective against colon cancer. Hemorrhoids are unrelated.

18-3. A. The Dukes' classification is based on the extent of colorectal tumor invasion into the bowel wall, and is designated A through D. However, despite the historical significance of using the Dukes' system in describing colorectal tumors, it is generally believed that the more detailed TNM staging system (tumor, nodes, metastases) should be preferentially used (Table 18-1).

TABLE 18-1 The TNM System Can Be Approximately Converted to the Dukes' System in the Following Way: Stage I = Dukes' A, Stage II = Dukes' B, Stage III = Dukes' C, and Stage IV = Dukes' D

Stage	Tnm Status		Tumor Invasion	Survival at 5 Years (%)
I	T1	N_0M_0	Limited to mucosa and submucosa	90–95
	T2	N_0M_0	Invasion into but not beyond the muscularis propria	
II	T3	N_0M_0	Through muscularis into subserosa (full thickness of bowel wall)	60–80
	T4	N_0M_0	Invasion into visceral peritoneum or adjacent organs	
III	Any T	N_1M_0	Involves lymph nodes	20–50
IV	Any T, N, M_1	Any	Metastatic disease	<5

18-4. B. The liver is the most common site of distant colorectal metastases. The lungs are the second most common. CEA can be used as a marker for colorectal tumor growth and is often followed in the postoperative patient as a means of recurrence surveillance. Although the CEA levels have little prognostic value on their own, trends can be important. Thus, in a patient in whom CEA is followed, a rising trend may herald the return of disease. If evaluation (e.g., by endoscopy) of the colon and rectum is negative for recurrence, the liver and lung will be the next most likely sites to harbor metastatic disease.

ADDITIONAL SUGGESTED READING

Boyle P, Leon ME. Epidemiology of colorectal cancer. Br Med Bull 2002;64:1–25.

Clinical Outcomes of Surgical Therapy Study Group. A comparison of laparoscopically assisted and open colectomy for colon cancer. N Engl J Med 2004;350:2050–2059.

Mandel JS. Screening of patients at average risk for colon cancer. Med Clin North Am 2005;89:43–59.

Nivatvongs S. Surgical management of malignant colorectal polyps. Surg Clin North Am 2002;82:959–966.

Smith R, Cokkinides V, Eyre H. American Cancer Society guidelines for the early detection of cancer. CA Cancer J Clin 2003;53:27–43.

CASE **19**

Anal Pain

CC/ID: 48-year-old woman with anal pain and bleeding.

HPI: The patient presents complaining of ~2 weeks of anal discomfort, usually worse after BMs. She says she sometimes feels like her "rectum is falling out," but notes that this sensation passes when she is no longer sitting on the toilet. She can sometimes feel what she perceives as a "mass" in her anus. She has also noted some blood on her toilet paper or streaked with her stools, but is not aware of any rectal bleeding except during BMs. She has no other abdominal complaints or h/o anorectal surgery. She has been passing one hard stool every 1 to 2 days but has been feeling a sense of incomplete evacuation. She has no problems with continence.

PMHx&
PSHx: G_3P_3. Recent casting for broken arm after fall. Otherwise
healthy.

Meds: MVI; Tylenol with codeine for pain

THOUGHT QUESTION

- Why does the sensation of her rectum "falling out" stop after she passes stool?
- What are likely causes of the blood streaking?
- What features on examination will help to differentiate these?
- What role may her medications be playing in her presentation?

DISCUSSION

The sensation of an intermittent anal mass or fullness is consistent with either prolapsing hemorrhoids or rectum (procidentia), the former of which is much more common. The increased abdominal pressure associated with straining can lead to both engorgement of rectal vessels and prolapse of redundant tissue (such as that with hemorrhoids or rectal prolapse). When rectal mucosa becomes inflamed, passage of stool can cause local trauma and bleeding. Consequently, anorectal bleeding of this nature will sometimes present as streaking of stools or staining of toilet paper without further evidence of frank bleeding.

On exam, rectal prolapse can often be elicited by having the patient strain or Valsalva, causing the tissue to push out in concentric rings (i.e., circumferential prolapse). Prolapsing hemorrhoids can be similarly elicited but will appear as piles (plump masses representing the engorged vessels covered by anorectal mucosa), separated by radial fissures. The patient's recent h/o narcotic-containing medications for pain may have led to constipation, increased straining, and hard stool trauma to the anorectal mucosa. However, cancer should never be overlooked in any patient with rectal masses, pain, and/or bleeding.

CASE CONTINUED

On exam, the patient has stable vital signs. Her rectal/anoscopic exam reveals a large inflamed pile in the left lateral position with minimal oozing and a smaller pile in the right anterior position, both with a base located proximal to the dentate line. You find no anal fissures, tags, or other pathology.

THOUGHT QUESTION

- What is the difference between internal and external hemorrhoids? Why does this matter?
- How are hemorrhoids graded?
- What would you recommend if you found a thrombosed hemorrhoid?

DISCUSSION

Internal hemorrhoids are those in which the base is located proximal to the dentate (or pectinate) line; external hemorrhoids arise distal to the dentate line and are covered with squamous epithelium. Because the mucosa proximal to the dentate line does not have somatic pain innervation, internal hemorrhoids can be manipulated, such as with in-office banding or injection sclerotherapy procedures. Attempting to rubber-band ligate an external hemorrhoid would cause the patient undue pain.

Hemorrhoids are graded I to IV (or first through fourth degrees) according to the criteria listed in Table 19-1.

TABLE 19-1 Hemorrhoid Grades

Grade/Degree	Bleeding?	Prolapse?	Reduction?
I/1st	+	−	NA
II/2nd	+	+	Spontaneous
III/3rd	+	+	Manual
IV/4th	+	+	Cannot

Thrombosed external hemorrhoids are excised if they are found within 24 to 48 hours of thrombosis (as diagnosed by onset of pain symptoms). Otherwise, they can be managed conservatively with analgesics and sitz baths, as the natural course is gradual resorption of the clotted blood, with attendant decrease in symptoms of pain.

QUESTIONS

19-1. You diagnose prolapsing, spontaneously reducing (grade II), internal hemorrhoids. After local treatment in the office, your management should be to
- A. Tell the patient to do nothing, because her symptoms will certainly pass.
- B. Discuss and encourage measures for improving stool softness and regularity.
- C. Encourage manual disimpaction of stools.
- D. Recommend tighter undergarments to prevent prolapse.
- E. Refer the patient for surgery.

19-2. Anal fissures are painful lesions that are anatomically most commonly found
   A. Right posterior.
   B. Right anterior.
   C. Left lateral.
   D. In the midline.
   E. In any orientation around the anal ring.

19-3. Recurrent anorectal abscesses are frequently associated with
   A. Intravenous drug abuse.
   B. Infectious stool.
   C. Anal fistulas.
   D. Insect bites.
   E. Chronic laxative use

19-4. Goodsall's rule states that a fistula-in-ano with an anterior external opening will have an internal opening
   A. In the anterior half of the anal canal, usually in a straight radial line from the external opening.
   B. In the anterior midline.
   C. In the posterior midline.
   D. Into the urethra.
   E. That ends in a blind pouch.

ANSWERS

19-1. B. The mainstay of hemorrhoid treatment is conservative medical management, including increased fiber and fluid intake, witch hazel and/or sitz baths for comfort, and possibly topical anti-inflammatory or anesthetic agents for pain. Most patients with grade I or II hemorrhoids will do well with improved bowel hygiene. In this patient's case, cessation of narcotics or addition of stool softeners will also likely be helpful. Symptoms can resolve spontaneously, but with large hemorrhoids, symptoms may recur unless long-term improvements in bowel habits are achieved. Banding and sclerosis may be helpful, but should not supplant behavioral modifications. Hemorrhoidectomy is generally reserved for symptoms refractory to medical management or in patients with larger (grade III) or nonreducible (grade IV) hemorrhoids.

19-2. D. Anal fissures are most commonly found in the midline, with most in the posterior position ($\sim 90\%$, versus $\sim 10\%$ anteriorly). Fissures found in atypical locations (i.e., off the midline) should raise suspicion for IBD, infection (such as tuberculosis), trauma, or neoplasm. Like hemorrhoids, treatment is usually conservative, with the expectation that the fissure will heal. When refractory to these measures, nitroglycerin cream, botulinum toxin injection, or lateral sphincterotomy may be used to relax the sphincter spasm thought to be the cause of fissure pain.

19-3. C. Anal crypts leading to fistulae are implicated in most cases of perirectal abscess. Patients with recurring abscesses and pain, followed by spontaneous drainage and relief of symptoms will often have fistula-in-ano. Examination may reveal a perianal sinus leading to an internal point (in an anal crypt) at the dentate line. Treatment is drainage of the abscess and, where applicable, unroofing of the fistula tract.

19-4. A. According to Goodsall's rule, an anal fistula with an external opening that is anterior will have an internal opening that is anterior, usually in a straight radial line. The other part of Goodsall's rule is that fistulas with posterior openings or openings >3 cm from the anal verge will open internally in the posterior midline. Fistulas defying this rule should raise the suspicion of IBD.

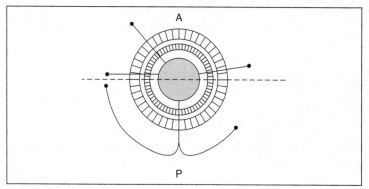

FIGURE 19-1. Goodsall's rule.

📖 *ADDITIONAL SUGGESTED READING*

Billingham RP, Isler JT, Kimmins MH, et al. The diagnosis and management of common anorectal disorders. Curr Probl Surg 2004;41:586–645.

Hardy A, Chan CL, Cohen CR. The surgical management of haemorrhoids—a review. Dig Surg 2005;22:26–33.

Nelson R. Anorectal abscess fistula: what do we know? Surg Clin North Am 2002;82:1139–1151.

Nisar PJ, Scholefield JH. Managing haemorrhoids. Br Med J 2003; 327:847–851.

Projectile Vomiting

CC/ID: 5-week-old male infant with 3 days of vomiting with feeds.

HPI: The infant is brought in by his parents with a report of persistent vomiting. He had been feeding and growing normally until 5 days ago, when the parents noted more frequent spitting up after feeds. Over the last 2 days, this has progressed to vomiting after every feed. He has been breast-fed since birth with no deviations.

THOUGHT QUESTION

- What else do you want to know about this infant's history?
- How does his age influence your differential diagnosis? What if he were 2 days old? Two years old?

DISCUSSION

Other important questions to ask in the evaluation of this infant would include an assessment of weight loss (as an indicator of nutritional/hydration status), the quality and appearance of the emesis (e.g., bilious/nonbilious, bloody, projectile), other GI symptoms (diarrhea, constipation), and the presence of constitutional symptoms (e.g., fever or lethargy).

Persistent emesis in a 5-week-old is suspicious for pyloric stenosis, because this entity tends to present in children who are about 1 month old (generally, ages 3 to 6 weeks). Newborns with persistent emesis should be evaluated for intestinal atresias. Toddlers (ages 6 to 18 months) comprise the age group that most commonly presents with intussusception. Viral syndrome/gastroenteritis is probably the most common cause of GI complaints in the pediatric population, but it is important to remember that this is a diagnosis of exclusion.

CASE CONTINUED

When questioned further, the parents state that the emesis appears to be partially digested milk with no evidence of any green bile or blood. The parents insist that the baby continues to have a vigorous appetite despite what seems to be an inability to digest his feeds. They have not noticed any change in the color, consistency, or frequency of his stools. He has not had any fevers, but he does seem to be a bit more cranky than usual. They are unsure if he has lost any weight.

PMHx: Full term, NSVD; normal growth and development to date; immunizations up to date

VS: Temp 36.5°C, HR 120, BP 75/50, RR 22, weight 6.3 kg

PE: *Gen:* Consolable infant, resting comfortably in his father's arms; skin turgor is poor. *HEENT:* Sunken fontanelle, mucous membranes are dry. *Chest:* Clear bilaterally. *Abdomen:* Soft, NT, ND, with a mobile, olive-shaped mass palpable in the mid-epigastrium.

THOUGHT QUESTION

- What tests will you obtain to confirm your diagnosis?
- What laboratory values would you expect to find in this infant?
- How will these values affect your management?

DISCUSSION

The finding of a palpable "olive" is nearly pathognomonic of pyloric stenosis. The imaging test of choice to confirm this diagnosis is abdominal ultrasound (US) to examine the pylorus. In particular, the goal will be to assess the dimensions of the pyloric sphincter, including both the length and the width.

The electrolyte picture most commonly seen in any vomiting patient is hypochloremic hypokalemic metabolic alkalosis (with paradoxical aciduria). The hypochloremia results from the loss of hydrochloric acid from the stomach. As acid is lost, the patient becomes alkalotic. To compensate, hydrogen ions are moved from the intracellular to the extracellular space in exchange for potassium. In addition, as the patient becomes more dehydrated, the kidneys compensate by retaining sodium and secreting potassium. The result of these actions is a net decrease in the extracellular potassium pool, causing hypokalemia. With progressive hypokalemia and hypovolemia, the kidneys must exchange increasingly more H^+ ions for sodium, exacerbating the alkalosis and producing the (paradoxical) aciduria.

Ultimately, pyloric stenosis is managed surgically. However, pyloric stenosis is *not* a surgical emergency, and any surgical intervention should be deferred until the patient has been adequately resuscitated (in terms of volume, acid-base status, and metabolic derangements). Therefore, treatment can always begin with aggressive medical management. Hydration is the first priority and should include replenishment of sodium and chloride. Potassium should also be administered after the baby has voided (i.e., has proven that kidney function is intact and that a potassium load can be handled). As a rule, NGTs should not be placed during the resuscitation phase in these patients, because they will only exacerbate the metabolic abnormalities.

CASE CONTINUED

An IV is started and a 1/2 NS (with K^+, after voiding) infusion begun. Labs are remarkable for a pH of 7.51, Na 128, K 3.0, Cl 90, and CO_2 32. An US is obtained, demonstrating a thickened pylorus. Labs drawn the next morning show near normalization of the alkalosis as well as the associated metabolic derangements. The baby is taken to the operating room where an uncomplicated pyloromyotomy is performed. He is eating by the end of the day and is discharged the following morning.

QUESTIONS

20-1. The pathology of pyloric stenosis involves
   A. Concentric hypertrophy of the gastric mucosa along the pyloric canal.
   B. Concentric hypertrophy of the pyloric muscle.
   C. Encroachment of small bowel musculature onto the pylorus.
   D. Inflammation of the entire pyloric apparatus.
   E. Impaction of food particles at the gastroduodenal junction.

20-2. Most common to least common sites of intestinal atresia are
A. Jejunum, ileum, colon.
B. Jejunum, colon, ileum.
C. Ileum, jejunum, colon.
D. Ileum, colon, jejunum.
E. Colon, jejunum, ileum.
F. Colon, ileum, jejunum.

20-3. Meconium ileus is associated with
A. Cystic fibrosis.
B. Trisomy 21.
C. Prematurity.
D. Fetal alcohol syndrome.
E. Maternal amniocentesis.

20-4. Imperforate anus will lead to feeding intolerance if unrecognized. Another anomaly that may be seen with imperforate anus is
A. Hepatomegaly.
B. Asplenia.
C. Situs inversus.
D. Facial dysmorphia.
E. Renal agenesis.

ANSWERS

20-1. B. Pyloric stenosis is caused by concentric hypertrophy of the muscular fibers of the pyloric sphincter leading to a narrowing of the gastric outlet.

20-2. C. Intestinal atresia occurs most commonly in the ileum and least commonly in the large bowel. It is usually diagnosed within the first days of life.

20-3. A. Meconium ileus results from obstruction of the terminal ileum by abnormal meconium. Ten to thirty-three percent of these patients have a family history and/or personal diagnosis of cystic fibrosis. Therefore, all patients who present with meconium ileus should be evaluated for cystic fibrosis.

20-4. E. Imperforate anus is associated with the VACTERL (vertebral, anal, cardiac, tracheoesophageal, renal, limbs) syndrome. The most common isolated association is genitourinary.

ADDITIONAL SUGGESTED READING

Blumer SL, Zucconi WB, Cohen HL, et al. The vomiting neonate: a review of the ACR appropriateness criteria and ultrasound's role in the workup of such patients. Ultrasound Q 2004;20:79–89.

Hajivassiliou, CA. Intestinal obstruction in neonatal/pediatric surgery. Semin Pediatr Surg 2003;12:241–253.

Upper Abdominal Pressure

CC/ID: Fullness and pressure in the upper abdomen.

HPI: Ms. X is a 32-year-old woman who has noticed a sensation of upper abdominal pressure and fullness for the past few months. She thinks this is slightly more noticeable when lying down. There does not appear to be any association with particular foods or eating. She denies nausea, vomiting, or diarrhea. There have been no constitutional symptoms.

PMH: none

PSH: wisdom tooth extraction

Meds: Tri-norinyl

All: NKDA

SH: glass of wine with dinner

FH: none

VS: Temp 37.6 °C, BP 98/45, HR 81

PE: *Gen:* Thin woman, no distress. *HEENT:* Eyes anicteric. *Chest:* CTA bilaterally. *Abdomen:* No scars; nondistended. Minimal tenderness to palpation over RUQ, no palpable mass. No rebound or guarding. *Pelvic:* No tenderness, masses, discharge. *Rectal:* Normal tone, nontender, no masses, heme negative.

THOUGHT QUESTION

- How do you initially workup a patient with such non-specific symptoms?

DISCUSSION

After a good physical exam, you should begin with a basic set of blood tests. In this patient, this should include a CBC and electrolytes. Given her vague RUQ tenderness, liver function tests should also be ordered. For imaging, either an abdominal ultrasound (US) or computed tomography (CT) scan of the abdomen would be appropriate.

CASE CONTINUED

Labs: WBC 4; Hct 41; Plts 255; Na 134; K 4.2; Cl 99 CO_2 23; BUN 18; Cr 0.6; glucose 98; AST 78; ALT 103; Alk Phos 120; Tbili 0.8.

Imaging: *Abdominal ultrasound:* 2 cm hypoechoic lesion in L lobe of liver, no biliary ductal dilation, gallbladder unremarkable, no gallstones. Pancreas WNL. *CT with and without IV contrast:* Liver with 2.3 × 1.9 cm mass in segment 4 of liver—hypodense on non-contrast images, irregularly enhancing on contrast images, no central scar. No ductal dilation. No other intra-abdominal abnormality.

THOUGHT QUESTION

- What is the differential for liver nodule in this patient?
- How does treatment vary by the diagnosis?
- What other studies might be helpful in making the diagnosis?

DISCUSSION

The majority of hepatic lesions found incidentally are benign and include hemangiomata, focal nodular hyperplasia (FNH), simple cysts, and hepatic adenoma (HA). Of course, malignancy, such as hepatocellular carcinoma, is always in the differential but is usually identified in the course of a workup for specific symptoms (i.e., jaundice, weight loss, abdominal mass).

For all tumors, symptoms and an inability to exclude malignancy are indications for resection. HA has a significant risk of spontaneous rupture and hemorrhage, which is an additional indication for elective resection. For FNH or hemangioma, enucleation is sufficient, while for HA, a formal resection is preferred given a risk of malignant transformation. For small or asymptomatic FNH and hemangiomata, close observation with serial imaging is most appropriate.

MRI is the most useful test to distinguish between cysts, hemangioma, FNH, and HA. ^{99}Tc-labeled red blood cell scintigraphy has been used to identify hemangioma. Similarly, ^{99}Tc-labeled sulfur colloid is taken up by Kupffer cells, which are present in FNH but not in HA, and forms the basis for this nuclear medicine study. Angiography can sometimes differentiate between FNH and HA. Lastly, percutaneous biopsy may be performed in select cases when considering malignancy but should be avoided when hemangioma is likely due to the risk of hemorrhage.

? QUESTIONS

21-1. Kasabach-Merritt syndrome is hemangiomata of skin, spleen, and liver associated with:

   A. Thrombocytopenia and afibrinogenemia.
   B. Hyperlipidemia and polycythemia vera.
   C. Pancytopenia.
   D. Retroperitoneal lymphadenopathy and deep venous thrombosis.

21-2. Which of the following appears to be related to the dosage and duration of estrogen use?

   A. Hemangioma.
   B. Focal nodular hyperplasia.
   C. Hepatic adenoma.
   D. Hepatocellular carcinoma.

21-3. Which of the following variants of hepatocellular carcinoma can be mistaken for HA?

   A. Clear-cell.
   B. Fibrolamellar.
   C. Lymphocytic.
   D. Giant cell.

21-4. Metastatic hepatic lesions are most likely due to which primary tumor?
- A. Breast.
- B. Lung.
- C. Melanoma.
- D. Colorectal.

ANSWERS

21-1. A. The clinical features of Kasabach-Merritt Syndrome are related to the consumptive coagulopathy which can occur in the setting of large hemangiomata. Treatment may include corticosteroids, interferon-alpha, radiation, and other antiproliferative agents.

21-2. C. 90% of patients with HA have used oral contraceptive pills (OCPs), often for longer than two years duration. Regression may occur with discontinuation of OCP use. All women with HA should stop use of OCPs. Pregnancy is associated with accelerated tumor growth and increased risk of rupture; therefore, elective resection should be recommended for women with known HA who are considering getting pregnant.

21-3. B. Well-differentiated, or fibrolamellar, hepatocellular carcinoma (HCC) has a better prognosis than other forms of HCC. Unlike other types of HCC, fibrolamellar HCC is infrequently associated with hepatitis B or cirrhosis. Other risk factors for HCC include hepatotoxins (i.e., aflatoxin B1), type 1 glycogen storage disease, (1-antitrypsin deficiency, hemochromatosis, tyrosinemia, and use of androgens.

21-4. D. Because of its unique dual blood supply and function as a filtering organ, the liver is a common site of metastases. Primary tumors that drain into the portal vein are most common (colorectal, carcinoid, and pancreatic).

SUGGESTED ADDITIONAL READING

Abdalla EK, Vauthey JN, Ellis LM, et al. Recurrence and outcomes following hepatic resection, radiofrequency ablation, and combined resection/ablation for colorectal liver metastases. Ann Surg 2004;239:818–825; discussion 825–827.

Alobaidi M, Shirkhoda A. Benign focal liver lesions: discrimination
from malignant mimickers. Curr Probl Diagn Radiol
2004;33:239–253.
Belli G, D'Agostino A, Ciciliano F, et al. Liver resection for hepatic
metastases: 15 years of experience. J Hepatobiliary Pancreat
Surg 2002;9:607–613.
Choi BY, Nguyen MH. The diagnosis and management of benign
hepatic tumors. J Clin Gastroenterol 2005;39:401–412.
Llovet JM. Updated treatment approach to hepatocellular
carcinoma. J Gastroenterol 2005;40:225–235.

III

Patients who Present with a Mass

Intermittent Abdominal Mass

CC/ID: 6-month-old girl with an abdominal bulge.

HPI: The parents of a healthy, growing infant girl tell you that for several weeks they have noted what appears to be a "bulge" in their daughter's mid-abdomen when she cries. They had not seen it previously but have noticed it regularly now that they have been looking for it. The bulge disappears once the baby is calm, and they have never not seen it go away. Her appetite and bowel habits appear to be unaffected.

PMHx: Former 36-week preemie, NSVD. Normal growth and development to date for adjusted age.

VS: Afebrile, HR 110

PE: *Gen:* Playful infant in no apparent distress; lying on the examining table causes her to cry. *Abdomen:* Soft, round; small ~2 × 2-cm periumbilical mass evident on Valsalva/crying, most easily reducible when the baby is calm; palpable ~1 × 1-cm umbilical defect.

THOUGHT QUESTION

- What is your diagnosis?
- What are risk factors for this condition in children and in adults?
- What will you tell the parents regarding treatment?

DISCUSSION

The baby has an umbilical hernia. Risk factors for umbilical hernia in children include prematurity, female sex, and African-American background. Unlike most other hernias, these congenital defects are at low risk for incarceration/strangulation. Furthermore, most umbilical hernias in infants will close spontaneously, particularly if the defect is smaller than 1.5 to 2 cm in diameter. Therefore, in this child without evidence of bowel compromise, observation is the recommended course of action. If the hernia is at any time irreducible or becomes otherwise problematic, prompt intervention would then be warranted.

In adults, umbilical hernias are noted to occur more frequently in women, with obesity and repeated pregnancies reported as common precursors. In addition, ascites is an exacerbating factor, and rupture has been reported in patients with chronic ascitic cirrhosis. Because strangulation of the colon and omentum is fairly common in adults (in contrast to children), early repair is encouraged. The classic repair is the "vest-over-pants" imbrication of the superior and inferior aponeuroses (Mayo hernioplasty). However, mesh-based repairs have become increasingly commonly used.

CASE CONTINUED

The child returns 2 years later for removal of a simple epidermal cyst diagnosed on a routine well-child visit. The parents mention that the abdominal mass is still present whenever she stands and/or strains. Though they do not believe she is having any pain or related ill effects, they are wondering whether they should be worried. Your examination of the periumbilical mass is essentially unchanged.

THOUGHT QUESTION

- What do you tell the parents now?

DISCUSSION

The diagnosis and recommended treatment plan are unchanged. Typically, operative intervention is reserved until the child is at least 4 to 5 years of age, at which time more than 80% will have spontaneously closed. After this time, the likelihood of spontaneous closure decreases, and the risk of incarceration begins to outweigh the risk of surgery. In this case, where the child is only 2 1/2 years old, remains asymptomatic, and has had no change in the size of her hernia, continued observation is a reasonable course of action.

CASE CONTINUED

When the child reaches ~5 years of age, she still has an evident hernia. The parents are anxious to see it fixed. She undergoes an uncomplicated primary repair of her defect.

QUESTIONS

22-1. A pediatric umbilical hernia is caused by
  A. A defect in the umbilical ring.
  B. A persistent umbilical vein.
  C. Failure of closure of the peritoneum.
  D. Perinatal ascites.
  E. Improper clamping of the umbilical cord at delivery.

22-2. *Gastroschisis* is associated with
  A. Uniform fatality.
  B. Cleft palate.
  C. A membrane-covered bowel.
  D. Chromosomal abnormalities.
  E. A tendency to be located to the right of midline.

22-3. Regarding *omphalocele*
  A. It is infrequently associated with other anomalies.
  B. It can involve herniation of intestines and other organs (e.g., liver).
  C. The defect tends to be located off of the midline.
  D. The overlying membrane is adequate to prevent moisture loss from the abdomen.
  E. It will resolve without operative intervention.

22-4. Closure of gastroschisis or omphalocele
  A. Should be deferred until the baby is proven to tolerate PO intake.
  B. Should be deferred if the baby's weight is not at least 2500 g.
  C. Should only be done if primary closure can be obtained.
  D. Should only be attempted if spontaneous closure does not occur.
  E. May be difficult because of bowel edema.

ANSWERS

22-1. A. Failure of timely closure of the umbilical ring leaves a central defect in the linea alba. The resulting umbilical hernia is covered by umbilical skin and subcutaneous tissue, but the fascial defect allows for protrusion of abdominal contents. Whereas this is a congenital defect in children, umbilical hernias in adults are acquired and are therefore considered to be a different pathologic entity.

22-2. E. Gastroschisis is a defect of the anterior abdominal wall that occurs lateral to the umbilicus, generally to the right side. In contrast to omphalocele, it is associated with *no* peritoneal sac, leading to evisceration with edema and foreshortening of the bowel. It is always associated with nonrotation of the gut. Other congenital defects are uncommon.

22-3. B. Anterior abdominal wall defects should be immediately covered after the baby has been delivered, because they can result in significant fluid losses for the child regardless of whether a membrane (i.e., peritoneal sac) is present. Omphalocele is associated with Beckwith-Wiedemann syndrome (macroglossia, macrosomia, hypoglycemia) and chromosomal defects. Gastroschisis usually involves herniation of intestine only; omphalocele is more likely to involve herniation of other intra-abdominal components. Operative repair is required.

22-4. E. Operative closure of these anterior abdominal wall defects should be performed shortly after diagnosis, because they represent a significant source of fluid loss. Infants with these defects do not need to demonstrate oral feeding tolerance before repair. Primary closure of the defect may be difficult or impossible at the time of the initial operation due to bowel edema and a relatively small abdominal cavity (which results from the decrease in intra-abdominal contents during development); therefore, staged repairs using a "silo" or temporary water-impermeable covering are often required. In this way, the abdominal wall can be gradually "stretched" as extruded abdominal contents are reintroduced into the abdominal cavity. Formal closure of the abdomen may not be possible for several days or even weeks.

ADDITIONAL SUGGESTED READING

Katz DA. Evaluation and management of inguinal and umbilical hernias. Pediatr Ann 2001;30:729–735.

Langer JC. Abdominal wall defects. World J Surg 2003;27:117–124.

CASE **23**

Pulsatile Abdominal Mass

CC: Pulsatile mass in the abdomen.

HPI: The patient is a 68-year-old man who presents to your office complaining of a "beating lump" in his abdomen. He says that he recently lost approximately 10 lbs and subsequently noticed this mass, particularly when lying supine. It is not painful and has not affected his appetite or bowel habits. His weight loss was intentional (he recently started spinning). He has no symptoms of claudication or cerebrovascular disease.

PMHx: Negative

PSHx: Inguinal hernia repair in his 20s

Meds: None

All: NKDA

SHx: Past smoker, no alcohol or other drugs

VS: Afebrile, BP 120/65, HR 65

PE: *Gen:* WD/WN man, fit-appearing, thin. *CV:* RRR, no murmurs/rubs/gallops. *Lungs:* CTA. *Abdomen:* Flat, soft, nontender, normoactive bowel sounds; pulsatile epigastric mass approx. 5 cm across; no bruits. *Ext:* No edema or cyanosis, 4+ distal pulses. *Rectal:* Normal tone, nontender, no masses, heme negative.

THOUGHT QUESTION

- You suspect an abdominal aortic aneurysm (AAA). What are the different imaging modalities for evaluating an AAA and what are their relative strengths and weaknesses?

DISCUSSION

Plain film radiography may show calcifications in the wall of the
aneurysm, but this provides little specific anatomic information. Ultrasonography (US) is readily available and inexpensive. Along with
aneurysm size, ultrasound can identify the renal and visceral vessels,
intraluminal thrombus, and areas of arterial occlusion. However, given
the much more detailed imaging provided by computed tomography
(CT) or magnetic resonance imaging (MRI), ultrasound is primarily
used for screening and serial follow-up of known aneurysms. CT is
currently the gold standard for diagnosis and operative planning, and
provides accurate information regarding size, intraluminal thrombus,
venous anomalies, and both proximal and distal extent. CT can also
detect inflammation and rupture. MRI provides the added advantages
of ability to reflect rate of blood flow, absence of ionizing radiation,
and avoidance of intravenous, potentially nephrotoxic, contrast.
Because it is an intraluminal study, arteriography may underestimate
aneurysm size, since mural thrombus and atherosclerotic plaque can
narrow the intraluminal diameter. Still, arteriography is the most accurate in determining proximal and distal extent of the aneurysm, in
identifying renal and visceral artery abnormalities, and in evaluating
for concomitant vascular occlusive disease.

CASE CONTINUED

You order a CT scan that shows a 6 cm AAA, originating just distal to
the renal arteries and extending into the R iliac artery. You counsel the
patient regarding an elective aortobi-iliac bypass graft. The patient
states that a buddy of his mentioned something about fixing his
aneurysm through his groin, and wants more information about that
approach. You acknowledge that the patient's aneurysm anatomy
does qualify him for consideration of an endovascular repair.

THOUGHT QUESTION

- What are the indications for AAA surveillance and
  repair?
- What is endovascular aneurysm repair? What are the
  advantages and disadvantages as compared to open
  repair?

DISCUSSION

The general treatment recommendation for AAAs <5 cm is annual US; if the patient becomes symptomatic, if the aneurysm enlarges >0.5 cm in a year, or if the aneurysm reaches >5 cm in size, then the aneurysm should be repaired.

For AAAs >5 cm in reasonable risk patients, most vascular surgeons would recommend an elective open repair. However, the development of endovascular stent grafting has provided an excellent alternative for patients with the appropriate aneurysm anatomy who are otherwise at high operative risk (e.g., age >80 years, significant coronary artery disease, renal failure). Using fluoroscopy, the graft is placed through the femoral artery and affixed to the aorta using hooked stents. The major advantage is avoidance of an open intra-abdominal operation in a patient with multiple comorbidities, for whom the risk of open surgery is prohibitive. The drawbacks of the endovascular approach include significant use of contrast arteriography (preoperative, intraoperative, and postoperative), potential for leak around the edges of the graft (requiring further procedures), and potential for migration of the graft (requiring life-long CT monitoring). Therefore, patients must be selected very carefully.

QUESTIONS

23-1. Other abdominal arterial aneurysms
A. Are most commonly found in the SMA.
B. Are usually found incidentally.
C. Are rarely associated with other somatic artery aneurysms.
D. Are associated with mesenteric ischemia.
E. Behave like AAAs.

23-2. A patient presenting with a ruptured AAA may be expected to have signs or symptoms of
A. Hypertension.
B. Epigastric ecchymosis.
C. Chest pain with deep inspiration.
D. Femoral or obturator neuropathy (e.g., leg numbness and weakness).
E. Dysuria.

23-3. Regarding aneurysm epidemiology
   A. In order of highest to lowest frequency: abdominal aorta > iliac > popliteal > common femoral.
   B. Juxtarenal AAA repair is associated with a lower morbidity and mortality than infrarenal repair.
   C. 15–20% of those over 65 years of age have an AAA.
   D. More than 50% of AAA patients have a family history of aneurysms.
   E. Hereditary coagulopathies are almost always associated.

23-4. Infected abdominal aortic aneurysms
   A. Are common.
   B. Are defined as mycotic when a result of cardiac emboli.
   C. Involve *Salmonella* in only 10%.
   D. Are frequently secondary to illicit drug injections.
   E. Are blood culture positive in 75%.

ANSWERS

23-1. B. Visceral artery aneurysms are associated with other somatic artery aneurysms in 30% to 40% of patients. Splenic artery aneurysms are most common (60%), followed by hepatic (20%), SMA, and then celiac (4%). Most are identified on abdominal imaging for other purposes. *Celiac artery aneurysms* are associated with a palpable mass and bruit in approximately 30% of patients and with rupture in 10% to 15%. They are likely secondary to atherosclerosis, medial degeneration, or trauma. *SMA aneurysms* tend to be symptomatic (90%) and palpable. The most common cause is infection due to subacute bacterial endocarditis. *Hepatic artery aneurysms* most frequently involve the common hepatic artery. Etiologies include atherosclerosis, medial degeneration, trauma (especially iatrogenic), and infection (commonly *Staphylococcus aureus*). Rupture occurs in 20%. *Splenic artery aneurysm* rupture in nonpregnant patients is rare (2%), but the incidence increases significantly when the aneurysm is diagnosed during pregnancy. Of note, multiparity is a significant etiologic factor for splenic artery aneurysm development. Other causative factors include pancreatitis, atherosclerosis, portal hypertension, and trauma. Because rupture of these aneurysms is associated with a high mortality rate, treatment is recommended in all reasonable risk patients in whom they are identified. This may be achieved surgically or via percutaneous embolization and occlusion techniques.

23-2. D. Risk factors for AAA rupture include size >5 cm, COPD, and hypertension. A pre-existing history of heart disease and hypertension, along with renal dysfunction, flank ecchymosis, and hematocrit <33% on presentation, are significant predictors of mortality in ruptured AAA. Mortality for ruptured AAA remains around 50% for patients undergoing *emergent* repair; this number approaches 90% if pre-hospital deaths are included. In contrast, operative mortality for *elective* AAA repair averages <5% in good risk patients. Patients with ruptured AAA present with *hypo*tension in 45%; hypertension would not be expected. Femoral and obturator neuropathy can occur with abdominal distension and subsequent pressure on these nerves by the expanding hematoma. Other symptoms referable to AAA include abdominal, back, or flank pain.

23-3. A. An aneurysm is defined as a focal dilation of a blood vessel to at least 50% greater than its normal diameter. The most common arterial aneurysm occurs in the infrarenal abdominal aorta. Suprarenal aneurysmal involvement occurs in <10% of patients, whereas iliac artery involvement occurs in almost 40%. Concomitant renal and visceral artery stenoses are found in 15% to 20%, and iliofemoral outflow occlusive disease is identified in up to 50%. Although these aneurysmal and occlusive lesions are frequently asymptomatic, this information is important in planning the operation.

Juxtarenal and suprarenal AAA repair is associated with a slightly higher morbidity and mortality than infrarenal AAA repair. It is estimated that approximately 3–5% of those over 65 years of age have an AAA. Only 15% of patients with AAA have a family history of aneurysm. Specific hereditary abnormalities associated with aneurysm formation include connective tissue genetic disorders such as Marfan's and Ehlers-Danlos syndromes.

23-4. B. Infected aneurysms are very rare and have an incidence of approximately 1%. The term "mycotic" is now commonly used to refer to all infected aneurysms, but it originally defined an aneurysm caused by infected cardiac valvular vegetations that embolized to, infected, and caused degeneration of a previously healthy aorta. Patients usually present with fever, abdominal or back pain, and evidence of peripheral emboli. *Salmonella* is involved in nearly 40% of infected aneurysms; other common organisms include *Staphylococcus, Streptococcus, Bacteroides, Escherichia coli*, and *Pseudomonas aeruginosa*. However, blood cultures are positive in <50%. Aneurysms infected with gram-negative bacteria are more prone to rupture and development of sepsis than those infected with other organisms. Tuberculous aneurysms have been found in patients previously vaccinated with BCG or treated with BCG for bladder cancer. Injection drug use can be the source of infected peripheral artery aneurysms (e.g., femoral artery at the site of injection) but is generally not associated with infected AAAs. All infected aneurysms should be treated surgically.

ADDITIONAL SUGGESTED READING

Brewster DC, Cronenwett JL, Hallett JW Jr., et al. Joint Council of the American Association for Vascular Surgery and Society for Vascular Surgery. Guidelines for the treatment of abdominal aortic aneurysms: Report of a subcommittee of the Joint Council of the American Association for Vascular Surgery and Society for Vascular Surgery. J Vasc Surg 2003;37:1106–1117.

Lederle FA, Johnson GR, Wilson SE, et al. Veterans Affairs Cooperative Study #417 Investigators. Rupture rate of large abdominal aortic aneurysms in patients refusing or unfit for elective repair. JAMA 2002;287:2968–2972.

Lederle FA, Wilson SE, Johnson GR, et al. Aneurysm Detection and Management Veterans Affairs Cooperative Study Group. Immediate repair compared with surveillance of small abdominal aortic aneurysms. N Engl J Med 2002;346:1437–1444.

Matsumura JS, Brewster DC, Makaroun MS, et al. A multicenter controlled clinical trial of open versus endovascular treatment of abdominal aortic aneurysm. J Vasc Surg 2003;37:262–271.

Messina LM, Shanley CJ. Visceral artery aneurysms. Surg Clin North Am 1997;77:425–442.

Breast Lump

 CC/ID: 43-year-old woman with a right breast lump.

HPI: The patient presents with a painless right breast lump noticed 2 weeks ago while taking a shower. She cannot recall having noticed it there before but does not perform self-exams on a routine basis. She has not felt anything similar in her left breast. She reports no related pain or nipple discharge. She feels otherwise well. A screening examination and mammogram 2 years ago was normal. She had an excisional biopsy of a right "benign" breast lump about 10 years ago.

PMHx: Mild HTN

PGynHx: G_4P_4, first pregnancy at age 26; menarche at age 11; premenopausal

PSHx: Appy in childhood, breast biopsy as in HPI

Meds: Lisinopril, birth control pills

FHx: Mother with ovarian cancer diagnosed at age 40; sister with breast cysts

THOUGHT QUESTION

- What are this patient's risk factors for breast cancer?
- Would your thinking be different if she had previously noted the lump and reported that it had subsequently disappeared? If she had bilateral lumps? If she was 20 years older? If she was 20 years younger? If she had bloody nipple discharge?

DISCUSSION

This patient's risk factors include early menarche; family history (particularly in a first-degree relative) of breast, ovarian, or prostate cancer; age; and prior breast pathology (specifically, there is an increased risk of developing breast cancer with a h/o benign proliferative disease or atypia on prior biopsy). Estrogen and progesterone use have not been conclusively linked to breast cancer risk. Other risk factors include a personal h/o breast cancer, h/o thoracic radiation, nulliparity, and late menopause. A lump that comes and goes, particularly with menses, is typical for a cyst. Bilateral lumps might suggest a diffuse process (e.g., fibrocystic disease) but would not exclude synchronous malignancies. Increasing age is a risk factor for breast cancer, although it can occur in younger patients with a familial predisposition. Fibroadenoma is more common in the young. Bloody nipple discharge is most commonly caused by intraductal papilloma, which is benign. Cytologic evaluation of the discharge can help with the diagnosis. Regardless of the risk factor profile, any dominant palpable mass requires further evaluation until there is clear knowledge of benign disease.

CASE CONTINUED

The patient has no constitutional symptoms.

PE: *Gen:* Well-appearing, NAD. *Breasts:* Symmetric, with no dimpling or skin changes. 15- to 20-mm mobile, nontender mass in the right upper outer quadrant, ~3 cm from the nipple. No nipple discharge. No dominant masses felt on the left. No axillary or clavicular lymphadenopathy.

THOUGHT QUESTION

- What studies will you order? What information will these give?

CASE CONTINUED

You send the patient for a mammogram to see whether there are other radiographic areas of concern that may not be palpable (Fig. 24-1). When she returns for follow-up, you tell her that suspicious calcifications were seen in the region of the palpable mass, but no other suspicious areas were found. An office ultrasound (US) shows the mass to be solid in nature, and so you do not attempt aspiration as you might with a cyst. Because the lesion is easily palpable, you then proceed with fine-needle aspiration (FNA). If this had been a nonpalpable mammographic finding (as in a screening exam), options for tissue diagnosis would have included mammographic/stereotactic needle biopsy (analogous to FNA) or excisional biopsy with mammographic needle localization. In the setting of a clinically and mammographically suspicious lesion, the sensitivity of FNA is 80% to 98%, with a false-negative rate of 2% to 10%. Thus, the clinician and patient need to be aware that a negative (i.e., noncancerous) finding on FNA in the presence of a palpable mass does not conclusively exclude carcinoma. False-positive results are rare, such that specificity approaches 100%. Excisional biopsy is the only *definitive* means of obtaining a tissue diagnosis.

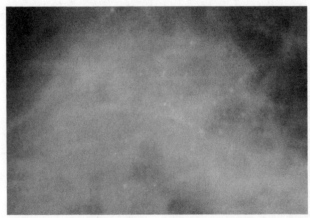

FIGURE **24-1.** In this mammogram, calcifications are seen as dense radiopaque specks, <1 mm in size. These are probably benign. Typically, "suspicious" calcifications would be spiculated and less regular-shaped than these. (*Image provided by Department of Radiology, University of California, San Francisco.*)

Cytology returns with invasive ductal carcinoma. The patient subsequently opts for and undergoes breast conservation therapy with lumpectomy, axillary node sampling, and adjuvant radiation therapy.

![?] *QUESTIONS*

24-1. Tamoxifen works via
A. Competitive antagonism of progesterone.
B. Competitive antagonism of estrogen.
C. Direct cytotoxicity to the tumor.
D. her-2/neu receptors.
E. Release of free radicals.

24-2. Which of the following anatomic associations is correct?
A. Long thoracic nerve → serratus anterior.
B. Intercostobrachial nerve → latissimus dorsi.
C. Thoracodorsal nerve → serratus anterior.
D. Long thoracic nerve → latissimus dorsi.
E. Thoracodorsal nerve → pectoralis major.

24-3. The estimated long-term risk of breast cancer for women is
A. Between 1 in 5 and 1 in 7.
B. Between 1 in 9 and 1 in 11.
C. Between 1 in 12 and 1 in 15.
D. Between 1 in 20 and 1 in 30.
E. Between 1 in 50 and 1 in 100.

24-4. Paget's disease is associated with invasion of tumor cells into
A. The epidermis.
B. Pectoralis major.
C. Pectoralis minor.
D. The clavicle.
E. The contralateral breast.

![!] *ANSWERS*

24-1. B. Hormonal therapy and chemotherapy are generally recommended based on lymph node positivity and estrogen and/or progesterone receptor status of the tumor. The hormonal therapy of choice in patients with breast cancer has long been tamoxifen, a competitive estrogen antagonist. Newer aromatase inhibitors (AI) may provide similar benefits, but studies are ongoing. Commonly used cytotoxic regimens include cyclophosphamide, methotrexate, and 5-fluorouracil (CMF) and cyclophosphamide, doxorubicin (Adriamycin), and 5-fluorouracil (CAF). There is increasing evidence to support a role for taxol-based therapies, which may soon replace these traditional regimens. Trastuzumab (Herceptin) is a relatively new agent that works by binding the *her*-2 receptors in tumors that overexpress the proto-oncogene *her*-2/*neu*.

24-2. A. Several important nerves are encountered in the course of axillary dissection. The *long thoracic nerve* innervates the serratus anterior; damage to this nerve leads to "winged scapula." The *thoracodorsal nerve* innervates the latissimus dorsi; damage to this nerve leads to weakness of shoulder abduction. The *intercostobrachial nerves* provide sensation to the medial arm; sacrifice of these nerves may lead to numbness or dysesthesia in the affected area.

24-3. B. The well-reported lifetime risk of a woman developing breast cancer is between 1 in 9 and 1 in 11. Risk is increased above this range in patients with risk factors as described in the case.

24-4. A. In relation to the breast, Paget's disease (often referred to as Paget's disease of the nipple) involves the *skin* of the nipple. It accounts for 1% to 3% of all breast malignancies and is usually associated with an underlying ductal carcinoma (invasive or in situ). Malignant cells invade the epidermal–epithelial junction, resulting in eczematous changes in the nipple–areola complex with scaling, crusting, erosion, or discharge. Pathognomonic of this entity is the presence of large, pale, vacuolated cells (Paget cells) in the epithelium.

ADDITIONAL SUGGESTED READING

Chlebowski RT, Col N, Winer EP, et al. American Society of Clinical Oncology Breast Cancer Technology Assessment Working Group. American Society of Clinical Oncology technology assessment of pharmacologic interventions for breast cancer risk reduction including tamoxifen, raloxifene, and aromatase inhibition. J Clin Oncol 2002;20:3328–3343.

Fisher B, Anderson S, Bryant J, et al. Twenty-year follow-up of a randomized trial comparing total mastectomy, lumpectomy, and lumpectomy plus irradiation for the treatment of invasive breast cancer. N Engl J Med 2002;347:1233–1241.

Fletcher SW, Elmore JG. Clinical practice. Mammographic screening for breast cancer. N Engl J Med 2003;348:1672–1680.

Kolb TM, Lichy J, Newhouse JH. Comparison of the performance of screening mammography, physical examination, and breast US and evaluation of factors that influence them: an analysis of 27,825 patient evaluations. Radiology 2002;225:165–175.

Neck Mass

CC/ID: 38-year-old woman with a neck mass.

HPI: The patient presents with a several month history of a "tightness" in her neck. She does not complain of any pain, hoarseness, or breathing difficulties, but is concerned about what she now senses as a discrete mass on the front of her neck. She also complains of fatigue and lethargy, but blames this on her recent 15-lb weight gain. She is otherwise healthy and feels generally well.

THOUGHT QUESTION

- What are possible sources of this patient's symptoms?
- Are there any specific questions you would like to have answered?

DISCUSSION

Neck masses can result from thyroid, parathyroid, lymphatic/neoplastic, or infectious causes. Patients may present with swelling, fevers, fluctuance, difficulty with speech, swallowing or respiration, cough, pain, or nonspecific constitutional symptoms or complaints.

Several questions may help direct examination and subsequent testing. For instance, patients with goiter (thyroid enlargement) may be hypo- or hyperthyroid, with related complaints of fatigue, temperature intolerance, weight loss or gain, etc. Patients with hyperparathyroidism may c/o symptoms related to disorders of calcium metabolism. Patients with lymphoma may have noticed masses in other nodal areas. Head and neck cancers have been associated with a h/o radiation exposure, iodide deficiency (specific to thyroid cancer), smoking, or alcohol use. Patients with infectious sources may have fevers or a h/o trauma or IV drug use (patients who inject into their neck can develop abscesses in this way). A family history of endocrinopathy would increase suspicion for thyroid or parathyroid causes. Some of the answers to these questions may not come up in the course of a routine history unless they are specifically elicited.

CASE CONTINUED

The patient denies any h/o tobacco, alcohol, or other drug use. She has no known exposures to radiation. She has noted no other masses. She does believe that perhaps she has felt a little cooler on average, but not markedly different than those around her. She has no abdominal, bone, or urinary complaints. She cannot recall any traumatic injury to the area.

PMHx: None

PSHx: None

Meds: None

All: NKDA

FHx: Negative for thyroid, parathyroid, MEN, or other endocrine syndromes.

VS: Temp 36.9°C, BP 110/70, HR 80, regular O_2 sat 99% on RA

PE: *Gen:* WD/WN woman, appearing slightly tired but otherwise in no apparent distress. *HEENT:* No exophthalmos, no oropharyngeal erythema or exudates. *Neck:* 5 × 7-cm firm, nontender, irregular mass in the anterior midline that moves with swallowing; no dominant nodules appreciated; no other cervical masses or lymphadenopathy. *Ext:* No myxedema. *Neuro:* Nonfocal exam. Mild global hyporeflexia.

THOUGHT QUESTION

■ What do you want to do next?

DISCUSSION

The exam is most consistent with diffuse thyroid enlargement, although the previously described other sources cannot be completely ruled out. The patient's history and findings are suggestive of hypothyroidism, and thyroid function tests will help to clarify this. Ultrasound (US) is a good study for characterizing the thyroid and for identifying suspicious nodules that may not be palpable. If a thyroid abnormality is confirmed, functional studies, such as with radioiodine scanning, may help to determine the metabolic activity of the lesion. "Cold" nodules have a somewhat higher likelihood of being malignant than "hot" nodules. Fine needle aspiration (FNA) can offer a tissue diagnosis in the setting of a discrete nodule or if there is a particular concern for malignant disease. It is useful to rule out parathyroid involvement as well, so calcium and parathyroid hormone levels should be checked.

CASE CONTINUED

The patient is found to have an elevated TSH and a depressed thyroid hormone (T_4) level. In addition, her serum tests positive for antimicrosomal and antithyroglobulin antibodies. You diagnose her with Hashimoto's thyroiditis and start her on thyroid replacement therapy. With these biochemical findings, radionuclide and US modalities are unlikely to provide useful additional diagnostic information. If there had been a dominant nodule, FNA would have been indicated.

Surgery is not indicated at this time, as there is no evidence of local compression or suspicion of malignancy. Generally, operation for nontoxic goiter is indicated if there are symptoms of airway, esophageal, or superior vena carva obstruction; if suspicious nodules show evidence of malignancy; if there is radiologic evidence of tracheal deviation or compression; if the goiter continues to grow despite thyroid hormone therapy; for substernal goiters (which are difficult to follow clinically); or if there is a significant cosmetic deformity (patient request).

QUESTIONS

25-1. A finding of follicular cells on FNA requires
  A. Thyroidectomy to determine malignancy.
  B. Repeat FNA.
  C. Thyroid suppressive medications.
  D. Observation.
  E. Genetic testing.

25-2. Graves' disease
  A. Is a premalignant disorder.
  B. Generally results in clinical hypothyroidism.
  C. Results from antibodies against the TSH receptor of the thyroid gland.
  D. Has no familial penetrance.
  E. Is an uncommon cause of hyperthyroidism.

25-3. Medullary thyroid cancer (MTC)
  A. Results in an increase in parathormone levels.
  B. Is associated with MEN-1.
  C. Is associated with MEN-2.
  D. Is treated by hemithyroidectomy.
  E. Is responsive to radioactive iodine.

25-4. Usual vascular supply to the thyroid involves a paired set of
  A. Three arteries and two veins.
  B. Three arteries and three veins.
  C. Two arteries and one vein.
  D. Two arteries and two veins.
  E. Two arteries and three veins.

ANSWERS

25-1. A. Follicular adenomas can be benign or malignant. Unfortunately, the diagnosis usually requires an intact architecture to ascertain, which cannot be acquired by needle biopsy. It is therefore important to rule out malignancy when a cytologic diagnosis of follicular cells is found. This is generally accomplished by a subtotal or hemithyroidectomy. Repeat FNA is not helpful, because if benign cells are found, malignancy still cannot be ruled out; if malignant cells are found, then thyroidectomy is required anyway. A common strategy is to perform hemithyroidectomy on the side with the concerning nodule. If it is confirmed to be benign, then the patient can be followed expectantly and will not require thyroid hormone replacement. If cancer is confirmed, then completion thyroidectomy may be indicated. Thyroid suppression and observation alone are inappropriate in the setting of possible cancer. Genetic testing is not necessary.

25-2. C. Graves' disease is the most common cause of *hyper*thyroidism in the United States and is antibody mediated. The constant stimulation of the thyroid-stimulating hormone (TSH) receptors leads to overproduction of thyroid hormone, resulting in the findings of hyperthyroidism. There seems to be a familial component to the disorder.

25-3. C. The findings in MEN-1 are parathyroid hyperplasia, pancreatic islet cell tumor, and pituitary adenoma. Medullary thyroid cancer (MTC) is a component of MEN-2, and is associated with an increase in calcitonin levels. Treatment is by total thyroidectomy. Unlike the well-differentiated tumors of papillary and follicular origin, MTC is not radioiodine-sensitive.

25-4. E. The right and left superior and inferior thyroid arteries are branches of the right and left external carotid and thyrocervical trunk, respectively. The thyroid drains to the right and left superior, middle and inferior thyroid veins. See Figure 25-1.

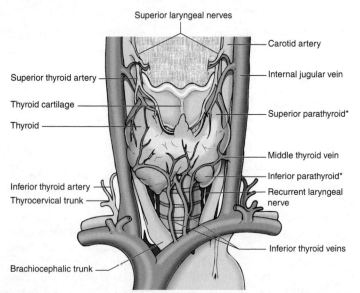

FIGURE 25-1. Anatomy of the thyroid gland. (*Used with permission from Karp SJ, Morris JPG, Soybel DI. Blueprints in Surgery, 2nd ed. Malden: Blackwell Science, Inc., 2001:111.*)

ADDITIONAL SUGGESTED READING

Castro MR, Gharib H. Continuing controversies in the management
of thyroid nodules. Ann Intern Med 2005;142:926–931.

Mandel SJ. Diagnostic use of ultrasonography in patients with
nodular thyroid disease. Endocr Pract 2004;10:246–252.

Pasieka JL. Hashimoto's disease and thyroid lymphoma: role
of the surgeon. World J Surg 2000;24:966–970.

Smith JR, Oates E. Radionuclide imaging of the thyroid gland:
patterns, pearls, and pitfalls. Clin Nucl Med 2004;29:181–193.

Thyroid Carcinoma Task Force. AACE/AAES medical/surgical
guidelines for clinical practice: management of thyroid carcinoma.
American Association of Clinical Endocrinologists. American
College of Endocrinology. Endocr Pract 2001;7:202–220.

Incidental Adrenal Mass

CC: 34-year-old woman with an adrenal mass found on CT.

HPI: The patient was brought to the ED 2 days ago after she fell from her bike. She had complained of abdominal pain (which has since resolved), and so a CT was performed. The CT showed no evidence of acute injury, but a 3-cm mass was seen in her left adrenal gland.

THOUGHT QUESTION

- Should this asymptomatic mass be worked up? What if it were 5 or 6 cm in size?
- What questions will you ask the patient to better evaluate this finding?
- What will you look for on physical exam?
- What tests, if any, will you order?

DISCUSSION

With the increasing number of CTs being performed, the finding of an incidental adrenal mass, often referred to as an adrenal "incidentaloma," has become more common (estimated at 0.6% of all abdominal scans). Size is an important consideration, because most would agree that surgical resection is warranted for any mass >4 to 6 cm in diameter, as masses of this size have an increased likelihood of being malignant. In all cases, biochemical evaluation is critical (discussed later), because a functional tumor, regardless of size, is also an indication for resection. Nonfunctioning tumors <4 to 6 cm in size can be followed with serial CTs.

History and examination should include questions and observations regarding weight change; family or personal history of MEN syndromes; hypertension; signs of hypokalemia, catecholamine excess, virilization, or feminization; changes in menstruation; other signs of Cushing's syndrome (truncal obesity, abdominal striae, moon facies, "buffalo hump"); and signs of occult malignancy. Laboratory evaluation should include serum potassium and 24-hour urine collection for free cortisol, vanillylmandelic acid (VMA), metanephrines, and catecholamines. Derangements in any of these values will guide further workup.

CASE CONTINUED

You learn that the patient has had some increase in recent headaches, but she believes this is related to anxiety about her job. She has otherwise been feeling well, with a stable weight, regular menses, and normal energy levels. She reports no other findings of concern on a recent routine physical exam for work, with the exception of "mild" hypertension. She tells you that there had been some discussion of starting her on medication if her blood pressure remained elevated, but that none had been started to date.

PMHx: Negative

PSHx: Right knee surgery ~10 years ago

Meds: Occasional ibuprofen for headache

FHx: No h/o malignancy or known endocrine disorder

VS: Temp 37°C, BP 155/90, HR 85

PE: *Gen:* Healthy, nonobese woman in NAD. *HEENT:* No facial dysmorphia, no exophthalmia, no neck masses. *Chest:* Clear bilaterally. *Heart:* RRR. *Abdomen:* Soft, flat; 3- to 4-cm ecchymosis over lower R ribs; no masses; no striae. *Ext:* Abrasions on R hand, elbow, and R lower leg; L/R strength equal and symmetric.

Labs: CBC within normal limits. Potassium 4.2. Urine and serum VMA is 1.5 to 2 times the upper limit of normal, with upper limit of normal metanephrines and normal catecholamines. You diagnose the patient with pheochromocytoma and schedule her for a laparoscopic adrenalectomy.

THOUGHT QUESTION

■ What will you do to prepare this patient for surgery?

DISCUSSION

Because of the potential for excess catecholamine release before or during their operation, these patients should receive preoperative alpha-blockade. Phenoxybenzamine is the agent of choice and is usually started 10 to 14 days before surgery. Patients are also encouraged to drink plenty of fluids during this time, as most are intravascularly depleted. The addition of beta-blockade (usually propranolol) is sometimes necessary to further control heart rate.

QUESTIONS

26-1. Pheochromocytoma is associated with
A. MEN-1.
B. MEN-2a/2b.
C. Pituitary adenomas.
D. Pancreatic neoplasms.
E. Hypercortisolism.

26-2. Pheochromocytoma is sometimes called the "10% tumor." Among the "10'"s this refers to are
A. 10% unilateral, 10% familial.
B. 10% benign, 10% extra-adrenal.
C. 10% sporadic, 10% benign.
D. 10% bilateral, 10% extra-adrenal.
E. 10% familial, 10% diagnosed in adults.

26-3. Primary hyperaldosteronism (Conn's syndrome) is marked by
A. Low renin levels.
B. Hyperkalemia.
C. Decreased total body sodium.
D. Increased urinary excretion of sodium.
E. Hypotension.

26-4. Which of the following associations regarding the difference between glucocorticoid production in Cushing's *disease* versus that in Cushing's *syndrome* is correct?

A. Cushing's disease = primary adrenal tumor.
   Cushing's syndrome = excess glucocorticoid administration.
B. Cushing's disease = malignant ectopic ACTH production.
   Cushing's syndrome = pituitary adenoma.
C. Cushing's disease = excess glucocorticoid production by the pituitary.
   Cushing's syndrome = excess ACTH production by the pituitary.
D. Cushing's disease = excess pituitary ACTH.
   Cushing's syndrome = any state resulting in hyperadrenocorticism.
E. Cushing's disease and Cushing's syndrome imply the same disease process, and should be used interchangeably.

ANSWERS

26-1. B. Pheochromocytoma is associated with MEN-2a (medullary thyroid cancer, pheochromocytoma, parathyroid hyperplasia) and MEN-2b (medullary thyroid cancer, pheochromocytoma, multiple mucosal neuromas), both genetic disorders with autosomal dominant transmission. It is also associated with other neuroectodermal diseases, including neurofibromatosis, von Hippel-Lindau disease, and tuberous sclerosis. MEN-1 describes a syndrome of pituitary adenoma, parathyroid hyperplasia, and pancreatic islet cell tumor. Hypercortisolism is associated with Cushing's syndrome.

26-2. D. Ten percent of pheochromocytomas are bilateral, 10% are familial, 10% are extra-adrenal, 10% are multiple (multiple sites or multiple tumors), 10% are diagnosed in children, and 10% are malignant. However, malignancy is difficult to define in the absence of overt extra-adrenal metastases, even with pathologic confirmation. Therefore, lifelong follow-up of these patients is critical.

26-3. A. In the case of *aldosteronoma*, there is high autonomous secretion of aldosterone with *low* renin levels. If renin levels are elevated, the increase in aldosterone is secondary to decreased renal blood flow (i.e., an appropriate renal response). An increase in aldosterone levels leads to increased urinary secretion of potassium with resultant *hypo*kalemia (leading to weakness and cramps) and *increased* total body sodium, leading to *hyper*tension.

26-4. **D.** Cushing's *disease* is due to excess pituitary ACTH, usually from a pituitary adenoma. The use of this term implies a primary pituitary pathology. Cushing's *syndrome* is any state of hypercortisolism, and may result from primary adrenal tumors (adenoma or carcinoma), ectopic ACTH (most notably from oat cell cancers of the lung), unusual cases of non–ACTH-dependent adrenal hyperplasia, or excess (i.e., iatrogenic) administration of glucocorticoids. Iatrogenic administration is the most common cause of Cushing's syndrome.

ADDITIONAL SUGGESTED READING

Duh QY. Adrenal incidentalomas. Br J Surg 2002;89:1347–1349.
NIH state-of-the-science statement on management of the clinically inapparent adrenal mass ("incidentaloma"). NIH Consens State Sci Statements 2002;19:1–25.

Groin Mass

CC: Two days of persistent R groin swelling, pain, and erythema.

HPI: The patient is an 83-year-old man who has noticed an intermittent right groin bulge that has been present for at least the past 10 years. However, he states that it has never stayed "out" for this long. He reports increased pain with coughing and slight improvement when lying down. In the past, the bulge has always disappeared with recumbency. He has not had any associated fever, dysuria, nausea, vomiting, or other GI complaints. He denies straining with urination or defecation, but does have a chronic smoker's cough.

PMHx: COPD, HTN, BPH, PVD

PSHx: Appendectomy as a child, TURP 5 years ago

Meds: Terazosin, atenolol, ASA, Ventolin

All: NKDA

SHx: 2 ppd smoker, no alcohol or other drugs

THOUGHT QUESTION

- What is your differential diagnosis at this point?

DISCUSSION

This history is classic for an inguinal hernia. However, other possibilities include femoral aneurysm or pseudoaneurysm, femoral hernia, lymphadenopathy, lipoma, testicular torsion, and epididymitis. Most hernias of any type (ventral/incisional, umbilical, lumbar) have a similar history, with gradual increase in size over time and worsened symptoms with increased intra-abdominal pressure.

CASE CONTINUED

VS: Temp 37.6°C, HR 84, BP 150/70

PE: *Gen:* Thin elderly man in no acute distress, cranky. *Abdomen:* Soft, flat, well-healed McBurney's scar, nontender and nondistended, normoactive bowel sounds; mildly erythematous 5 to 6 cm bulge overlying the R inguinal ligament, extending into the top of the scrotum—firm and slightly tender to touch; no change with cough; no impulse or defect in the L inguinal canal through the scrotum. *GU:* Bilateral descended testes, nontender, no masses. *Rectal:* Normal tone, no masses, heme negative.

Labs: CBC, lytes, and UA within normal limits.

THOUGHT QUESTION

- Do you think this is an incarcerated or a strangulated hernia? What is the difference? Why does it matter?

DISCUSSION

An incarcerated hernia is one that is not reducible and implies that there is no evidence of vascular compromise. A strangulated hernia involves tissue ischemia and possibly necrosis. A suspected strangulated hernia should not be reduced because return of necrotic bowel to the abdominal cavity may lead to bowel perforation and intra-abdominal sepsis. Incarceration is a surgical urgency, whereas strangulation is a surgical emergency. In this case, the patient shows no evidence of bowel at risk or impending sepsis (fever, tachycardia, leukocytosis), but the hernia has not spontaneously reduced in 2 days. This suggests that it is likely incarcerated but not strangulated.

This hernia should not go untreated. An attempt at reduction using Trendelenburg positioning (for gravity assistance), IV sedation (for pain control and muscle relaxation), and gentle pressure should be made. If it is successful, the patient may be scheduled for a prompt elective repair. If the attempt fails, however, the patient should be taken urgently to the operating room.

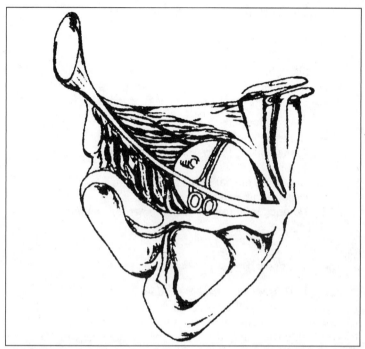

FIGURE 27-1. Anatomy of the Groin. (*Image provided by Shawn Girsberger Graphic Design.*)

QUESTIONS

27-1. The borders of Hesselbach's triangle are
A. Inguinal ligament, transversalis fascia, spermatic cord.
B. Scarpa's fascia, pectineal line, rectus sheath.
C. Inferior epigastric vessels, arcuate line, anterior superior iliac spine.
D. Inguinal ligament, femoral vein, lacunar ligament.
E. Inguinal ligament, rectus sheath, inferior epigastric vessels.

27-2. Appropriate hernia nomenclature includes
A. Pantaloon—hernia involving the mesenteric bowel wall.
B. Richter—hernia involving an extra-abdominal structure.
C. Spigelian—hernia through the linea semilunaris.
D. Littre—hernia containing the appendix.
E. Sliding—hernia involving both direct and indirect inguinal components.

27-3. Which of the following hernia repairs involves the use of mesh?
- A. McVay.
- B. Bassini.
- C. Shouldice.
- D. Lichtenstein.
- E. Transscrotal.

27-4. Femoral hernias
- A. Are more common in men.
- B. Are less likely to present with incarceration than inguinal hernias.
- C. Are found medial to the femoral vein.
- D. Occur as a result of infection.
- E. Do not communicate with the peritoneal space.

ANSWERS

27-1. E. Hesselbach's triangle is defined by the inferior epigastric artery superiorly, the border of the rectus sheath medially, and the inguinal ligament inferolaterally. Hernias that occur through this anatomic triangle and the floor of the inguinal canal are considered *direct* hernias. They are most often associated with tissue laxity and strain (as with increased age and abdominal pressure). Therefore, direct hernias are usually considered "acquired" hernias and frequently occur in older patients. Hernias found lateral to the inferior epigastric vessels are called *indirect* and are due to persistence of the congenital processus vaginalis, which leads into the scrotum or labia. Indirect hernias can be found in any age patient. The hernia sac of an indirect hernia generally lies on the anteromedial surface of the spermatic cord. It is difficult to determine which type of hernia is present by physical exam alone. The *iliohypogastric* and *ilioinguinal nerves* can be found running through Hesselbach's triangle and should be identified and preserved during hernia repair. See Figure 27-2.

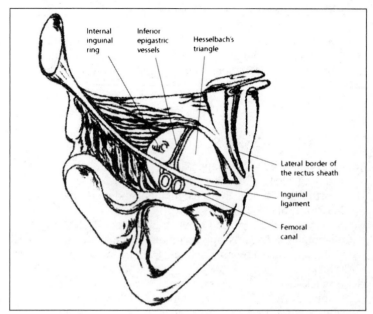

FIGURE 27-2. Anatomy of the Groin. (*Image provided by Shawn Girsberger Graphic Design.*)

27-2. C. A Richter hernia involves herniation of the *anti*-mesenteric bowel wall into an abdominal wall defect. A pantaloon hernia has both a direct and an indirect component, causing the hernia with its two "legs" to lie with one leg on either side of the inferior epigastric vessels. A Littre hernia contains a Meckel's diverticulum. Sliding inguinal hernias have a sac that is partially formed by the wall of a viscus.

27-3. D. There is no such technique as a transscrotal hernia repair. The traditional Bassini repair, like the Shouldice and McVay techniques, involves anatomic reapposition of the tissue planes. The Lichtenstein, laparoscopic, and other mesh plug techniques emphasize "tension-free" repair and use polypropylene mesh sheets or plugs to cover or fill the tissue defects. Laparoscopic approaches are growing in popularity, although a recent study suggests a significant increase in recurrence rates with those techniques. Currently, recurrence rates for traditional open repairs average <10%, whereas the Lichtenstein group claims near 1% recurrence. Laparoscopic centers average 2% to 6% recurrence rates. Estimates of recurrence rates are often inaccurate or incomplete because patients may not return to the same physician for repair of a recurrent hernia.

27-4. C. Femoral hernias are less common than inguinal hernias but have a 20% incidence of incarceration at presentation (compared with 10% for inguinal). They are found medial to the femoral artery and vein and inferior to the inguinal ligament. They are more common in women and do communicate with the peritoneal space.

ADDITIONAL SUGGESTED READING

Awad SS, Fagan SP. Current approaches to inguinal hernia repair. Am J Surg 2004;188(6A Suppl):9S–16S.

Kingsnorth A, LeBlanc K. Hernias: inguinal and incisional. Lancet 2003;362:1561–1571.

McCormack K, Scott NW, Go PM, et al. EU Hernia Trialists Collaboration. Laparoscopic techniques versus open techniques for inguinal hernia repair. Cochrane Database Syst Rev 2003;(1): CD001785.

McCormack K, Wake BL, Fraser C, et al. Transabdominal pre-peritoneal (TAPP) versus extraperitoneal (TEP) laparoscopic techniques for inguinal hernia repair: a systematic review. Hernia 2005;9:109–114.

Nathan JK, Pappas TN. Inguinal hernia: an old condition with new solutions. Ann Surg 2003:238(6 Suppl):S148–157.

Hip Swelling and Pain

CC: Swelling, redness, and tenderness on R hip × 1 day.

HPI: Ms. X is a 48-year-old woman with a long history of IV drug abuse and multiple abscesses, who c/o swelling, redness, and pain over her R hip for the past day. She last injected heroin into her R hip 1 week prior. She reports fever and chills for 2 days and says she is unable to lie on her R side due to pain. She denies diabetes or HIV.

PMHx: Hepatitis B+; hepatitis C+

PSHx: Multiple incision and drainage (I&D) procedures

Meds: None

All: NKDA

SHx: 1 ppd cigarette smoker, occasional alcohol, 2 g heroin IV per day—last used this morning into her L shoulder (she states it has been too painful to inject into her R hip)

VS: Temp 39.5°C, HR 108, BP 90/50

PE: *Gen:* Thin disheveled woman; somnolent but arousable. *Lungs:* Fine crackles at bases. *CV:* RRR. *Abdomen:* Soft, nondistended, mild tenderness over the liver with tip felt 2 cm below costal margin. *Ext:* Shoulders, arms, buttocks, hips, and thighs with multiple I&D scars; R hip with 8 × 10-cm area of erythema and induration with 4-cm central area of fluctuance.

Labs:

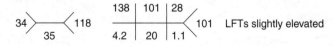

34 > < 118
    35

138 | 101 | 28
4.2 | 20 | 1.1 > 101 LFTs slightly elevated

THOUGHT QUESTION

- What terminology is used to describe different types/ depths of soft tissue infections? How are they treated?
- What is your assessment of this woman's presentation?

DISCUSSION

Erythema with superficial infection is considered simple *cellulitis*. Involved organisms are generally gram-positive bacteria from skin flora and can be treated with IV or oral first-generation cephalosporins. Diabetics and immunocompromised patients should be treated with broader spectrum antibiotics, to include better coverage of gram-negative and anaerobic organisms as well. Infection spreading via the lymphatics can appear as red "streaks" leading proximally from the original infection and is termed *lymphangitis*. This is treated more aggressively with parenteral antibiotics and extremity elevation until improvement is seen. Deep soft tissue infections (*necrotizing fasciitis* or *myositis* and *pyomyositis*) are rapidly progressive and can occur in the presence or absence of an overlying superficial infection. Patients often present in septic shock. These infections can be caused by single organisms (e.g., α-hemolytic streptococcus, *Clostridium perfringens*), but are more often polymicrobial with gram-positive and gram-negative aerobes, in addition to anaerobes. Signs of a necrotizing infection include woody or brawny induration; drainage of watery, gray, or brown fluid from the wound (classically described as "dishwater fluid"); crepitus ("gas gangrene"); and skin blebs. Markedly elevated WBC (e.g., >20,000) and fever are frequently seen. Soft tissue gas can sometimes be detected on plain films, whereas CT can show not only soft tissue air, but also fluid and inflammation. However, absence of any of these signs and symptoms does not exclude a deep infection.

This woman has a fever of 39.5°C and a WBC of 24. Both values are higher than would be expected for a simple soft tissue infection or abscess. Superficial abscesses alone (i.e., no cellulitis or deep tissue infection) should not cause a very elevated WBC, because the contamination in those cases is localized and walled off. The patient also has a slight gap acidosis, tachycardia, and possibly hypotension (depending on her baseline blood pressure). These are worrisome for necrotizing fasciitis and sepsis.

CASE CONTINUED

You plan immediate operative debridement, close monitoring in the ICU, aggressive fluid resuscitation, and intravenous antibiotics. Her blood pressure increases slightly to 105/55 with a 1-L NS bolus. In the OR, you find about 60 cc of superficial pus overlying brownish, nonbleeding, and poorly contractile (in response to stimulation with the electrocautery) gluteal muscles. Skin, fat, and muscle are debrided circumferentially from this region until healthy bleeding tissue is encountered. You pack the wound open and take the patient back to the ICU with plans for a second-look procedure in 12 hours.

THOUGHT QUESTION

- How would your treatment differ if the patient had been a healthy non-IV drug user who had recently slept in a cabin where spiders may have been present?

DISCUSSION

Soft tissue infection after a spider bite is generally limited to cellulitis alone. However, dermonecrosis with deeper infection can occur, most notoriously with the *brown recluse spider*, found primarily in the South and Midwest. The wound often appears as a crater-like ulcer with induration and eschar. Treatment involves analgesia, oral dapsone, and operative debridement only if absolutely necessary.

QUESTIONS

28-1. Mortality of deep soft tissue infections is at least 50% and is related to
- A. Delay in diagnosis.
- B. Inadequate debridement.
- C. Inadequate antibiotic coverage.
- D. All of the above.

28-2. Fournier's gangrene is a soft tissue infection of the
- A. Perineum.
- B. Face.
- C. Breast.
- D. Buttocks.

28-3. Suppurative hidradenitis is a chronic infection of the apocrine sweat glands that
  A. Most commonly involves staph, strep, and *Escherichia coli* bacterial species.
  B. Should be treated first with debridement.
  C. Usually involves the extremities.
  D. Leads to sepsis if untreated.

28-4. Pilonidal cysts
  A. Occur most frequently in young men (3:1 male–female ratio).
  B. Can only be treated operatively.
  C. Are a congenital defect.
  D. Can be caused by local illicit drug injection.

ANSWERS

28-1. D. Deep soft tissue infections such as necrotizing fasciitis are rapidly progressive and require immediate and aggressive treatment. This should include immediate broad-spectrum antibiotics and wide debridement. If clinical suspicion is high, imaging is not necessary before proceeding to the operating room. Intraoperatively, tissue should be examined for viability, and devitalized tissue should be excised until healthy bleeding tissue is reached. Scheduled re-exploration is often necessary to ensure that the remaining tissue is unaffected. Diabetics, the elderly, and others whose immune systems are compromised are particularly at risk, because they are less able to mount an immune response to these complex infections.

28-2. A. Fournier's gangrene requires the same treatment as any other deep soft tissue infection—debridement and antibiotics. Urologic reconstruction may be required in cases with extensive tissue loss.

28-3. C. Suppurative hidradenitis most often involves the axillary (more common in females), perineal (more common in men), areolar and inframammary, inguinal, and periumbilical regions. Risk factors include acne, obesity, and excessive sweating. Treatment consists of avoidance of sweating and local irritants (e.g., deodorants, talcum powder, creams), and the use of antibiotics, hot compresses, and incision and drainage if necessary. Chronic, recurring disease may ultimately require wide excision of local apocrine tissue and skin grafting.

28-4. A. Nonoperative treatment of pilonidal cysts involves meticulous perineal hygiene and shaving of the gluteal cleft if appropriate. Operative treatment begins with abscess unroofing and removal of granulation tissue and inspissated hair follicles. Chronic disease or sinuses can be treated with tract excision and rotational flap coverage. Previously, pilonidal cysts were considered congenital, deriving from an epithelialized tract of the gluteal cleft. However, the current belief is that they originate from obstruction of a cleft hair follicle with abscess formation and involvement of surrounding follicles. The differential diagnosis includes perianal Crohn's, suppurative hidradenitis, and actinomycosis.

ADDITIONAL SUGGESTED READING

Endorf FW, Supple KG, Gamelli RL. The evolving characteristics and care of necrotizing soft-tissue infections. Burns 2005;31:269–273.

Mitchell KM, Beck DE. Hidradenitis suppurativa. Surg Clin North Am 2002;82:1187–1197.

Slade DE, Powell BW, Mortimer PS. Hidradenitis suppurativa: pathogenesis and management. Br J Plast Surg 2003;56:451–461.

Swanson DL, Vetter RS. Bites of brown recluse spiders and suspected necrotic arachnidism. N Engl J Med 2005;352:700–707.

Tillou A, St Hill CR, Brown C, et al. Necrotizing soft tissue infections: improved outcomes with modern care. Am Surg 2004;70:841–844.

Wong CH, Wang YS. The diagnosis of necrotizing fasciitis. Curr Opin Infect Dis 2005;18:101–106.

Testicular Mass

CC/ID: Swollen right testicle

HPI: Mr. X is a 28-year-old man who noted recently in the shower that his right testicle felt somewhat swollen. He has not felt any pain in the testicle but on questioning has had a heavy sensation in the scrotum off and on over the past few months. He had attributed this to a new weight lifting regimen. He has had no weight loss, anorexia, cough, back pain, or bony pain.

PMH: none

PSH: none

Meds: none

All: penicillin → hives

SH: beer on weekends

FH: none

VS: Temp 37.2°C, BP 133/70, HR 64

PE: *Gen:* Muscular man, no distress. *HEENT:* Eyes anicteric, no supraclavicular lympadenopathy. *Chest:* CTA bilaterally. *Abdomen:* No scars; nondistended. Nontender, no palpable mass. *GU:* circumcised penis, left testicle normal size and consistency, right testicle with 2-cm ovoid rubbery mass at apex. *Rectal:* normal tone, nontender, small prostate, heme negative.

THOUGHT QUESTION

- What is the differential diagnosis?
- What is the initial workup?

DISCUSSION

A solid testicular mass is testicular cancer until proven otherwise. However, the differential also includes testicular torsion, which is a surgical emergency. Other possible testicular abnormalities are epididymitis, hydrocele, varicocele, hernia, hematoma, and spermatocele.

The evaluation of a testicular mass begins with a bimanual exam of the scrotum, as well as abdominal and chest exam for evidence of metastatic disease and gynecomastia. Radiologic tests should begin with a scrotal ultrasound (US) and may continue with a CT scan of the abdomen and pelvis and a CXR if indicated. CT is the best study to evaluate the retroperitoneum. Blood should be sent for baseline labs and serum tumor markers, including alpha fetoprotein (AFP), beta subunit of human chorionic gonatdotropin (beta-hCG) and lactated dehydrogenase (LDH). Lastly, radical inguinal orchiectomy provides both histologic identification of the tumor and local tumor control.

CASE CONTINUED

Labs: CBC and basic metabolic panel normal, AFP normal, b-hCG 8500 mIU/ml, normal <5 mlU/ml, LDH 253.

Imaging: *Scrotal ultrasound:* 2.2 cm solid mass on right, *CT with and without IV contrast:* Solid organs without evidence of metastases, 5-mm pelvic retroperitoneal lymphadenopathy. *CXR:* no nodules.

Pathology: Right testicle obtained during orchiectomy showed well-differentiated seminoma.

THOUGHT QUESTION

- What is the treatment plan now?

DISCUSSION

After resection of the involved testicle, early stage seminoma is usually treated with radiation therapy directed towards the para-aortic lymph nodes. Cure rates are well over 95%, with recurrence in

3–15%. Alternatively, surveillance with close follow-up may be selected for small (<3 cm) seminomas with favorable histologic features and negative post-operative serum tumor markers. For higher stage tumors, radiation therapy is still the treatment of choice, although chemotherapy may be considered and is certainly the indicated therapy for bulky, advanced, or recurrent disease.

QUESTIONS

29-1. Compared to seminomas, non-seminomatous germ cell tumors (NSGCT) are:
A. More indolent with late relapses.
B. More likely to be localized at presentation.
C. More sensitive to radiation therapy.
D. More often associated with elevated beta-hCG and AFP.

29-2. Which of the following is true regarding testicular cancer?
A. Most common solid malignancy in men ages 15–35 years.
B. Acute testicular pain occurs in 50%.
C. Pulmonary metastases are rare.
D. Associated with gonadal dysgenesis and impaired spermatogenesis in 80%.

29-3. Paraneoplastic syndromes that may occur with testicular tumors include which of the following?
A. Syndrome of inappropriate ADH secretion.
B. Hyperthyroidism.
C. Diabetes insipidus.
D. Hypercortisolism.

29-4. Cryptorchidism
A. is associated with a higher incidence of testicular cancer
B. is seen in 10% of full-term newborn boys
C. generally leads to improved fertility
D. is commonly manifest as a completely intraabdominal testis

ANSWERS

21-1. D. Because NSGCT are relatively radioresistant, retroperitoneal lymph node dissection is a more likely choice for treatment of early disease. Surveillance is still an option for tumors that have no lymphovascular invasion or are not embryonal carcinoma type. High risk and higher stage tumors are treated with chemotherapy. Cure rates with these modalities are excellent (>95%). Germ cell tumors account for 95% of testicular cancers.

29-2. A. Testicular pain is rare as a presenting symptom and occurs in 10%. Low semen quality is found in approximately 50% of patients. However, sperm cryopreservation is recommended before starting treatment.

29-3. B. Beta-hCG shares a common alpha-subunit and a similar beta-subunit with thyroid stimulating hormone (TSH). Thus, beta-hCG has a weak thyroid-stimulating action, and tumors that secrete large amounts of hCG can lead to hyperthyroidism. Similarly, many testicular tumors express Ma2 antigen, and patients form anti-Ma2 or anti-Ta antibodies. Ma2 antigen is also found in neuronal nucle-oli, and some patients may develop limbic encephalitis. Gyneco-mastia is found in only 5% of men with testicular GCTs; however, it occurs in 20–30% of patients with Leydig cell tumors. Gynecomas-tia is usually associated with beta-hCG production by the tumor, although elevated serum levels may or may not occur.

29-4. A. Cryptorchidism places the affected patient at increased risk for testicular tumor development. The risk is approximately 50 in 100, 000, which is 20 times the risk seen in the general population. Orchidopexy is not protective against subsequent testis cancer and approximately 15–20% of tumors occur in a contralateral descended testis. Cryptorchidism is seen in 3% of newborn boys, decreasing to 1% in boys aged 6 months to 1 year. Men who previously had bilat-eral cryptorchidism have greatly reduced fertility compared to those who had unilateral cryptorchidism and those of the general male population. Most undescended testicles are in the inguinal canal.

ADDITIONAL SUGGESTED READING

Albers P, Albrecht W, Algaba F, et al. Guidelines on testicular cancer. Eur Urol 2005;48:885–894.

Horwich A, Shipley J, Huddart R. Testicular germ-cell cancer. Lancet 2006 4;367:754–765.

Husmann DA. Cryptorchidism and its relationship to testicular neoplasia and microlithiasis. Urology 2005;66:424–426.

Yoon GH, Stein JP, Skinner DG. Retroperitoneal lymph node dissection in the treatment of low-stage nonseminomatous germ cell tumors of the testicle: an update. Urol Oncol 2005;23:168–177.

CASE **30**

Flank Pain

CC/ID: 62 year-old man with L flank pain and fullness.

HPI: The patient states that the "ache" has been persistent for the last several weeks. He cannot remember any particular inciting event, but since the onset, he has been constantly aware of it. Nothing seems to specifically make it better or worse. He denies any history of trauma. He has not had any fevers, nausea, vomiting, weight loss, or change in his bowel habits. He has no history of similar pain previously.

PMH: asthma, "heartburn", arthritis

PSH: "ulcer surgery" ~ 30 years ago; cataract removal; inguinal hernia repair

MEDs: protonix, ibuprofen, inhalers, prn NKDA

SH/H: smoked while enlisted, none for >35 years; drinks "sometimes." Retired cook.

EXAM: *Gen*: pleasant thin man in NAD, appearing his stated age. *Chest*: rare scattered expiratory wheezes *Abd*: soft, flat; well-healed upper midline scar; minimal TTP in the L flank with a firm fullness that moves with respiration. *Groins*: bilateral descended testicles, well healed R groin scar; L scrotal varicocele that does not empty with recumbency. *Ext*: warm, well-perfused; symmetric, with no edema.

THOUGHT QUESTION

- What is your working differential for this patient?
- What is the significance of the scrotal varicocele?
- Is there any other directed history that might be useful?
- What will you do next?

DISCUSSION

An older patient with a mass should be considered to have cancer until proven otherwise. Despite the fact that his presenting complaint was pain, the finding of a mass is certainly worrisome. In considering what might present in the L flank, anatomic considerations should make you think of colon, pancreatic tail, kidney, adrenal, or perhaps spleen. Inquiring as to tumor-specific risk factors would be appropriate (e.g., family history, exposures). It would be possible to have an inflammatory process such as diverticulitis or pancreatic pseudocyst causing both pain and a palpable L-sided mass, though he gives no other history of symptoms to suggest this. Determining whether he has had a colonoscopy or a history of pancreatitis in the past may help in deciding if those disease processes should be pursued. In addition, questions pertaining to functional adrenal tumors (see Chapter 26) may be in order.

The scrotal varicocele should perhaps direct a more thorough evaluation of a primary renal problem, as this finding may be seen in instances where the gonadal vein is obstructed as it enters into the renal vein. This is more commonly seen on the L side, though certainly any mass in the area may lead to this effect.

Given the fairly broad differential, it would be reasonable to proceed with screening biochemical studies (looking for electrolyte abnormalities, anemia, signs of infection, etc), as well as some sort of imaging study. Ultrasound, computed tomography (CT), and magnetic resonance imaging (MRI) are all good options.

CASE CONTINUED

The patient gives no family or personal history of malignancy. Review of systems is generally unremarkable. You order labs and decide to start with a screening ultrasound.

Labs:

	11		138	104	10	Ca++ 11.5	TBili 1.1
7 >	----------	< 212	--------------------		< 95		AST 80
	33		3.9	25	1.1		ALT 92
							AlkP 200

ESR 20　　　　　　　　PT/PTT/INR 13.1/30/1.2

UA: 4+ hematuria

Imaging: *Abdominal ultrasound*—8 cm mostly solid, irregular, heterogeneous mass in the lower pole of the L kidney; pancreas, spleen, liver, gallbladder, adrenals, and R kidney appear normal.

THOUGHT QUESTION

- How do you interpret the laboratory findings?
- How will you work up the renal mass? What is the differential? What if this were a child?

DISCUSSION

The most notable lab findings are the anemia, hypercalcemia, elevated liver function tests (LFTs), and hematuria. All of these may be accounted for by renal cancer, which is notoriously associated with a number of paraneoplastic syndromes. The most common findings are anemia, cachexia/weight loss/fatigue, fever, hypertension, hypercalcemia, hepatic dysfunction (Stauffer syndrome), amyloidosis, erythrocytosis, enteropathy, and neuromyopathy. Other findings include dermatomyositis and elevated ESR. Hypercalcemia is seen in up to 15% of patients with renal cancer, and generally suggests a poor prognosis. Other less common findings are thrombocytosis, as well as increases in hCG, ACTH, renin, glucagon, insulin, or PTH-related protein (which may contribute to hypercalcemia). In this setting, the hematuria suggests invasion (of the tumor) into the collecting system.

When evaluating a renal mass, it is important to note whether it is cystic or solid. If a mass meets US criteria for a simple cyst (smooth walls, sharp demarcation, anechoic), then no further evaluation is required. If these criteria are not met, then CT or MRI should be obtained. CT is preferred as it has a >90% sensitivity and specificity for characterizing renal masses. MRI is often good if caval involvement is suspected. Bone scans may be helpful in staging, though the yield is fairly low in the absence of bony complaints or elevated alkaline phosphatase. Renal arteriography is infrequently used.

Renal lesions are more likely to be metastatic than primary in origin. The most common primary tumor is renal cell carcinoma (RCC), which originates from the proximal tubular epithelium of the renal cortex, and accounts for ~3% of all adult malignancies and 80–85% of primary renal neoplasms. Transitional cell cancer (TCC) is the next most common primary renal tumor, accounting for ~8%. Wilms' tumor is common in children. Benign lesions include abscess, angiomyolipoma, oncocytoma, and xanthrogranulomatous pyelonephritis, each of which can usually be distinguished on CT. Adenoma may be difficult to distinguish from carcinoma, so resection is usually required. Fine needle aspiration (FNA) is not usually performed, because of low specificity and concerns about possible seeding.

CASE CONTINUED

You order a CT scan to confirm and stage your suspected diagnosis. Findings include: thick, irregular walls with septae, enhancement post-contrast, and local invasion into the perinephric fat. You obtain further staging with chest CT, and order a bone scan, both of which are negative for signs of metastatic disease. Based on your findings, the patient is scheduled for L radical nephrectomy. You explain that this will involve early ligation of the vascular pedicle, and resection of the kidney and Gerota's fascia. Classically, this operation also includes resection of the ipsilateral adrenal gland, though most contemporary surgeons will perform this only for upper pole lesions > 4 cm, tumor stage T3 or higher (i.e., not organ-confined), or for evidence of adrenal metastases on preoperative staging studies. The extent of lymph node dissection required is controversial. Laparoscopic approaches are acceptable in selected patients. RCC is poorly chemo- or radio-sensitive, but immunotherapy has been promising.

QUESTIONS

30-1. The percent of patients with RCC who have distant metastases or significant locoregional disease at presentation is
   A. <10.
   B. 25.
   C. 50.
   D. 75.
   E. >90.

30-2. The "classic triad" of RCC symptoms comprises
   A. Flank pain, hematuria, palpable abdominal mass.
   B. Flank pain, dysuria, fever.
   C. Umbilical pain, urinary frequency, palpable abdominal mass.
   D. Umbilical pain, hematuria, groin adenopathy.
   E. Pelvic pain, pyuria, palpable bladder.

30-3. Nephron sparing surgery for renal cancer (partial nephrectomy) may be considered

- A. In tumors confined to the renal capsule that are <4 cm in diameter.
- B. In tumors that extend beyond the renal capsule, but are confined to Gerota's fascia and are <3 cm in diameter.
- C. In any tumor with only isolated metastases.
- D. In patients younger than 40 years of age.
- E. The technique of partial nephrectomy should not be used in the setting of cancer.

30-4. For which of the following patients might RCC screening be beneficial?

- A. 40-year-old with a history of benign adrenal adenoma.
- B. 10-year-old with unilateral renal agenesis.
- C. 60-year-old with a history of fungal urinary tract infections (UTI).
- D. 50-year-old with long-standing diabetes.
- E. 30-year-old with end stage renal disease (ESRD) on hemodialysis for the past 5 years.

ANSWERS

30-1. B. Approximately one-quarter of patients with RCC will have metastatic or locally advanced disease at the time of diagnosis. Symptoms can be very variable. Patients may present with symptoms related to their metastases, such as pathologic fractures, cough, dyspnea, or lymphadenopathy. In those cases, diagnosis is often made by biopsy of the affected area (e.g., lymph node biopsy), or by the finding of a kidney mass seen on CT. The most common sites of metastatic spread are regional lymphatics, lung, bone, liver, brain, ipsilateral adrenal, and contralateral kidney. Up to 5% will have IVC involvement at the time of diagnosis.

30-2. A. The "classic triad" of RCC is flank pain, hematuria, and a palpable abdominal renal mass. Although individually these remain the most common complaints at the time of diagnosis, contemporary series now report that this triad is found in fewer than 10% of patients who present with a new diagnosis of renal cancer. This is thought largely to be due to increased incidental diagnoses being made on imaging studies performed for other purposes (incidentaloma). Other commonly seen symptoms are fever, weight loss, hypertension, night sweats, malaise, varicocele, and sequelae of hypercalcemia.

30-3. A. Nephron sparing surgery for renal cancer has been accepted for T1 tumors (confined to the renal capsule) that are less than 4 cm in diameter. This has been shown to result in adequate resection margins and rates of disease recurrence that are comparable to those seen after radical nephrectomy; this has not been the case for T2 or greater disease (tumor outside of the renal capsule). Partial nephrectomy is also considered in patients who have small multiple and/or bilateral tumors, tumor in a solitary kidney, or compromised renal function. Cryoablation and radiofrequency ablation (RFA) techniques are being studied, but long-term data are lacking.

30-4. E. Renal cancer is not common enough to warrant widespread screening programs (i.e., is not cost effective), but it is thought that certain patients at increased risk might benefit from early detection procedures (such as US). These patients include those with von Hippel-Lindau syndrome (among whom up to 40% will develop RCC, usually multiple); tuberous sclerosis; strong family history of RCC (including the syndromes of hereditary papillary renal carcinoma [HPRC], familial renal oncocytoma [FRO], and hereditary renal carcinoma [HRC]; end-stage renal disease (ESRD) on dialysis for more than 3–5 years (especially in young patients); and possibly those with a history of kidney irradiation. Other risk factors that might be taken into consideration include cigarette smoking, obesity, hypertension, unopposed estrogen therapy, history of renal transplantation with associated immunosuppression, and exposure to petroleum products, heavy metals, solvents, or asbestos. There is no known increase in cancer risk in patients with adrenal adenoma, unilateral kidney, fungal UTI, or diabetes.

SUGGESTED ADDITIONAL READING

Dunn MD, Portis AJ, Shalhav AL, et al. Laparoscopic versus open radical nephrectomy: a 9-year experience. J Urol 2000;164:1153–1159.

McLaughlin JK, Lipworth L. Epidemiologic aspects of renal cell cancer. Semin Oncol 2000;27:115–123.

Pantuck AJ, Zisman A, Dorey F, et al. Renal cell carcinoma with retroperitoneal lymph nodes. Impact on survival and benefits of immunotherapy. Cancer 2003;15(97):2995–3002.

Patard JJ, Shvarts O, Lam JS, et al. Safety and efficacy of partial nephrectomy for all T1 tumors based on an international multicenter experience. J Urol 2004;171(6 Pt 1):2181–2185.

Russo P. Renal cell carcinoma: presentation, staging, and surgical treatment. Semin Oncol 2000;27:160–176.

IV

Thoracic Complaints

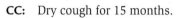

Persistent Cough

CC: Dry cough for 15 months.

HPI: Mr. X is a 56-year-old man who has noted a dry hacking cough for more than a year. The cough seems to have gotten worse in the past few months despite multiple courses of antibiotics for "walking pneumonia" and "bronchitis." At one point, he coughed up some blood-tinged phlegm. He currently smokes 2 packs of cigarettes a day and has done so since he was a teenager. He has lost 25 pounds in the last 6 months.

PMHx: Pneumonia twice in the last year

PSHx: None

Meds: Currently day 3 of a 7-day course of erythromycin for "bronchitis"

All: NKDA

SHx: As above, no alcohol

VS: Unremarkable, O_2 sat 94% on RA, RR 17

PE: *Gen:* Thin man, no acute distress, nicotine stains on fingers and teeth, voice slightly hoarse. *CV:* RRR, no murmur/rub/gallop. *Lungs:* Barrel chest, trace wheeze over R upper lung field; otherwise clear, no supra/infraclavicular lymphadenopathy. *Abdomen:* Soft, NT/ND, no hepatosplenomegaly, no masses. *Ext:* No edema, no clubbing or cyanosis. *Neuro:* Grossly nonfocal, AO × 4.

THOUGHT QUESTION

- What is your next step in trying to diagnose this man's problem?

DISCUSSION

Given that the patient has already been treated for bronchitis and pneumonia without improvement, and in light of his significant smoking history, one must exclude lung neoplasm before entertaining more rare diseases such as pneumonitis or bronchiectasis. Thus, the first step in this case should be to obtain a *chest x-ray*. Comparison with previous films, if they exist, is extremely helpful in determining whether a nodule is new. If a new nodule is found, or if the CXR is nondiagnostic, a *chest CT* is the most appropriate next step. If an effusion is identified, *thoracentesis* can be performed for cytology to rule out a malignant effusion.

CASE CONTINUED

Labs: WBC 8; Hct 39; Plts 405; Lytes WNL; LFTs WNL; Ca 11.2.

Imaging: *CXR:* 2-cm spiculated nodule in the R apex; fullness in the R hilum suggestive of lymphadenopathy. There is no pleural effusion. (Note: CXR 1 year ago was normal.) A chest CT is obtained that confirms a R apical nodule with hilar lymphadenopathy but no other obvious lesions.

THOUGHT QUESTION

- Of what significance is this patient's hoarseness?
- What are other signs of advanced disease that might be noted on physical exam?

DISCUSSION

A hoarse voice can result from tumor involvement of the recurrent laryngeal nerve with subsequent vocal cord paralysis. *Superior vena cava syndrome,* with neck, arm, and face swelling and pain, is caused by compression of the superior vena cava by a mass. *Pancoast's syndrome* is the involvement of the cervical sympathetic plexus and local blood vessels by an apical tumor, resulting in arm pain and swelling, reduced distal pulse, and Horner's syndrome. Tracheal deviation or stridor can denote airway involvement and impending obstruction.

QUESTIONS

31-1. Which of the following is *true* regarding lung cancer?
- A. The adrenal gland is the most common site of recurrence after resection.
- B. Non-small cell cancers include squamous, adenocarcinoma, and large cell cancers.
- C. Associated paraneoplastic syndromes are rare.
- D. The majority are small cell tumors.

31-2. Which of the following associations is *true*?
- A. Squamous—originates centrally in the bronchi.
- B. Adenocarcinoma—originates in the chest wall.
- C. Bronchioloalveolar—subtype of squamous cell tumor.
- D. Carcinoid—typically peripheral.

31-3. Which of the following is a suspected cause of lung cancer?
- A. Alpha-1 antitrypsin deficiency.
- B. Inhaled steroids.
- C. Vinyl chloride exposure.
- D. Betel-nut ingestion.

31-4. Which of the following is *true* regarding pleural effusions?
- A. Pleural fluid drains via the diaphragm into the peritoneal space.
- B. Chemical pleurodesis causes increased expression of adhesion molecules between the visceral and parietal pleura.
- C. Massive bloody effusions are caused by a leaking arteriovenous fistula in the pleura.
- D. Empyema can lead to a draining chest wall sinus or a systemic abscess.

ANSWERS

31-1. A. Lung cancer is the second most prevalent type of cancer but the number one cause of cancer-related death. Eighty percent of lung cancers are non-small cell and 20% are small cell. Recurrences tend to occur within 2 years of resection. The most common site of recurrence following resection of non-small cell cancers is the brain. Local recurrence is more frequent with squamous cell tumors than with nonsquamous tumors. Small cell tumors usually metastasize early to regional lymph nodes and are associated with Cushing's syndrome, SIADH, and myasthenia. Large cell tumors tend to produce distant metastases and increased gonadotropin secretion with resultant gynecomastia.

It is essential to determine the pathologic cell type of the tumor before making any treatment plan, because non-small cell cancers are treated with resection, whereas small cell tumors are generally treated with chemoradiation before considering surgery. Almost half of non-small cell cancers show more than one cell type. Small cell cancers are part of the family of neuroendocrine tumors. Tissue diagnosis can be made via bronchoscopy with biopsy or bronchial washing for central lesions, or CT-guided percutaneous needle biopsy for peripheral lesions. However, surgery (open or thoracoscopic) may be required to obtain a tissue diagnosis in cases where these biopsy techniques are unable to adequately access the tumor.

31-2. A. Carcinoid tumors originate from the neuroendocrine cells of the bronchial epithelium and typically are found in the central or lobar airways. Adenoid cystic carcinoma originates from the submucosal glands of the trachea or bronchi. Central tumors tend to present with hemoptysis, atelectasis, or postobstructive pneumonia. Peripheral tumors, often adenocarcinoma, may present with pain if extension occurs to the chest wall, spine, or brachial plexus. Squamous tumors tend to metastasize to regional lymph nodes and can cause Pancoast's syndrome, hypercalcemia, and hypertrophic pulmonary osteoarthropathy. Adenocarcinoma often leads to distant metastases and is associated with nonbacterial endocarditis, thrombophlebitis, and also hypertrophic pulmonary osteoarthropathy. Bronchioloalveolar type tumors are a subtype of adenocarcinoma that grows along alveolar walls and are often bilateral.

31-3. C. Environmental exposures associated with lung cancer include tobacco, radon, and asbestos. In addition to vinyl chloride, occupational carcinogens include arsenic, chromium, nickel, copper, beryllium, benzene, and uranium. It is also believed that there may be a genetic predisposition to lung cancer, such as a decreased ability to detoxify carcinogens. Betel-nut ingestion is associated with the development of gastric cancer.

31-4. D. Pleural fluid normally is absorbed by the visceral pleura and lymphatics. Malignant effusions are most commonly caused by lung cancer and lymphoma in men, and breast, genital tract, and lung cancers in women. Bloody effusions are generally caused by malignant tumor involving the pleura. Very large benign pleural effusions are often caused by tuberculosis, empyema, CHF, or cirrhosis. *Chemical pleurodesis* is used to treat recurrent effusions by causing an inflammatory pleuritis that reapposes the visceral and parietal pleural surfaces and obliterates the pleural space. Nonloculated parapneumonic empyemas tend to be posterior and lateral, extending to the diaphragm. A chest wall sinus resulting from an intrathoracic infection is called an *empyema necessitatis*.

ADDITIONAL SUGGESTED READING

Jackman DM, Johnson BE. Small-cell lung cancer. Lancet 2005;366:1385–1396.

Juergens RA, Brahmer JR. Adjuvant therapy for resected non-small-cell lung cancer: past, present, and future. Curr Oncol Rep 2005;7:248–254.

Krupnick AS, Kreisel D, Hope A, et al. Recent advances and future perspectives in the management of lung cancer. Curr Probl Surg 2005;42:540–610.

Sahn SA. Malignant pleural effusions. Semin Respir Crit Care Med 2001;22:607–616.

Spiro SG, Silvestri GA. One hundred years of lung cancer. Am J Respir Crit Care Med 2005 1;172:523–529.

Shaw P, Agarwal R. Pleurodesis for malignant pleural effusions. Cochrane Database Syst Rev. 2004;(1):CD002916.

Thomas L, Doyle LA, Edelman MJ. Lung cancer in women: emerging differences in epidemiology, biology, and therapy. Chest 2005;128:370–381.

Thomas L, Kwok Y, Edelman MJ. Management of paraneoplastic syndromes in lung cancer. Curr Treat Options Oncol 2004;5:51–62.

Shortness of Breath

CC: Shortness of breath after procedure.

HPI: Ms. X is a 48-year-old woman who presents to the ED with fever and altered mental status. She was found to have thrombotic thrombocytopenic purpura (TTP) and was admitted for emergent plasmapheresis. The admitting team inserted a right internal jugular (IJ) central line. During line placement, the patient was noted to cough. She subsequently complained of right-sided chest pain on inspiration and shortness of breath. Placement was otherwise uneventful; there was good blood return, and the line flushed easily. After the procedure, however, the patient was found to have an oxygen saturation of only 89% on RA, after having had O_2 sats of 98% to 99% before the procedure. You are consulted to help manage this patient.

THOUGHT QUESTION

- Why might this patient be having respiratory distress?
- What do you do next?
- How did this happen?

DISCUSSION

Although acute pulmonary embolus is a remote possibility because patients with TTP are coagulopathic, the first three diagnoses on your differential in this particular setting should be pneumothorax, pneumothorax, and pneumothorax. The first things you should do are 1) get a set of vital signs, 2) place the patient on oxygen, and 3) order a stat portable CXR. This pneumothorax likely resulted from an inadvertent needle injury to the lung during line placement. Needle injury during line placement is usually more common with the subclavian approach because the subclavian vein lies very close to the apex of the expanded lung; however, pneumothoraces resulting from the IJ approach can occur with improper or inexperienced technique. Other causes of pneumothorax include spontaneous (both primary and secondary) and posttraumatic.

CASE CONTINUED

VS: Temp 39°C, HR 105, BP 112/60, O$_2$ sat 89% on RA, 94% on 6 L NC, RR 22

PE: *Gen:* Thin pale woman, mildly tachypneic, not cyanotic. *Neck:* No JVD, trachea midline, R internal jugular line in place. *CV:* RRR, heart sounds not muffled, no murmurs/rubs/gallops. *Lungs:* Clear bilaterally, slightly diminished on right, hyperresonant to percussion on right, no egophony.

Imaging: *Upright CXR:* 50% pneumothorax on the R, otherwise lung fields clear. See Figure 32-1 for an example.

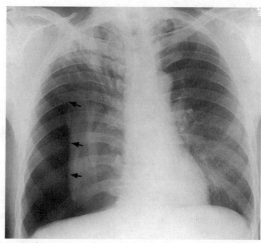

FIGURE **32-1.** Right pneumothorax: there are no visible lung markings beyond the lung edge (arrows). (*Used with permission from Patel PR. Lecture Notes on Radiology. Oxford: Blackwell Science, Ltd., 1998:40.*)

THOUGHT QUESTION

- How should a simple pneumothorax be treated?
- Would the presence of JVD or tracheal deviation alter your management?

DISCUSSION

Small, simple pneumothoraces will often be asymptomatic. If there is no ongoing air leak, pleural air is reabsorbed slowly over time and somewhat more quickly with oxygen administration. Although many asymptomatic pneumothoraces (usually <30% in size) can be observed and followed with serial CXRs, this pneumothorax is moderately sized and symptomatic—the patient is short of breath, tachypneic, and slightly tachycardic. Thus, a *tube thoracostomy* (chest tube) should be performed. Simple *needle aspiration* is also an option. The chest tube should be left in until the lung has been re-expanded, thereby sealing any lung injury; this may take hours or even days. Occasionally, a patient will not present immediately with the pneumothorax; therefore, any patient who complains of acute chest pain or persistent shortness of breath within 1 week of central line placement should have a CXR to rule out this complication.

JVD and tracheal deviation are suggestive of a *tension pneumothorax* with mediastinal shifting to the contralateral side and impaired venous return. This is caused by a lung or chest wall injury that creates a "one-way valve" air leak, leading to the rapid accumulation of air under tension in the pleural cavity. This kind of injury is exemplified by a "sucking chest wound" in a trauma situation and should be treated by covering the wound with an occlusive dressing (to close the "valve") and proceeding with chest tube placement. In a nontrauma situation, a tension pneumothorax should be treated immediately with needle thoracostomy to relieve the intrathoracic pressure, followed by conventional tube thoracostomy for lung re-expansion. If left untreated, a large tension pneumothorax will cause impaired venous return, which can lead to cardiac arrest.

QUESTIONS

32-1. Which of the following is *true* regarding line placement complications?
   A. Mediastinal hemorrhage is usually self-limited.
   B. Hemorrhage can occur only into the ipsilateral hemithorax.
   C. Horner's syndrome is often permanent.
   D. Carotid puncture is always treated operatively.

32-2. Spontaneous pneumothorax
   A. Occurs six times more frequently in men than women.
   B. Results from defective alveolar membranes.
   C. Tends to occur in the elderly.
   D. Is less likely to occur in smokers.

32-3. Which of the following is *true* regarding pneumothorax?
   A. It can be a presenting sign of esophageal perforation.
   B. It is always identifiable on a supine CXR, as long as it is >20% in size.
   C. It is not a problem as long as the patient is emergently intubated.
   D. It occupies a smaller proportion of the pleural cavity at the end of expiration than inspiration.

32-4. Bleeding risk during procedures is normal for which of the following situations?
   A. Platelets <50,000.
   B. INR >1.5.
   C. Renal failure.
   D. PTT <40.

ANSWERS

32-1. A. Pneumothorax during central line placement is a known complication that occurs in 1% to 4% of cases. Hemorrhage resulting from perforation of the blood vessel or heart wall can occur into either side of the chest. Puncture of the carotid sheath and injury to the sympathetic nerve plexus can cause a Horner's syndrome, which usually resolves spontaneously with time. If air embolus occurs and the patient is hemodynamically stable, one can attempt to aspirate the air back through the catheter. The patient should be placed in the left lateral decubitus and Trendelenburg (head down) position. This keeps the air bubble in the right atrium or ventricle (rather than obstructing RV outflow) where it will gradually dissolve. Air embolus can occur during central line removal as well as placement; therefore, patients should always be in the supine or Trendelenburg position during either of these procedures. An inadvertent carotid puncture can often be managed with manual compression alone, but this should always be done in consultation with a vascular surgeon.

32-2. A. Spontaneous pneumothorax results from rupture of subpleural blebs and most often occurs in persons aged 25–35. Tobacco use seems to follow a dose–response curve with spontaneous pneumothorax: light smokers have a 7× risk and heavy smokers have up to a 100× risk of spontaneous pneumothorax compared with nonsmokers.

32-3. A. The ideal plain film for identifying a pneumothorax is an upright CXR taken at end-expiration when the pneumothorax occupies a relatively greater proportion of the pleural cavity. In an upright film, the pleural air collects at the apices and around the periphery, where it can be distinguished from the parenchyma. With a patient in the supine position, however, the air collects anteriorly and does not form a border with the parenchyma that can be easily seen from an anteroposterior view. Intubation is not automatically indicated for respiratory distress resulting from a pneumothorax. Prompt evacuation of the pleural air and re-expansion of the lung is usually adequate to relieve the distress. In a trauma situation where the patient may require intubation for other reasons, a chest tube should be inserted before the patient is placed on positive pressure ventilation or immediately thereafter, because positive airway pressure can convert a simple pneumothorax to a tension pneumothorax. The tube size does not need to be more than 28 Fr and may even be a percutaneous 9 to 12 Fr pigtail catheter, provided you are evacuating only air. In the case of chest tube placement for hemothorax or other effusion, the chest tube should be at least 36 Fr to minimize the possibility of the tube becoming obstructed by clot or other cellular debris.

32-4. D. Invasive procedures are usually not performed in patients with impaired hemostasis unless absolutely necessary. This includes patients with platelets <50,000 and INR >1.5, often found in liver failure and inherited coagulation factor deficiencies. If possible, these deficiencies should be corrected with blood products (platelets, fresh frozen plasma, cryoprecipitate, or specific factor replacements, etc.) before any invasive procedure. Renal failure causes impaired platelet function, and this can be treated with variable success using platelet infusion, estrogen, and/or 1-desamino-8-D-arginine vaso-pressin (ddAVP). Thrombotic thrombocytopenic purpura (TTP) can involve platelet counts <10,000. Operations such as laparoscopic splenectomy have been done successfully and with minimal blood loss in these patients using meticulous surgical technique and platelet infusions at the time of splenectomy. The internal jugular (IJ) approach for central line placement is preferred in coagulopathic patients because of the superficial location of the vein and the compressibility of the carotid artery if an arterial puncture is inadvertently made.

ADDITIONAL SUGGESTED READING

Agee KR, Balk RA. Central venous catheterization in the critically ill patient. Crit Care Clin 1992;8:677–686.

Bailey SH, Shapiro SB, Mone MC, et al. Is immediate chest radiograph necessary after central venous catheter placement in a surgical intensive care unit? Am J Surg 2000;180:517–21; discussion 521–2.

Baumann MH, Strange C, Heffner JE, et al. AACP Pneumothorax Consensus Group. Management of spontaneous pneumothorax: an American College of Chest Physicians Delphi consensus statement. Chest 2001;119:590–602.

Devanand A, Koh MS, Ong TH, et al. Simple aspiration versus chest-tube insertion in the management of primary spontaneous pneumothorax: a systematic review. Respir Med 2004;98: 579–590.

Fatigue and Shortness of Breath with Exertion

CC: Fatigue and shortness of breath with exercise ×2 months.

HPI: Ms. X is a 32-year-old woman who has been told she has a heart murmur "all her life." It has never been an issue, and she has been otherwise healthy until the past few months. She reports getting tired very easily now and even gets short of breath when walking up the two flights of stairs at her office. She had a bout of "bronchitis" a few months ago, but these symptoms have lingered long past the resolution of her cough. She denies any palpitations or "racing" heartbeats, angina, or syncope.

PMHx: As above

PSHx: None

Meds: None

All: NKDA

SHx: Social EtOH and smoking; tried marijuana in college but none since; no IV drug use; no occupational exposures (asbestos, etc.)

FHx: No known cardiac problems, no cancers

THOUGHT QUESTION

- What is in your differential?
- What studies might you order to help in making a diagnosis?

DISCUSSION

A history of heart murmur should make you consider congenital heart disease or valvular disease (e.g., mitral valve prolapse, rheumatic heart disease). However, the heart murmur may be a "red herring"; therefore, the history of respiratory infection is important and may suggest recurrent or persistent infection, chronic lung disease, and asthma. Although the patient is young and says she smokes only socially, lung neoplasm is also a possibility. Evaluation of this patient should begin with a physical exam, basic blood work, and a CXR.

CASE CONTINUED

VS: Afebrile, HR 92, normal sinus rhythm, BP 110/54, RR 18, O_2 sat 93% on RA

PE: *Gen:* WD/WN woman in no acute distress, AO ×4. *HEENT:* Normocephalic, PERRL, EOMI. *Lungs:* CTA bilaterally, no crackles or wheezes, no dullness to percussion. *CV:* RRR, left parasternal heave, mid-systolic ejection murmur over left upper sternal border, mid-diastolic rumble over left lower sternal border, widely split and fixed S_2 with prominent pulmonary sound, no clicks. *Abdomen:* Soft, NT/ND, no hepatosplenomegaly. *Ext:* Slight cyanosis of fingerbeds, no clubbing or edema.

Labs: lytes WNL

Imaging: *CXR:* Increased pulmonary vascular markings, enlarged RA and RV, prominent PA

THOUGHT QUESTION

■ What is the most likely diagnosis at this point? Why? How will you confirm this?

■ What is the significance of the patient's cyanosis?

DISCUSSION

This constellation of findings is most consistent with an *atrial septal defect (ASD)*. There is no evidence of primary lung disease by examination or CXR. ASDs are the most common congenital cardiac lesion in adults and account for 10% to 15% of all congenital heart lesions. ASDs are (initially) left-to-right intracardiac shunts (due to the greater compliance of the right ventricle compared with the left) that lead to increased pulmonary blood flow. There are three types of ASDs: ostium secundum (70%), ostium primum (20%), and sinus venosus (10%). Symptoms generally occur when the ratio of pulmonary blood flow to systemic blood flow (Q_p/Q_s) is >2. In addition to fatigue, shortness of breath, and recurrent respiratory infections, atrial dysrhythmias are common. Large defects tend to be symptomatic early and are often repaired in childhood. Repair may be via open heart surgery or more recently via cardiac catheterization with an umbrella closure device.

Arterial desaturation occurs when the patient develops a right-to-left shunt. In adults, this results when the chronically increased pulmonary blood flow leads to the development of decreased RV compliance, pulmonary hypertension, and subsequent reversal of shunt flow. In adults with an unrepaired ASD, pulmonary hypertension develops in 35% to 50% (in children, the incidence is only 5% to 8%). This pathologic change is called *Eisenmenger's syndrome* and leads to significant and progressive congestive heart failure. It is generally irreversible and can be cured only with a combined heart–lung transplant. Once this syndrome develops, repair of the septal defect is often contraindicated because it could result in severe RV overload and worsened CHF.

QUESTIONS

33-1. Which of the following is *true* regarding ASD?
   A. More common in males (2:1).
   B. Does not require antibiotic prophylaxis against endocarditis.
   C. ECG may show left bundle branch block and left axis deviation.
   D. Complications include paradoxical emboli.

33-2. Ventricular septal defects
  A. Are the least common congenital cardiac lesion.
  B. Usually become apparent during childhood.
  C. Are rarely associated with other systemic and cardiac anomalies.
  D. Can be suggested by a harsh pansystolic murmur.

33-3. Coarctation of the aorta is associated with which of the following?
  A. Klinefelter's syndrome.
  B. Atrial septal defect.
  C. Hypoplastic limb growth.
  D. Differential cyanosis.

33-4. Tetralogy of Fallot involves which of the following?
  A. Atrial septal defect.
  B. Congestive heart failure.
  C. Aortic stenosis.
  D. Cyanosis.

ANSWERS

33-1. D. ASD is more common in females (2:1 predominance). Although the likelihood of endocarditis with ASD is low, prophylaxis is still recommended, especially if associated with mitral valve prolapse or anomalous pulmonary venous return. Generally, the ECG shows *right* axis deviation with incomplete right bundle branch block. Spontaneous closure or decrease in the size of an ASD can occur in the first 5 years of life. Paradoxical emboli can occur when the intracardiac shunt becomes right-to-left; rather than lodging in the pulmonary circulation, emboli originating from the venous system travel across the cardiac defect and "paradoxically" become arterial emboli. Of note, 20% of normal individuals will have a patent foramen ovale, which is asymptomatic unless the patient develops increased right atrial pressure leading to a right-to-left shunt.

33-2. D. Ventricular septal defects are the most common congenital cardiac lesion (20% to 25%) and are found in 1 in 1000 live births. They are often associated with other systemic and cardiac anomalies. Large lesions tend to become apparent early in infancy when the pulmonary vascular resistance falls, leading to increased left-to-right shunting and congestive heart failure. Symptoms in children include tachypnea, tachycardia, poor feeding with diaphoresis, and failure to thrive. Small ventricular septal defects may close spontaneously, but those still present after 6 months of age rarely do.

33-3. D. Coarctation is associated with Turner's syndrome (although coarctation is actually more common in males), bicuspid aortic valve, ventricular septal defect, and aortic stenosis. Ninety-eight percent of cases occur at the level of the ligamentum arteriosum and often leads to both pre- and poststenotic dilatation of the aorta ("figure of 3" on CXR). Collaterals commonly develop, particularly via the intercostal arteries, which results in "rib notching" on CXR. Hypertension is found in the upper extremities, with diminished lower extremity pulses and possibly even claudication. Other complaints include headache and nosebleeds. Differential (upper body) cyanosis is found in neonates when the ductus arteriosus is still patent, and blood flows from the pulmonary artery through the patent ductus arteriosus to the aorta distal to the coarctation. Treatment involves open resection of the stenotic area or balloon angioplasty. In neonates, prostaglandin E_1 can be used to temporarily dilate and keep open the ductus arteriosus.

33-4. D. Tetralogy of Fallot is the most common *cyanotic* congenital heart defect (accounting for 10% of all congenital heart defects), is slightly more common in boys, and may have a familial association with other congenital cardiac lesions. The components of Tetralogy of Fallot are as follows: 1) large nonrestrictive ventricular septal defect, 2) overriding aorta, 3) RV outflow tract obstruction, and 4) RV hypertrophy. It results in cyanosis early in infancy (depending on the degree of RV outflow tract obstruction) but rarely leads to CHF. "Tet spells" are cyanotic episodes that are theorized to occur with spasm of the RV outflow tract or increased pulmonary vascular resistance (e.g., with crying or dehydration). They are often self-treated with squatting (which increases systemic vascular resistance and decreases right-to-left shunting, improving central venous return and cardiac output). On CXR, the classic finding is of a boot-shaped heart and decreased pulmonary vascularity. Repair involves ventricular septal defect closure and repair of the RV outflow tract obstruction (i.e., pulmonary valve replacement). Palliative or temporizing therapy includes creation of a Blalock-Taussig shunt (subclavian artery to pulmonary artery) to increase pulmonary blood flow.

📖 *ADDITIONAL SUGGESTED READING*

Brown MD, Wernovsky G, Mussatto KA, et al. Long-term and developmental outcomes of children with complex congenital heart disease. Clin Perinatol 2005;32:1043–1057.

Corno AF. Surgery for congenital heart disease. Curr Opin Cardiol 2000;15:238–243.

Dore A, Glancy DL, Stone S, et al. Cardiac surgery for grown-up congenital heart patients: survey of 307 consecutive operations from 1991 to 1994. Am J Cardiol 1997 1;80:906–913.

Morris CD, Menashe VD. 25-year mortality after surgical repair of congenital heart defect in childhood. A population-based cohort study. JAMA 1991;266:3447–3452.

Warnes CA. The adult with congenital heart disease: born to be bad? J Am Coll Cardiol 2005 5;46:1–8.

Shortness of Breath with Presyncope

CC: Fatigue and shortness of breath ×2 months.

HPI: Mr. X is a 52-year-old man who reports tiring easily at the end of the day and often gets short of breath when walking on the golf course. He has noticed this change in his exercise tolerance for at least the past 2 months. He denies any episodes of chest pain or pressure (angina), but he does remember "feeling faint" once or twice at the end of a golf round. He denies nocturnal dyspnea or orthopnea but admits to his feet being more swollen than normal lately, especially at night.

PMHx: "Heart murmur" since childhood

PSHx: None

Meds: None

All: NKDA

SHx/FHx: Noncontributory

VS: Afebrile, HR 76, BP 133/87, O_2 sat 99% on RA

PE: *Gen:* WD/WN man, no acute distress, slightly overweight. *HEENT:* PERRL, EOMI, no JVD, systolic murmur heard in both carotid arteries. *CV:* RRR, harsh crescendo-decrescendo systolic murmur at right upper sternal border, faint diastolic blowing murmur, forceful nondisplaced apical impulse. *Lungs:* CTA bilaterally except for fine crackles at bases. *Abdomen:* Soft, NT/ND, no hepatosplenomegaly. *Ext:* 1+ pedal edema, palpable pulses.

THOUGHT QUESTION

- What is in your differential?
- What is the triad of symptoms normally found with this diagnosis?
- What studies should be obtained at this point?

DISCUSSION

In a patient of this age and with symptoms of CHF and exercise intolerance, ischemic heart disease is of primary concern, even without symptoms of angina. However, given the history of heart murmur and the patient's cardiac exam, the patient likely has aortic stenosis with a component of aortic insufficiency. The triad of symptoms normally found with aortic stenosis is angina, syncope, and CHF. Other causes of syncope (e.g., arrhythmia, carotid disease) must be ruled out before attributing those episodes entirely to aortic stenosis. Aortic stenosis is the most common fatal valvular lesion, with sudden death occurring in up to 20%. The most common cause of aortic stenosis is rheumatic heart disease (30% to 40%). Nonrheumatic aortic valve disease can be congenital (bicuspid aortic valve), degenerative (involving extensive calcification), or infectious (endocarditis).

Any patient being evaluated for cardiac disease should have an ECG and CXR. When assessing for valvular disease, *echocardiography* with Doppler ultrasound is useful for visualizing valve and leaflet motion and configuration, and for measuring the pressure gradient across the valves. *Cardiac catheterization* is important in ruling out concomitant coronary disease and for measuring valve area. It can also clarify the presence of supravalvular or subvalvular obstructions.

CASE CONTINUED

Imaging: *ECG:* Normal sinus rhythm (NSR), left atrial enlargement, LV hypertrophy, no ST segment or T wave changes, no Q waves. *CXR:* LV prominence, otherwise normal. *Echo:* LA and LV hypertrophy, increased LV end-diastolic pressure, thickened aortic valve leaflets, aortic valve area 0.9 cm^2 (moderate aortic stenosis), mild aortic regurgitation, mild mitral valve stenosis; tricuspid and pulmonary valves normal. *Cath:* normal coronary arteries, aortic valve pressure gradient 120 mm Hg, ejection fraction 40%, no wall motion abnormalities.

THOUGHT QUESTION

■ What are the indications for aortic valve replacement?

DISCUSSION

Surgery is recommended for symptomatic patients or for asymptomatic patients with an aortic valve area <0.7 cm². Aortic valve area <1.0 cm² is generally associated with symptoms, whereas that <0.7 cm² is considered severe disease. Normal aortic valve area is 2.5 to 3.5 cm². A pressure gradient of 90 to 200 mm Hg across the valve can be present in severe disease. The left ventricle adapts to the outflow obstruction by developing concentric hypertrophy, which may result in decreased diastolic compliance. In advanced disease, the left atrium may also become hypertrophied, while the ventricle will become dilated. If valvular dysfunction develops acutely, the patient will have none of these compensatory adaptations and may die of sudden severe heart failure.

For mild to moderate valvular disease, there are treatment options other than complete valve replacement. Open repair (i.e., annuloplasty) or catheter-based therapies (i.e., commissurotomy) are possible depending on the valvular anatomy and specific pathology.

CASE CONTINUED

This patient has symptoms of CHF and syncope with moderate aortic stenosis and mild aortic regurgitation. He is scheduled for elective aortic valve replacement. Given the patient's relatively young age and absence of risk factors for anticoagulation, a mechanical valve replacement is planned.

QUESTIONS

34-1. Which of the following definitions is *true*?
   A. Systolic dysfunction—impaired ventricular filling.
   B. Diastolic dysfunction—contractility (pump) failure.
   C. Quincke sign—head bobbing in time with heartbeat.
   D. Janeway lesion—erythematous lesions on palms and soles.

34-2. Bacterial endocarditis
   A. Rarely affects prosthetic valves.
   B. Has low associated mortality.
   C. Is diagnosed primarily on echocardiogram.
   D. Is treated initially with intravenous antibiotics.

34-3. Which of the following is a known complication of prosthetic valve placement?
   A. Thrombocytopenia.
   B. Valvular thrombosis.
   C. Metabolic acidosis.
   D. Coagulopathy.

34-4. Long-term anticoagulation is recommended for which of the following?
   A. Atrial fibrillation after cardiac surgery.
   B. Porcine valve replacement.
   C. Atrial fibrillation with mitral valve disease.
   D. Mitral valve replacement.

ANSWERS

34-1. D. Systolic dysfunction refers to pump failure, while diastolic dysfunction results in impaired ventricular filling. Head bobbing with the pulsations of the heart is called a Musset sign; the Quincke sign is capillary pulsations in the fingertips. Both are found in aortic insufficiency. Janeway lesions are associated with infective endocarditis. They vary in size, may be flat or raised, and last for variable time periods. Osler's nodes are similar to Janeway lesions but are painful. The etiology of these lesions is unclear and is believed likely related to embolic or immune complex phenomena.

34-2. D. Prosthetic valves and diseased native valves are at high risk for endocarditis. Use of IV drugs can lead to infection of normal native valves. Presenting symptoms of endocarditis include fever, chills, sweats, and peripheral emboli. Most patients develop a murmur at some point during the disease process; however, almost one-third have no murmur at presentation. Blood cultures are the cornerstone of making the diagnosis. Medical treatment of endocarditis involves long-term intravenous antibiotics (4 to 6 weeks); however, the mortality rate is high and is most often a result of aortic insufficiency. Surgery is indicated for antibiotic failure, valvular insufficiency, perivalvular abscess, and pericarditis. Because of the morbidity and mortality related to endocarditis, patients with diseased or prosthetic valves are advised to use prophylactic antibiotics before invasive procedures (e.g., dental work, colonoscopy).

34-3. B. Calcific degeneration occurs primarily with bioprosthetic valves (hetero- or homografts). Hemolysis tends to occur with mechanical valves but usually resolves over time. Other complications associated with valve replacement include atrial and ventricular arrhythmias. Mechanical valves have various designs, including ball in cage (Starr-Edwards), tilting disk (Bjork-Shiley), and tilting disk with a bileaflet mechanism (St. Jude). Most bioprosthetic valves are porcine heterografts fixed in glutaraldehyde. Mechanical valves are more resistant to structural failure, but require lifelong anticoagulation (which increases bleeding risk) and have a higher rate of endocarditis, thromboembolism, and perivalvular leakage compared with bioprosthetic valves. The main drawback of bioprostheses is poor durability (50% to 80% at 10 years) compared with mechanical valves. Overall, the rates of valve-related complications and survival are similar between the two groups.

34-4. C. Atrial fibrillation after cardiac surgery is usually a transient event related to fluid overload, hypoxia, and other factors causing sympathetic discharge and tachycardia (fever, anxiety, pain, etc.). Anticoagulation in that setting is generally not recommended unless the atrial fibrillation is prolonged for more than several days. Other indications for anticoagulation are atrial fibrillation with cardiomyopathy and, more controversially, bioprosthetic valve placement (often only for a short time after surgery). Contraindications to anticoagulation are presence of a bleeding diathesis, high risk of trauma (via either occupation or recreation), history of medication noncompliance, and women of child-bearing age who wish to become pregnant.

ADDITIONAL SUGGESTED READING

Baddour LM, Wilson WR, Bayer AS, et al. Infective endocarditis: diagnosis, antimicrobial therapy, and management of complications. Circulation. 2005 (14);111:e394–434.

Bonow RO, Carabello B, de Leon AC, et al. ACC/AHA Guidelines for the Management of Patients With Valvular Heart Disease. J Heart Valve Dis. 1998;7:672–707.

Butchart EG, Gohlke-Barwolf C, Antunes MJ, et al. Working Groups on Valvular Heart Disease, Thrombosis, and Cardiac Rehabilitation and Exercise Physiology, European Society of

Cardiology. Recommendations for the management of patients after heart valve surgery. Eur Heart J 2005;26:2463–2471.

Dajani AS, Taubert KA, Wilson W, et al. Prevention of bacterial endocarditis. Recommendations by the American Heart Association. JAMA 1997;277:1794–1801.

Rahimtoola SH. Valvular heart disease/cardiac surgery. J Am Coll Cardiol 2005;45(11 Suppl B):20B–23B.

Salem DN, Stein PD, Al-Ahmad A, et al. Antithrombotic therapy in valvular heart disease—native and prosthetic: the Seventh ACCP Conference on Antithrombotic and Thrombolytic Therapy. Chest 2004;126(3 Suppl):457S–482S.

Chest Pressure

CC: Substernal chest pressure ×2 hours.

HPI: Mr. X is a 56-year-old man with h/o HTN and hyperlipidemia, who reports two hours of chest pressure and tightness associated with left arm and neck pain. It began early this morning as he was walking his dog. There was no diaphoresis, nausea, or vomiting. This happened once before about a month ago at the start of the winter weather. During that episode, the pain had gone away after a few minutes when he had warmed up inside. This time, the symptoms did not lessen when he returned home. He tried one of his wife's sublingual nitroglycerin, which helped somewhat but did not completely relieve the pain. He denies dyspnea on exertion, orthopnea, or paroxysmal nocturnal dyspnea. He has no history of peptic ulcer disease or heartburn.

PMHx: As above

PSHx: None

Meds: Atenolol, Zocor

All: NKDA

SHx: 2 ppd smoker for past 20 years, no alcohol or illicit drugs

FHx: Mother died of heart attack, father with high cholesterol

VS: Afebrile, HR 67, BP 177/89, RR 14, O_2 sat 95% on RA

PE: *Gen:* WD/WN man in no acute distress. *HEENT:* PERRL, ocular xanthomas, EOMI, no JVD, no carotid bruits. *Lungs:* CTA bilaterally. *Abdomen:* Soft, NT/ND, no hepatosplenomegaly. *CV:* RRR, no murmurs/rubs/gallops. *Ext:* Palpable pulses, no clubbing/cyanosis or edema.

THOUGHT QUESTION

■ Which initial studies may help you with a diagnosis?

DISCUSSION

This patient presents with substernal chest pain, and although the most concerning diagnosis is angina and myocardial ischemia, the differential also includes gastroesophageal reflux, peptic ulcer disease, biliary colic, esophageal spasm, and costochondritis. Evaluation should begin with an ECG to look for ischemic changes (i.e., T wave inversion, ST segment elevation or depression, Q waves). Basic blood tests and a CXR may also be helpful to rule out cardiac risk factors (hyperlipidemia, hyperthyroidism, anemia, diabetes) and cardiomegaly. Angina can be precipitated by exercise, cold exposure, eating, and emotional stress. An *exercise treadmill test* can screen for myocardium at risk and, if positive, identify a need for further testing (i.e., coronary angiography). *Thallium scan* is another screening stress test that may provide more specific information (i.e., ejection fraction, specific wall motion or perfusion abnormalities), although its accuracy is still only 75% to 85%.

CASE CONTINUED

Labs: Thyroid function tests normal

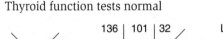

Imaging: *CXR:* No pulmonary edema or cardiomegaly. *ECG:* NSR 65, normal axis, no ST or T wave changes.

THOUGHT QUESTION

- What are the indications for coronary artery bypass grafting (CABG)?
- What are some alternatives to CABG?

DISCUSSION

Mortality increases with increasing number of coronary vessels involved by occlusive atherosclerosis but is highest with left main involvement. Left ventricular dysfunction is also correlated with mortality. Therefore, CABG is recommended for progressive or unstable angina on maximal medical therapy, significant left main coronary disease or multivessel disease, reduced ejection fraction, and reversible ischemia. Notably, CABG without the use of cardiopulmonary bypass (off-pump bypass) is a recent development that has been performed successfully on both single and multivessel disease.

The role of *percutaneous transluminal coronary angioplasty* and stenting has grown steadily over the last several years and is no longer limited to high risk patients or those with single-vessel disease. The long-term patency and durability of these interventions has been the main concern, with restenosis and reintervention rates of up to 40% within the first year. However, current research shows promising results in the use of drug-eluting stents (e.g., rapamycin) to reduce the incidence of intimal hyperplasia and restenosis. Other investigational procedures include transmyocardial laser revascularization.

CASE CONTINUED

Additional sublingual nitroglycerin and intravenous morphine are able to resolve the patient's symptoms. He then undergoes an exercise treadmill test. He is able to reach his target heart rate and exercise for the full duration of the test without ECG evidence of ischemia. Therefore, no surgery is indicated at this time, and treatment involves sublingual nitroglycerin PRN and a daily aspirin. His atenolol dose is increased for better blood pressure management. He is encouraged to start exercising regularly (i.e., three times a week) and is referred to a smoking cessation program. If his symptoms recur, the patient should be scheduled for a cardiac angiogram.

QUESTIONS

35-1. Myocardial blood flow
   A. Occurs primarily during systole.
   B. Involves oxygen extraction rates of <50%.
   C. And oxygen delivery are increased mainly by vasodilation.
   D. Is determined by sympathetic stimulation.

35-2. Which of the following is most often involved by coronary artery disease?
- A. Left main.
- B. Right coronary.
- C. Anterior descending.
- D. Left circumflex.

35-3. Which of the following is most frequently used as a coronary bypass conduit?
- A. Greater saphenous vein.
- B. Internal mammary artery.
- C. Radial artery.
- D. Right gastroepiploic artery.

35-4. The most common complication of cardiopulmonary bypass is
- A. Atrial dysrhythmias.
- B. Horner's syndrome.
- C. Myocardial infarction.
- D. Sternal wound infection.

ANSWERS

35-1. C. Coronary blood flow occurs primarily during diastole. In the setting of adequate arterial perfusion pressure, myocardial blood flow is determined by autoregulation of the regional arterioles in response to local metabolic demand. Oxygen extraction in the coronary bed is 75% to 100%. However, when perfusion pressure decreases or diastolic intramyocardial pressure increases, myocardial blood flow is redistributed away from the subendocardium where intramural compressive forces are the greatest. In this way, patients can develop subendocardial ischemia (i.e., non-Q wave MI). Persistence or worsening of this perfusion deficit can lead to transmural ischemia (i.e., Q wave MI).

35-2. C. In order of most to least frequently involved is anterior descending > right coronary > left circumflex > left main > posterior descending. The most severe atherosclerotic changes tend to occur in the *proximal* third or half of the coronaries. The cross-sectional area of a vessel must be decreased by >75% to result in increased resistance to blood flow. It is possible, however, to have angina without atherosclerosis or in the setting of minimal disease. This phenomenon is known as coronary arterial spasm and is referred to as atypical angina, or *Prinzmetal's* variant. Patients are generally managed medically. After CABG, improvement in anginal symptoms is noted in more than two-thirds of patients. Moreover, there is a decreased incidence of MI, improved LV function, and stabilization of exercise tolerance. Perioperative morbidity and mortality is <2%, and long-term survival is better than 95% at 5 years (for elective CABG, ejection fraction >40% or age <65).

35-3. A. The most widely used autogenous conduit is saphenous vein, followed by internal mammary artery. Radial artery grafts are increasingly used, because it has been found that arterial conduits have greater long-term patency rates than venous bypass grafts (85% to 90% of internal mammary arteries patent at 10 years versus only 50% of saphenous veins). Postoperative medical therapy (for high blood pressure, diabetes, and hyperlipidemia) and risk factor modification (diet, smoking cessation, and exercise) are imperative, because bypass grafts and the remaining native vessels are still susceptible to atherosclerotic changes and disease progression.

35-4. A. Other complications of bypass are stroke (2%) and renal dysfunction (due to acute tubular necrosis). Atrial arrhythmias are very common (10% to 30% in myocardial revascularization and up to 75% in valve replacement), whereas sternal infection and MI are both rare (1% to 2% each). Platelet dysfunction, fibrinolysis, coagulation factor depletion or dysfunction, and inadequate heparin reversal are common "medical" causes of bypass-related bleeding. Unfortunately, the incidence of these complications has not definitively been reduced in CABG cases performed "off-pump" or without the cardiopulmonary bypass machine.

ADDITIONAL SUGGESTED READING

Bakhai A, Hill RA, Dundar Y, et al. Percutaneous transluminal coronary angioplasty with stents versus coronary artery bypass grafting for people with stable angina or acute coronary syndromes. Cochrane Database Syst Rev 2005;(1):CD004588.

Deedwania PC, Amsterdam EA, Vagelos RH. Evidence-based, cost-effective risk stratification and management after myocardial infarction. California Cardiology Working Group on Post-MI Management. Arch Intern Med 1997;157:273–280.

Hoffman SN, TenBrook JA, Wolf MP, et al. A meta-analysis of randomized controlled trials comparing coronary artery bypass graft with percutaneous transluminal coronary angioplasty: one- to eight-year outcomes. J Am Coll Cardiol 2003;41:1293–1304.

Lipinski MJ, Fearon WF, Froelicher VF, et al. The current and
    future role of percutaneous coronary intervention in patients
    with coronary artery disease. J Interv Cardiol 2004;17:283–294.
Rihal CS, Raco DL, Gersh BJ, et al. Indications for coronary artery
    bypass surgery and percutaneous coronary intervention in chronic
    stable angina: review of the evidence and methodological
    considerations. Circulation 2003; 108:2439–2445.

Acute Chest Pain

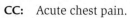

CC: Acute chest pain.

HPI: Ms. X a 42-year-old woman with a h/o HTN and drug abuse, presents to the ED c/o sudden onset of substernal chest pain after a cocaine binge. She has been high for several days and does not remember the last time she took her blood pressure pills. She describes the pain as a "tearing" sensation that shoots through to her back. The pain has been constant for the past three hours.

PMHx: As above, no operations

PSHx: As above, no operations

Meds: "A pink pill"

All: NKDA

SHx: 1 ppd tobacco, occasional EtOH, daily crack cocaine, past heroin

FHx: No known CAD, no known connective tissue disease

THOUGHT QUESTION

- What should you include in your differential diagnosis?

DISCUSSION

This patient may be having an acute MI, esophageal spasm or rupture, or an acute aortic dissection. This presentation (including the cocaine use) is classic for aortic dissection, but the patient should always also be ruled out for an MI. The chest pain associated with an aortic dissection is often abrupt with a rapid peak, whereas that related to MI can be vague, intermittent, and slow to peak. In addition, dissection pain may migrate as the flap extends distally.

CASE CONTINUED

VS: Temp 37.6°C; HR 117; BP R arm 223/115, L arm 220/117; O_2 sat 95% RA; RR 18

PE: *Gen:* Thin disheveled woman, moaning and agitated, diaphoretic, AO × 3. *CV:* RRR, no murmurs/rubs/gallops; no sternal tenderness to palpation. *Lungs:* CTA bilaterally. *Abdomen:* Soft, NT/ND, no pulsatile masses or bruits. *Ext:* Warm, well-perfused, 4+ peripheral pulses throughout, no edema or cyanosis.

Labs: WBC 9, Hct 37, Plts 180, K 4.4, BUN 29, Cr 1.3, first troponin is negative, LFTs WNL, coags WNL, Upreg neg.

Imaging: *ECG:* Sinus tachycardia, no acute ST-T segment changes.

THOUGHT QUESTION

- How should you manage this patient initially?
- What imaging study should you perform to make the diagnosis?

DISCUSSION

This very hypertensive patient should be admitted to the ICU for close monitoring. This includes an arterial line, central line for central venous pressure, Foley catheter, and cardiac rhythm monitoring. Serial labs, 12-lead ECG, and CXR are also important in detecting any ischemic or anatomic (i.e., leak, rupture) changes. There are two hemodynamic forces involved in the initiation and propagation of a dissection: the impulsive "tearing" force generated by acceleration of the cardiac output (dp/dt) in systole and forces related to the mean arterial pressure. Therefore, *blood pressure control* is essential for limiting further dissection.

There are three primary means of diagnosing an aortic dissection: transesophageal echocardiogram, MRI, and CT. *Transesophageal echocardiogram* can provide excellent evaluation of cardiac function and the aortic annulus and can be done at the bedside. However, it does not provide any information about the infrarenal aorta or its branches. *MRI* can provide information regarding the entire aorta, its branches, and even possibly the coronary arteries as well;

however, this is very time consuming and study quality can be affected significantly by patient cooperation and the skill of the interpreting radiologist. *CT* is believed to be reliable, reproducible, and readily obtainable, and it provides similar information as an MRI. Therefore, CT is generally the first imaging study performed to diagnose an aortic dissection and clarify its proximal and distal involvement. Its only relative contraindication is renal insufficiency, which may prohibit the use of IV contrast. *Angiography* is also an option for imaging a dissection, and endovascular interventions can be performed in appropriate situations. However, because transesophageal echocardiogram and CT are more easily performed and are both highly sensitive and specific, angiography is generally reserved for confirming the diagnosis if necessary and for possible interventions when indicated.

CASE CONTINUED

The patient is brought to the ICU where she is started on a continuous infusion of blood pressure medication. CT scan shows a dissection of the descending thoracic aorta.

QUESTIONS

36-1. An aortic dissection
A. Untreated has very low mortality.
B. Occurs only in patients with connective tissue disorders, congenital heart disease, and young, pregnant women.
C. Can be treated with primary aortic repair, flap fenestration, or endovascular stenting.
D. Results from atherosclerotic degeneration of the intima.

36-2. Which of the following drugs would you be most likely to use in this case?
A. Neo-Synephrine.
B. Esmolol.
C. Nitroglycerin.
D. Dobutamine.

36-3. An absolute indication for immediate surgical intervention is
   A. Recurrent chest pain.
   B. Headache.
   C. Urinary retention.
   D. Widened mediastinum with pericardial rub.

36-4. Aortic dissections are classified by
   A. Antegrade or retrograde propagation.
   B. Need for surgical or medical therapy.
   C. Location in the thoracic aorta.
   D. Presence or absence of associated aneurysm.

ANSWERS

36-1. **C.** Aortic dissections tend to occur in men 50 to 70 years of age. They are rare in patients <40 years of age except in conditions such as connective tissue disorders, congenital heart disease (particularly bicuspid aortic valve), and pregnant women. Untreated acute aortic dissections are lethal in 21% within 24 hours, 60% within 2 weeks, and 90% at 3 months. Aortic dissections are not a direct result of atherosclerotic disease but are generally associated with long-standing hypertension. Repair that restores continuity of the primary, or true, lumen is often sufficient; decompression of the false lumen is generally not necessary.

36-2. **B.** The first-line treatment for aortic dissection is *β-adrenergic antagonists*. If beta-blockers are contraindicated or not well tolerated, other agents such as calcium channel blockers or sodium nitroprusside can be used as well. Although nitroglycerin can reduce blood pressure, it is solely a vasodilator, does not alter cardiac output force, and is not the drug of choice for management of an acute dissection. Once patients are pain free, blood pressure is well controlled, and there is no evidence of end-organ ischemia, the IV drugs can be converted to an oral regimen for long-term management.

36-3. **D.** Although most dissections provide adequate perfusion through both true and false lumens, 30% will develop peripheral ischemic complications. Oliguria, refractory hypertension, and rising BUN and creatinine are all suggestive of renal artery compromise. Elevated liver function tests may indicate hepatic ischemia.· Acute abdominal pain, acidosis, nausea, vomiting, and bloody diarrhea are symptoms of acute bowel ischemia. A change in distal pulse exam or blood pressure indicates extremity involvement, and neurologic

changes can reflect cerebral or spinal ischemia. Widened mediastinum or increasing pleural effusion on CXR, and pericardial or
pleural rub are signs suggestive of intrathoracic leak or rupture of the
aortic dissection. A new cardiac murmur may herald involvement of
the aortic annulus and detachment of an aortic valve cusp. Any of
these findings is an indication for immediate surgical intervention.

36-4. C. Aortic dissections are classified according to involvement
of the thoracic aorta in relation to the left subclavian artery and the
ligamentum arteriosum. Stanford type A dissections involve the
ascending aorta (proximal to the left subclavian) with or without
involvement of the descending aorta, whereas type B dissections
involve only the descending thoracic aorta (distal to the left subclavian) with or without extension below the diaphragm into the
abdomen. In type A patients, surgical repair is undertaken emergently
to avoid cardiac tamponade, coronary occlusion, or acute valvular
dysfunction. On the other hand, for type B patients in the absence of
impending rupture or organ ischemia, aortic reconstruction has not
been found to provide significant survival benefit over medical management. Therefore, the mainstay of therapy in type B dissections is
pharmacologic blood pressure control. A dissection can propagate
antegrade or retrograde. Occasionally, a second intimal tear can occur
that restores luminal continuity and is called "re-entry." This is most
often found at branch points of the aorta. Chronic aortic dissections
should be followed with CT or ultrasound, because they are at risk for
aneurysmal degeneration (Fig. 36-1).

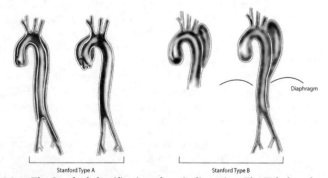

Stanford Type A   Stanford Type B

FIGURE 36-1. The Stanford classification of aortic dissection. The Debakey classification is another system for describing dissections (I, ascending and
descending aorta; II, ascending aorta only; III, descending aorta only). Stanford
A encompasses both Debakey I and II, whereas Stanford B corresponds to
Debakey III. The Stanford classification is more commonly used because it
easily distinguishes which line of therapy is indicated for the dissection (medical versus surgical). (*Illustration by Shawn Girsberger Graphic Design.*)

📖 *ADDITIONAL SUGGESTED READING*

Fann JI, Smith JA, Miller DC, et al. Surgical management of aortic dissection during a 30-year period. Circulation 1995 1;92 (9 Suppl):II113–121.

McGee EC Jr, Pham DT, Gleason TG. Chronic descending aortic dissections. Semin Thorac Cardiovasc Surg 2005;17:262–267.

O'Gara PT. Acute aortic dissection. Curr Treat Options Cardiovasc Med 1999;1:11–18.

Sandridge L, Kern JA. Acute descending aortic dissections: management of visceral, spinal cord, and extremity malperfusion. Semin Thorac Cardiovasc Surg 2005;17:256–261.

Suzuki T, Mehta RH, Ince H, et al. International Registry of Aortic Dissection. Clinical profiles and outcomes of acute type B aortic dissection in the current era: lessons from the International Registry of Aortic Dissection (IRAD). Circulation 2003;108 (Suppl 1):II312–317.

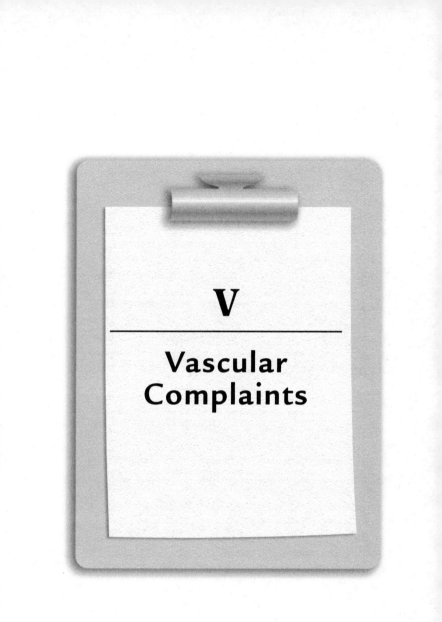

V

Vascular Complaints

CASE **37**

Leg Cramping

CC: Progressive leg cramping with walking.

HPI: Mr. X is a 65-year-old man with a h/o HTN, hyperlipidemia, and smoking who presents to your office and states that he is only able to walk one block before getting cramping in his calves, R > L. This cramping forces him to stop walking for several minutes before he can continue. He describes the cramping as a dull ache without radiation up the leg. He denies proximal (thigh, buttock) cramping, impotence, or rest pain. There are no neurologic deficits. One year ago, he had been able to walk four blocks without symptoms. He denies shortness of breath or chest pain while walking.

PMHx: As above

PSHx: s/p CABG with R saphenous vein harvest

Meds: Atenolol, ASA, simvastatin

All: NKDA

SHx: 80 pack-year smoker, currently smoking 1 ppd; denies alcohol or other drug use

VS: Afebrile; HR 65; BP R arm 153/70, L arm 149/72

PE: *Gen:* Slightly overweight man, no acute distress. *CV:* RRR, no murmurs. *Lungs:* CTA. *Abdomen:* Soft, NT/ND, no pulsatile masses, no bruits over the aorto-ilio-femoral regions. *Ext:* No edema or clubbing; hairless skin over lower legs; feet are cool and slightly cyanotic, become pale with elevation and ruborous with dependency; toenails are thickened.

Pulses:

	carotid	brachial	femoral	popliteal	DP	PT
right	4	4	4	0	0	0
left	4	4	4	2	1	0

No bruits heard in any position.

Bilateral DP/PT heard by Doppler, monophasic R, biphasic L.

ABIs: R DP 110, R PT 100, L DP 120, L PT 120 → R ABI = 110/153, L ABI = 120/153

THOUGHT QUESTION

- What is your next step in evaluating this patient's disease?
- What treatment would you recommend?

DISCUSSION

Pulse volume recordings and segmental pressures are a noninvasive means of assessing for both disease location and severity. In combination with duplex ultrasound, these studies can be very useful in the initial evaluation of peripheral vascular disease. If resting studies show only mild disease but the symptoms are suggestive, they should be repeated after exercise to unmask flow-limiting disease. *CT and MR angiograms* are non-invasive imaging studies for evaluating arterial anatomy. *Conventional arteriography* is, of course, the gold standard; however, given its invasive nature, it is usually reserved until symptoms are significant enough to merit intervention. Intervention can be performed at the time of arteriography if the lesion is appropriate, or bypass may be planned.

Smoking cessation reduces symptom progression by 25%, operative rate by 75%, and mortality by more than 50%. Daily exercise (to just beyond the limits of claudication symptoms) is thought to promote collateral blood vessel development and is also known to improve outcome. Therefore, *risk factor modification* in these patients is essential. Diligent medical care is important; cholesterol, blood pressure, and blood glucose levels should all be checked and carefully controlled if abnormal. *Aspirin* or other platelet-inhibiting agents should be prescribed when there is evidence of atherosclerotic disease. Finally, the patient should be instructed to wear comfortable well-fitting shoes and to maintain meticulous foot hygiene.

This is particularly important in diabetic patients who have impaired wound healing beyond that due to poor circulation.

This patient has a right ABI of 0.65, and a left ABI of 0.78. He has no evidence of tissue loss (e.g., nonhealing foot ulcers) or rest pain. Intervention is indicated for significant impairment of activities of daily living due to symptoms or for critical ischemia (manifested by tissue loss, rest pain, or threatened limb). If his claudication is not disabling to either his lifestyle or occupation, then a recommendation for an organized exercise regimen, smoking cessation, and follow-up visit in 4 to 6 months could be made.

QUESTIONS

37-1. Which of the following is more true of neurogenic leg pain as compared with claudication?
   A. Brought on by standing, relieved by sitting.
   B. Localized to the thigh.
   C. Occurs over the distribution of the saphenous nerve.
   D. Associated with abnormal ABIs.

37-2. Which of the following is *true*?
   A. Rest pain indicates inadequate perfusion at rest and is a precursor to claudication.
   B. Gangrene indicates insufficient perfusion to support tissue survival and is a precursor to limb loss.
   C. Atherosclerotic lesions tend to occur in straight, nonbranching segments of arteries.
   D. Most patients with claudication will eventually require amputation.

37-3. Acute ischemia is typified by pain, pallor, paresthesia, pulselessness, and _____?
   A. Paralysis.
   B. Priapism.
   C. Pulsus paradoxus.
   D. Poikilothermia.

37-4. Which of the following is associated with Leriche syndrome?
   A. Rest pain.
   B. Ischemic colitis.
   C. Iliac aneurysm.
   D. Impotence.

ANSWERS

37-1. A. Generally, claudication is reproducible pain in a muscle group brought on by exercise and relieved by rest. In contrast, neurogenic symptoms are often produced while standing and relieved by sitting. Moreover, this type of pain is often in the distribution of the sciatic nerve rather than being localized to the calves, thighs, or buttocks, as occurs with claudication. The vascular exam is likely to be normal in neurogenic pain with a normal *ABI*. ABIs are calculated by dividing the lowest systolic blood pressure at the ankle (either the dorsalis pedis or the posterior tibial arteries) by the highest systolic pressure at the brachial artery (checked in both arms using Doppler). A ratio of 0.9 to 1.2 is considered normal. An ABI of 0.5 to 0.89 is associated with claudication, and an ABI <0.5 is associated with severe ischemia and often tissue loss or rest pain. If distal pulses or the ABI is normal at rest in a symptomatic patient, repeating these assessments after a period of exercise will likely unmask a flow-significant lesion. ABIs can be used to follow patients over time; a decrease in ABI is associated with symptom progression and increased likelihood of requiring operation.

37-2. B. Atherosclerosis is a diffuse disease but tends to have accelerated development at bifurcations in the arterial system, likely due to hemodynamic changes and shear forces. Bruits represent turbulent flow, usually resulting from a partial obstruction of the arterial lumen by atherosclerotic disease. As a stenosis progresses to complete obstruction, the bruit may disappear with loss of blood flow. *Rest pain* is often localized to the forefoot, is induced when the patient lies down, and is relieved by hanging the foot over the side of the bed (the dependent position allows gravity to facilitate forward blood flow). The prevalence of claudication is 15% in patients over 50 years of age. Fortunately, 70% experience no change in symptoms over 5 to 10 years, whereas 20% to 30% will eventually require an intervention for progression to rest pain or tissue loss. <10% will require amputation. Amputations occur seven times more frequently in diabetics than nondiabetics.

37-3. D. Acute peripheral ischemia is most frequently the result of thromboembolism. The source of an embolus can be cardiac in nature (as from atrial fibrillation) or vascular (e.g., atheroemboli from a diseased aorta, thrombus from an aortic or popliteal aneurysm). Depending on the underlying disease and time course of ischemia, an arteriogram may be performed first or the patient may be taken directly to the OR. Treatment options include catheter-directed thrombolysis, operative thromboembolectomy, or bypass. Although acute ischemia, if unrelieved, can progress to the point of weakness or paralysis of the affected limb, paralysis is not one of the characteristic "5 Ps" of ischemia. The fifth P is poikilo-thermia, or coolness to touch.

37-4. D. The symptom triad originally defined by Leriche included intermittent claudication, impotence, and absence of femoral pulses. This syndrome is highly suggestive of significant aortoiliac occlusive disease and often involves infrainguinal disease as well. Ischemic colitis is not a common finding in aortoiliac disease but is a potential complication when performing an aortoiliac or aortofemoral bypass. This patient has normal femoral pulses and no buttock claudication or impotence; therefore, he most likely has infrainguinal disease without significant aortoiliac disease.

ADDITIONAL SUGGESTED READING

Beebe HG. Intermittent claudication: effective medical management of a common circulatory problem. Am J Cardiol 2001 28;87(12A):14D–18D.

Comerota AJ. Endovascular and surgical revascularization for patients with intermittent claudication. Am J Cardiol 2001; 87(12A):34D–43D.

Dormandy J, Heeck L, Vig S. The natural history of claudication: risk to life and limb. Semin Vasc Surg 1999;12:123–137.

Feinglass J, McCarthy WJ, Slavensky R, et al. Functional status and walking ability after lower extremity bypass grafting or angioplasty for intermittent claudication: results from a prospective outcomes study. J Vasc Surg 2000;31(1 Pt 1):93–103.

Transient Weakness

CC: Transient arm weakness and L eye blindness this morning.

HPI: Ms. X is an 80-year-old woman with a h/o HTN. She reports a 15-minute episode this morning of a "shade" falling over her left eye (*amaurosis fugax*) and weakness in her right arm. She currently has no residual deficits. She has not experienced this before. She has no h/o MI or atrial fibrillation.

PMHx: As above

PSHx: As above

Meds: Diltiazem, ASA

All: NKDA

SHx: Noncontributory (not a smoker)

THOUGHT QUESTION

- What are the possible etiologies of this patient's symptoms?

DISCUSSION

Neurologic symptoms that present and resolve this quickly most likely represent a transient ischemic attack (TIA). Other possibilities include migraine, intracranial mass lesion, and multiple sclerosis. If the visual changes are isolated or involve more than transient blindness, one must consider ophthalmologic disorders. The etiology of a TIA includes cardiac embolism (1/3), lacunar infarct due to arteriolar occlusion in hypertensive patients (1/4), and vascular embolic source (1/3). Vascular emboli generally result from carotid artery plaque rupture, but aorta or vertebral artery-based emboli can also occur. Other more rare etiologies of TIA include hypercoagulable disorders and fibromuscular dysplasia. The incidence of cerebrovascular accident increases with age and is associated with atherosclerotic disease.

CASE CONTINUED

VS: Afebrile; BP R arm 174/65, L arm 170/65; HR 85

PE: *Gen:* Well-nourished elderly woman, no acute distress. *Neuro:* Alert and oriented, intact and nonfocal sensorimotor exam. *HEENT:* PERRL, EOMI, L carotid bruit. *CV:* Regular, no murmurs or gallops. *Resp:* CTA bilaterally. *Abdomen:* Soft, NT/ND, no abdominal bruits. *Ext:* No clubbing, cyanosis, or edema; 4+ distal pulses.

THOUGHT QUESTION

- What is the imaging study of choice at this point?
- What are the treatment guidelines?

DISCUSSION

Head CT or MRI is reasonable to assess for acute stroke, particularly in a setting where thrombolytic therapy may be considered. However, since the most likely cause is TIA due to carotid atherosclerotic disease, *ultrasonography* is the study of choice for initial evaluation and serial follow-up of the carotid arteries. Increased peak systolic and end-diastolic velocities reflect arterial stenosis. Specificity is 84% and sensitivity is 99% compared with arteriography. *Arteriography* is useful when the anatomy is atypical or when the ultrasound is inconclusive. In addition, arteriograms can be helpful when there is ultrasound evidence of a very proximal or distal (i.e., intracranial) stenosis and in the setting of bilateral disease. The primary risk of arteriography is that of a catheter-induced stroke (<1%). An alternative to conventional arteriogram is *MR* or *CT* angiography.

There are two important randomized prospective trials that examined the role of carotid endarterectomy in both symptomatic and asymptomatic patients. The North American Symptomatic Carotid

Endarterectomy Trial (NASCET, 1991) showed that in patients with nondisabling stroke or TIA and ipsilateral stenosis >70%, surgical treatment (carotid endarterectomy) resulted in a 9% incidence of ipsilateral stroke at 2 years compared with 26% for best medical management alone. The Asymptomatic Carotid Artery Study (ACAS, 1995) reported that for asymptomatic patients with unilateral carotid stenosis >60%, incidence of stroke at 5 years was 5% in the carotid endarterectomy group compared with 11% in the medically treated group. These studies showed that surgical management is superior for the prevention of stroke in patients with significant carotid artery stenosis. Endovascular approaches (angioplasty and stent) are now being evaluated for carotid occlusive disease.

CASE CONTINUED

A duplex ultrasound is performed and shows an 80% to 95% stenosis of the L internal carotid artery and a 50% stenosis in the R internal carotid artery. There is moderate disease in both external carotid arteries. Because this patient is symptomatic with an ipsilateral high grade stenosis, the standard of care dictates that an elective carotid endarterectomy be scheduled within the next few weeks. Her right-sided carotid disease should be followed by ultrasound at yearly intervals, and if the degree of stenosis progresses or if she becomes symptomatic, she should be advised to have the right side fixed at that time.

QUESTIONS

38-1. Which of the following is correct?
A. TIA—deficit that resolves in less than 48 hours.
B. Stroke—fixed neurologic deficit (>24 hours).
C. Calcification is rare in carotid atherosclerotic plaques.
D. Carotid bruit is indicative of severe stenosis.

38-2. In evolving stroke or crescendo TIAs,
A. Recovery occurs in 50% without treatment.
B. Anticoagulation is the first line of treatment.
C. Carotid endarterectomy is contraindicated.
D. Thrombolysis is dangerous.

38-3. Which of the following is true about vertebrobasilar insufficiency?
- A. Vertebrobasilar insufficiency is primarily due to hemodynamic causes.
- B. The right subclavian and vertebral arteries are more prone to plaque formation than the left.
- C. Subclavian steal syndrome involves proximal subclavian artery occlusion and reversed blood flow in the ipsilateral vertebral artery.
- D. Posterior cerebral insufficiency occurs in subclavian steal syndrome when exercising the arm on the contralateral side.

38-4. Which of the following structures are found within the carotid sheath?
- A. The glossopharyngeal nerve.
- B. The spinal accessory nerve.
- C. The vagus nerve.
- D. The hypoglossal nerve.

ANSWERS

38-1. B. A TIA, by definition, resolves within 24 hours of the onset of symptoms and is usually resolved in less than 1 hour. The risk of stroke is approximately 25% during the first 5 years after a TIA, and the risk appears to be even higher when associated with a carotid stenosis >70%. Although carotid bruits are generally associated with some degree of carotid disease, only one-third signify a severe stenosis.

38-2. B. The natural history of evolving stroke or crescendo TIA is poor, and without treatment good recovery is expected in <10%. Anticoagulation with heparin is recommended as the initial treatment, but for a carefully selected group of patients, thrombolysis can improve outcome. Candidates for thrombolysis should have no evidence of intracranial hemorrhage or other pathology by CT or MRI. Arteriography is then performed, and if discrete thrombo-embolus is found in the cerebral circulation, thrombolytic therapy can be applied. Carotid endarterectomy is undertaken when both the patient and the neurologic deficit are stable; however, timely operation is important to avoid the risk of recurrent stroke, which is 5% to 10% per year.

38-3. C. Vertebrobasilar insufficiency can have both hemodynamic and thromboembolic sources. Left-sided subclavian and vertebral artery lesions are more common than on the right,
presumably because of the early bifurcation and takeoff of the left
subclavian artery leading to turbulent blood flow in this area. In
subclavian steal syndrome, dizziness, "drop attacks," and other
symptoms of posterior (vertebrobasilar) cerebral insufficiency are
classically associated with exercise of the arm on the affected *ipsilateral* side. However, symptoms actually occur more often with
head rotation or extension, which temporarily occludes the unaffected vertebral artery and further decreases posterior circulation.
Subclavian artery stenosis can be detected by physical exam; thus,
blood pressure should be measured and pulses checked on both
arms of all vascular patients. A differential finding is suggestive of
subclavian stenosis; however, more distal obstruction cannot be
ruled out without arteriography (Fig. 38-1).

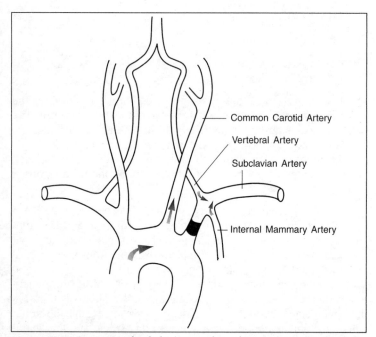

FIGURE **38-1.** Anatomy of subclavian steal syndrome. A proximal subclavian artery occlusion leads to retrograde flow in the ipsilateral vertebral
and internal mammary arteries. This maintains perfusion to the arm at the
expense of perfusion to the posterior cerebral circulation. (*Illustration by
Shawn Girsberger Graphic Design.*)

38-4. C. The hypoglossal nerve lies anterior to the carotid artery, crossing it obliquely at about the level of the carotid bifurcation. At that level, the carotid sheath is indistinct.

ADDITIONAL SUGGESTED READING

Beneficial effect of carotid endarterectomy in symptomatic patients with high-grade carotid stenosis. North American Symptomatic Carotid Endarterectomy Trial Collaborators. N Engl J Med 1991;325:445–453.

Endarterectomy for asymptomatic carotid artery stenosis. Executive Committee for the Asymptomatic Carotid Atherosclerosis Study. JAMA 1995;273:1421–1428.

Halliday A, Mansfield A, Marro J, et al. MRC Asymptomatic Carotid Surgery Trial (ACST) Collaborative Group—Prevention of disabling and fatal strokes by successful carotid endarterectomy in patients without recent neurological symptoms: randomised controlled trial. Lancet 2004; 363:1491–1502. Erratum in: Lancet. 2004;364:416.

Mayberg MR, Wilson SE, Yatsu F, et al. Carotid endarterectomy and prevention of cerebral ischemia in symptomatic carotid stenosis. Veterans Affairs Cooperative Studies Program 309 Trialist Group. JAMA 1991;266:3289–3294.

Randomised trial of endarterectomy for recently symptomatic carotid stenosis: final results of the MRC European Carotid Surgery Trial (ECST) Lancet 1998;351:1379–1387.

Yadav JS, Wholey MH, Kuntz RE, et al. Stenting and Angioplasty with Protection in Patients at High Risk for Endarterectomy Investigators. Protected carotid-artery stenting versus endarterectomy in high-risk patients. N Engl J Med 2004;351:1493–1501.

Foot Drainage

CC: Foul-smelling green drainage from L foot ×5 days.

HPI: Mr. X is a 77-year-old man, h/o DM, HTN, and CAD, who comes to you complaining of a foul-smelling greenish discharge from his left foot for the past 5 days. He denies any recent trauma to the foot. He denies any fever or chills. He reports cramping in both legs after walking four blocks but denies rest pain.

PMHx: As above, MI 30 years ago, bilateral cataracts and glaucoma

PSHx: Five-vessel CABG 20 years ago; L femoral-below knee popliteal bypass 8 years ago (reversed saphenous vein); R femoral-above knee popliteal bypass 5 years ago (ePTFE); R 2nd toe amputation 2 years ago for similar infection

Meds: Glipizide, atenolol, Isordil, ASA, occasional albuterol inhaler, "eye drops"

All: NKDA

SHx: Past smoker (100 pyh)—quit 2 years ago, no EtOH or other drugs

VS: Temp 37.2°C, HR 65, BP 144/76, O_2 sat 93% on RA

PE: *Gen:* WD/WN elderly man in no acute distress. *HEENT:* No carotid bruits, no JVD. *CV:* RRR, no murmurs or gallops, well-healed sternotomy scar. *Lungs:* Trace expiratory wheeze bilaterally, otherwise clear. *Abdomen:* Soft, NT/ND, no pulsatile masses felt or abdominal bruits heard: *Ext:* Well-healed bilateral saphenous vein harvest scars, bilateral lower extremities shiny, hairless skin with hypertrophic toenails and dependent rubor, skin cool, peripheral neuropathy of bilateral forefeet, R foot s/p 2nd toe amputation, L foot with 2 × 1-cm ulceration between great and 2nd toe and 3 × 4-cm ulcer over lateral aspect of 5th toe and forefoot—both draining greenish malodorous pus; bone visible in base of both wounds; erythema and edema across toes and forefoot.

Pulses:

	carotid	radial	femoral	popliteal	DP	PT
right	4	4	3	2	0	0
left	4	4	2	0	0	0
+L femoral bruit						
Bilateral DP/PT heard by Doppler, monophasic						

ABIs: R DP 90, R PT 100, L DP 40, L PT 35 → R ABI = 90/144 = 0.63, L ABI = 40/144 = 0.28

THOUGHT QUESTION

- What is your diagnosis?
- What are this patient's risk factors?
- What is your plan?

DISCUSSION

This man has evidence of arterial insufficiency with infection (a purulent open foot wound with surrounding cellulitis), or *wet gangrene*. *Dry gangrene* occurs when there is severe arterial insufficiency in the absence of infection and generally presents with a blackened mummified digit or forefoot that can be allowed to autoamputate. This patient has many relevant risk factors: age, diabetes, peripheral vascular disease, and history of smoking.

Wet gangrene should be treated aggressively to prevent systemic spread of infection. Broad-spectrum IV antibiotics should be initiated presuming a polymicrobial infection (wound cultures may be taken first but are often contaminated or nonspecific). X-rays should be obtained to look for foreign body, fracture, soft tissue gas, and evidence of osteomyelitis. The patient should be taken to the operating room for debridement of the wound back to healthy bleeding tissue.

CASE CONTINUED

Left foot x-rays show bony degeneration of the L 2nd phalanx and 5th metatarsal bones with no foreign body or fracture. The patient has a WBC of 12 and a creatinine of 1.1. The wound Gram stain shows gram-positive cocci and gram-negative rods; all cultures are pending. The patient is started on antibiotics and taken to the operating room.

THOUGHT QUESTION

- What are the general indications for amputation?

DISCUSSION

Amputation is performed in the settings of gangrene, persistent and unreconstructable rest pain, nonhealing ulcers, and significant extremity trauma (i.e., crush or other complex injury). The goal is to remove any nonviable tissue, relieve the source of (rest) pain, and facilitate primary wound healing and rehabilitation. Given the likely osteomyelitis of several foot bones and the involvement of the entire forefoot by infection, you decide to perform a guillotine transmetatarsal amputation (no formal closure of the stump). Because this patient has marginal ABIs, his lower extremity blood supply will likely be insufficient to fight the infection and heal the wound. Therefore, he will need to have an aortogram with runoff to evaluate his previous bypass and to determine the options for revascularization versus formal amputation (i.e., with flap closure of the stump).

QUESTIONS

39-1. Postoperative care after an amputation involves which of the following?
- A. Antibiotics.
- B. Bed rest.
- C. Aspirin.
- D. Maintenance of full range of joint motion.

39-2. Which of the following complications of amputation may require reoperation?
   A. Phantom limb pain.
   B. Joint contracture.
   C. Pseudoaneurysm formation.
   D. Wound hematoma.

39-3. Syme amputations
   A. Are technically difficult procedures.
   B. Do not require preservation of the epiphyseal growth plates in children.
   C. Have no wound healing problems.
   D. Are indicated for trauma or infection of single digits in the foot.

39-4. Below-knee amputations
   A. Rely on adequate tibial length to approximate a normal gait.
   B. Cost less than vascular reconstruction.
   C. Are an uncommon procedure in vascular surgery.
   D. Utilize minimal soft tissue coverage of the bone.

ANSWERS

39-1. D. Aspirin is not specifically indicated after amputation. Patients may be kept at bed rest with DVT prophylaxis to avoid dependent edema and potential stump trauma, but this is not essential. Avoidance of stump edema is also facilitated by the use of compressive dressings (e.g., Ace wrap) or even rigid (cast) dressing. Early physical therapy with bedside range of motion and strengthening exercises is the rule. Nutrition is important for wound healing and overall muscle strength and endurance. Antibiotics are not indicated unless there is evidence of systemic infection.

39-2. D. Pseudoaneurysms are unlikely to form, because the vessels are ligated and there is no anastomosis involved. *Phantom extremity pain* is a central pain syndrome that is distinct from *neuroma*, which results from regenerative nerve tissue causing pain when trapped within the scar or near the skin surface. Flexion joint contracture is a serious problem, because it can preclude the fitting of a prosthesis. Prevention is the key, with active and passive range of motion exercises early in the postoperative course and knee (or hip) immobilization in the extended position when not exercising. Skin ulceration over bony prominences is often a result of a poorly fitting prosthesis. The wounds generally heal with local care and non-weight bearing on the affected pressure point. The prosthesis should be refitted, or perhaps even the amputation itself may need to be revised. Wound hematomas should be avoided with meticulous hemostasis intraoperatively, but once they develop, they can be a nidus for bacterial infection and should be treated with evacuation and reclosure of the wound.

39-3. A. Selection of amputation level depends on the indication for surgery, rehabilitation potential, and wound healing potential. Indicators of wound healing potential are nutritional status, absence of local infection, and adequate muscle and skin blood flow (which can be quantified by transcutaneous oxygen measurements). Generally, a normal palpable pulse at the level just above the proposed amputation site will predict wound healing; however, absence of a pulse does not necessarily mean the wound will not heal with time. Syme's operations (i.e. amputation at the level of the ankle joint) are technically difficult procedures most often used for trauma involving the forefoot where a transmetatarsal amputation would be inadequate. They are troublesome wounds to maintain and heal and are rarely used for patients with diabetes or significant peripheral vascular disease. Single or isolated digit wounds can be adequately addressed with toe or ray amputations without needing to remove the entire foot.

39-4. A. Below-knee amputations are the most common major amputation performed. The overall cost of amputation (hospitalization and rehabilitation) is greater than the cost of vascular reconstruction. Adequate tibial length allows weight to be dispersed onto the patellar tendon and the quadriceps when walking with a prosthesis. The energy required to walk on a prosthesis increases as the level of amputation moves more proximally. Soft tissue coverage of the residual bone should be achieved without tension to avoid exacerbation of any tissue ischemia. Dead space should be obliterated using deep sutures to avoid wound hematoma. The mortality rate associated with below-knee amputation is high (>12%) and is related to the patient's underlying cardiovascular disease.

ADDITIONAL SUGGESTED READING

Apelqvist J, Larsson J. What is the most effective way to reduce incidence of amputation in the diabetic foot? Diabetes Metab Res Rev 2000;(16 Suppl 1):S75–83.

Frykberg RG. An evidence-based approach to diabetic foot infections. Am J Surg 2003;186(5A):44S–54S; discussion 61S–64S. Review.

Miyajima S, Shirai A, Yamamoto S, et al. Risk factors for major limb amputations in diabetic foot gangrene patients. Diabetes Res Clin Pract 2006;71:272–279.

Treiman GS, Oderich GS, Ashrafi A, et al. Management of ischemic heel ulceration and gangrene: An evaluation of factors associated with successful healing. J Vasc Surg 2000;31:1110–1118.

Leg Heaviness

CC/ID: Right leg heaviness when walking

HPI: MP is a 51-year-old woman who has noted right leg heaviness and a dull ache with walking over the past six months. It seems to be worse at night and better in the mornings. She works as a bank teller and stands all day long. She has had three children and remembers that, when pregnant with her last two children, she had swelling of her right labia.

PMH: none

PSH: none

Meds: none

All: NKDA

SH: former social smoker

FH: mother and aunt have varicose veins

THOUGHT QUESTION

- What may be causing this patient's symptoms?
- What tests can be done to confirm the diagnosis?

DISCUSSION

In any patient who complains of discomfort with walking, it is important to differentiate between vascular and neurogenic causes. Spinal canal stenosis and intervertebral disk disease can cause pain and paresthesias associated with walking, standing for long periods of time, or going between sitting and standing positions. Vascular causes include both arterial and venous insufficiency. Arterial insufficiency can be assessed by a thorough history and physical exam, including peripheral pulses. This patient's symptoms are typical for venous insufficiency. Varicose veins can be found in 15–30% of adults and is more common with increasing age. Varicose veins may be primary in nature, or secondary to venous scarring and inflammation (i.e., after deep venous thrombosis). In addition to describing the varicosities themselves (tenderness, bleeding, firmness), physical exam focuses on lower leg edema or swelling, ulcerations or skin breakdown, and presence of infection. Patients should be examined in both the standing and supine positions.

A *Trendelenberg test* consists of leg elevation to drain venous blood, followed by placement of a tourniquet at various levels on the leg. The patient is then made to stand, and the speed and direction of venous refilling is noted. Normal arterial flow should fill the veins from below upward in 30–35 seconds. Any rapid filling from above suggests proximal venous valvular incompetence. *Duplex ultrasound* is the definitive test for venous reflux and can accurately identify the involved vein. It can also establish the presence of deep venous thrombosis. *Phlebography* and *direct measurement* of venous pressures are invasive methods that are rarely used today. *Photoplethysmography* records reflect infrared light from the subepidermal venous pool, which represents the blood content in the skin. *Magnetic resonance venography* may be used to clarify the anatomy in preparation for a venous reconstruction or valve repair.

CASE CONTINUED

On examination, the woman has large varicose veins along the right medial thigh and posterior calf, as well as "spider veins" along the lateral thigh and ankle. She has minimal edema of the lower legs and no evidence of ulceration. She has never used compression stockings before. She is prescribed compression stockings and directed to keep her legs elevated as much as possible above the level of her heart.

222

THOUGHT QUESTION

- If this patient returns with persistent symptoms despite compliance with the stockings and elevation, what are her surgical options?

DISCUSSION

Sclerotherapy is used for small (1–4 mm) varicosities or spider veins. It involves injection of a sclerosing agent such as hypertonic saline into the vein to cause chemical irritation and scarring of the vein. Saphenofemoral junction ligation is used to treat an incompetent greater saphenous vein (GSV). This involves a small groin incision with dissection of the confluence of the common femoral and greater saphenous veins and any local branches. The GSV is divided from the common femoral vein and ligated. A similar procedure can be performed at the saphenopopliteal junction for incompetent lesser saphenous veins. The GSV can also be completely removed by a vein stripping procedure in conjunction with high ligation. Alternatively, there are now endovenous devices which utilize radiofrequency or laser ablation to sclerose the GSV or LSV via an intraluminal catheter. Stab phlebectomy is performed on individual varicose branches, usually in the lower leg where stripping is less common. This involves serial, small incisions overlying each identified varicosity and manual extraction of the branch. Lastly, incompetent perforators can be divided by a subfascial endoscopic procedure or open ligation and division.

QUESTIONS

40-1. Venous claudication is a bursting pain which is:
A. Brought on by walking and relieved with standing.
B. Brought on by walking and relieved with sitting.
C. Brought on by standing or sitting and relieved with walking.
D. Related to insufficient blood flow to the leg muscles.
E. Caused by thrombosed varicose veins.

40-2. Venous neuropathy is a burning pain caused by:
A. Dilated veins exerting pressure on somatic nerves.
B. Substance P released from engorged venous endothelium.
C. Lower leg ischemia related to impaired venous return.
D. Fascial inflammation.
E. Excess blood flow to the skin.

40-3. Varicose veins are:
   A. Deep to the superficial fascia.
   B. Located within the dermis.
   C. Found only in the greater saphenous distribution.
   D. Rarely incompetent.
   E. Superficial to the superficial fascia.

40-4. Venous stasis ulcers:
   A. Always require skin grafting.
   B. Result from local tissue ischemia related to edema and fibrotic changes.
   C. Rarely respond to local wound care and elevation.
   D. Occur primarily around the knee.
   E. Often lead to amputation.

ANSWERS

40-1. C. Muscular activity, as in walking, activates the pump action of the calf muscles and increases emptying of the lower leg veins. This is in contradistinction to arterial claudication, which is brought on by exercise and relieved by rest. Thrombosed varicose veins are firm rather than soft and may be tender to palpation. Overlying erythema suggests superficial thrombophlebitis and should be treated with warm compresses and NSAIDs.

40-2. A. Other symptoms of varicose veins include aching and tiredness of the legs, which is usually improved with elevation and therefore is less noticeable in the morning than at night. Symptoms may be worse at the start of a woman's menstrual period, related to elevated progesterone levels. Symptoms do not necessarily correlate with the size of the varicosities. Varicose veins include intracuticular telangiectasias (spider veins), subdermal reticular veins, and subcutaneous varices.

40-3. E. Venous insufficiency may be present in the deep veins of the leg, as well as the superficial veins. It is critical to determine a history of deep venous thrombosis (DVT) as a cause of venous insufficiency. Duplex ultrasound is also useful for documenting the presence of DVT prior to consideration of vein stripping. Vein stripping is contraindicated in the presence of DVT, as the superficial veins then act as collateral venous outflow for the leg.

40-4. B. Chronic venous stasis ulcers typically occur over perforating veins (connecting the deep and superficial venous systems). These are inframalleolar or retromalleolar, along Linton's line related to the posterior arch vein. Venous ulcers are often surrounded by hyperpigmentation and hemosiderin deposition. Conservative measures are the initial treatment of choice and include leg elevation, compression, and local wound care.

ADDITIONAL SUGGESTED READING

Bergan JJ, Kumins NH, Owens EL, et al. Surgical and endovascular treatment of lower extremity venous insufficiency. J Vasc Interv Radiol. 2002;13(6):563–568.

Felty CL, Rooke TW. Compression therapy for chronic venous insufficiency. Semin Vasc Surg. 2005;18(1):36–40.

Mundy L, Merlin TL, Fitridge RA, et al. Systematic review of endovenous laser treatment for varicose veins. Br J Surg. 2005; 92(10):1189–1194.

Nicolaides AN; Cardiovascular Disease Educational and Research Trust; European Society of Vascular Surgery; The International Angiology Scientific Activity Congress Organization; International Union of Angiology; Union Internationale de Phlebologie at the Abbaye des Vaux de Cernay. Investigation of chronic venous insufficiency: A consensus statement (France, March 5–9, 1997). Circulation. 2000;102(20):E126–E163.

Tran NT, Meissner MH. The epidemiology, pathophysiology, and natural history of chronic venous disease. Semin Vasc Surg. 2002;15(1):5–12.

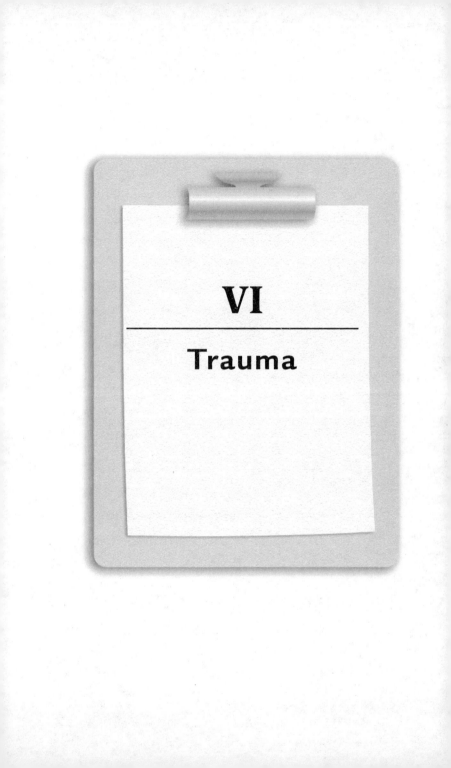

VI

Trauma

House Fire

CC: Caught in fire.

HPI: Mr. X is a 55-year-old man who was caught in a house fire. It appears that he was trying to escape when a burning ceiling panel fell on him. He is brought to the ED where you are the treating physician.

PMHx: HTN, CAD

PSHx: None

Meds: Atenolol, Lipitor, Imdur

All: NKDA

VS: BP 104/65, HR 112, RR 28; weight 82 kg; O_2 sat 87% on 100% non-rebreather FM

PE: *Gen:* WD/WN slightly overweight man, tachypneic, moaning. *HEENT:* Eyebrows singed, PERRL, TMs clear, nares with soot, oropharynx clear, trachea midline, no C-spine tenderness or deformities. *Lungs:* Diffuse wheezes bilaterally, no crackles/rales. *CV:* RRR, no murmurs. *Abdomen:* Soft, NT/ND, pelvis stable. *Ext:* Full-thickness burns over backs of arms and legs, partial thickness burns on hands and feet, no bony deformities. *Back:* Full-thickness burns over upper back and shoulders, no bony deformities or tenderness. *Neuro:* Opens eyes spontaneously but moans only, moves all extremities.

THOUGHT QUESTION

- How are burns described (graded) in terms of depth? What are the associated clinical characteristics?

DISCUSSION

Traditionally, burns have been described as first, second, and third degree. *First-degree* burns involve only the epidermis and are characterized by erythema and pain. *Second-degree* burns involve the epidermis and a variable amount of the dermis. Superficial second-degree burns are characterized by blister formation and minimal scarring. Deeper second-degree burns result in hypertrophic scarring and thin, fragile overlying epithelium. *Third-degree* burns look white and waxy and lack sensation and capillary refill. These burns require skin grafting, because all of the epithelial elements that could serve as a source of re-epithelialization have been destroyed. A more functional classification is to describe burns as either *partial thickness* (first and second degree), which heal spontaneously, or *full thickness* (third degree), which require skin grafting.

CASE CONTINUED

Given this patient's poor oxygen saturation and evidence of possible inhalational injury (sooty nares, wheezes on exam), you decide to intubate him. On direct laryngoscopy, you do not see any erythema, edema, or sooty staining of the larynx. An arterial blood gas performed before intubation is 7.55/28/46/–7/84%. An initial carboxyhemoglobin level is 15% (normal is <10% in nonsmokers and <20% in smokers). Meanwhile, two large-bore IVs and a Foley catheter have been placed. There is no evidence of any trauma other than the burns. After an hour, there is only 50 mL of urine in the Foley bag despite the fact that the patient has already received 2 L of lactated Ringer solution.

THOUGHT QUESTION

- How do you manage this patient's fluid resuscitation?

DISCUSSION

Severe burn patients require an aggressive fluid resuscitation, and even though this patient has received 2 L, he probably still has a significant deficit and ongoing fluid requirement. The *Parkland formula* is one of several used to calculate the fluid requirements of an acute burn patient. It is based on burn size rather than depth. The formula is 4 mL/kg/% total body surface area (TBSA) burn to be given in the first 24 hours. Half of this volume should be given in the first 8 hours, and the remainder is given over the subsequent 16 hours. (For this patient, 4×82 kg $\times 40\%$ TBSA = 13,120 mL expected requirement in the first 24 hours.) This means that the patient should receive approximately 820 mL/hour of lactated Ringer for the first 8 hours (6560 mL) and 410 mL/hour for the following 16 hours (the other 6560 mL). This formula is a guideline; patient response and clinical status should be reassessed frequently and fluid resuscitation adjusted accordingly, e.g., increasing the IV rate in the setting of low urine output or adjusting for pulmonary edema or renal failure. Nutrition (ideally enteral) should be initiated once the initial resuscitation is completed. Colloid administration to replace protein losses is controversial.

QUESTIONS

41-1. The "Rule of 9s" in burn management refers to:
A. Body surface area.
B. Calculation of hypermetabolism.
C. Time intervals of cellular injury.
D. Calculation of evaporative water loss.

41-2. Which of the following injuries is common with electrical burns?
A. Small bowel edema.
B. Cardiac arrhythmias.
C. Antegrade amnesia.
D. Shoulder dislocation.

41-3. Which of the following treatments and their indications is correct?
A. Escharotomy/fasciotomy for burns across joints.
B. Ocular lubrication and topical antibiotic for corneal ulceration.
C. Sulfamylon (mafenide acetate) cream for facial burns.
D. 30 minutes of irrigation with neutralizing agent for chemical burns.

41-4. A common complication after burn injury is
  A. Gastroduodenal ulceration.
  B. Pneumonia.
  C. DVT.
  D. Delirium.

ANSWERS

41-1. A. In the first 6 to 8 hours, gaps develop between endothelial cells in the area of injury, resulting in a significant loss of fluid and protein into the interstitium and into the burn wound itself. Changes in vascular permeability occur even in nonburned tissues, most likely as a result of the release of inflammatory cytokines. Capillary integrity begins to normalize within 18 to 24 hours, and fluid shifts are decreased. Although an initial *hypo*metabolic state can be found after a burn, within 24 to 48 hours *hyper*metabolism develops. This persists until the wound is covered with epithelium from skin grafting or the patient's own healing process. Contributing to an increased metabolism is evaporative water loss, which is normally 15 mL/m^2/hr but can be up to 300 mL/m^2/hr in an open burn wound. This can be minimized by covering the wound with an impermeable membrane and keeping the patient in a warm environment.

The body is divided into regions, each of which is assigned a % surface area. The "Rule of 9s" is perhaps the easiest way to quickly remember these values (arm = 9%, head = 9%, trunk = 18% anterior +18% posterior, leg = 18%) (Fig. 41-1). The patient's open hand is also approximately 1% of his total body surface area. This patient has approximately 4% total body surface area partial-thickness burns and 36% total body surface area full-thickness burns. Estimation of total body surface area burn can help predict prognosis and guide treatment. Patients with >2–5% total body surface area full-thickness or >15% total body surface area partial-thickness burns should be admitted for inpatient therapy. Moreover, burns involving the hands, feet, face, or perineum can result in significant disability if not properly treated; therefore, these patients are also usually automatically admitted. Finally, patients with electrical, chemical, or inhalational injuries and all patients <2 or >60 years old are admitted for observation and treatment regardless of total body surface area burn, because there is a higher morbidity and mortality in these two age groups.

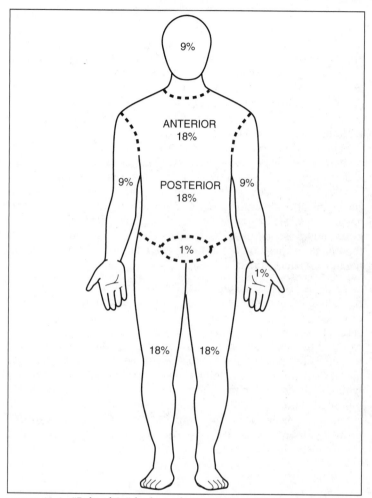

FIGURE 41-1. "Rule of 9s" body surface area map. (*Illustration by Shawn Girsberger Graphic Design.*)

41-2. B. In addition to local tissue injury, electrical burns can cause deep tissue destruction which is not obvious on visual inspection. Moreover, electrical current can travel across joints, and therefore one should always be vigilant in looking for extremity swelling and compartment syndrome. Spine fractures can occur when the paravertebral muscles contract with the passage of electrical current. Patients should be monitored for at least 24 to 72 hours for cardiac arrhythmias following electrical injury.

41-3. B. Facial burns are generally treated with mild topical antibiotic ointments only. Sulfamylon is used on exposed cartilage (e.g., ears) and on eschar, because it is able to penetrate these poorly perfused surfaces. It is not usually used on the face, because it can be very painful on partial thickness injuries, which characterize the majority of facial burns. Any evidence of compartment syndrome (i.e., impaired neurologic function, increased pain, elevated compartment pressure) is an indication for escharotomy with or without fasciotomy. Full thickness circumferential burns of the extremities will sometimes be treated prophylactically with an escharotomy. Significant burns involving the chest or torso can cause an increase in required ventilation pressure and should also be treated with escharotomy if respiratory distress or difficulty with (mechanical) ventilation occurs. Chemical burns should be irrigated with water or normal saline. Neutralizing acid or alkali solutions should not be used. Extremities are elevated and splinted in the functional position to minimize edema and contractures and to maximize potential rehabilitation.

41-4. A. DVT is uncommon. Gastrointestinal tract dysfunction (including hepatic and pancreatic dysfunction) can occur as a result of early transient splanchnic blood flow deficits. This altered visceral blood flow, in conjunction with the systemic stress response, can lead to impaired gastric mucosal defenses and peptic ulcer formation. All burn patients should be placed prophylactically on antiulcer medication. Pneumonia can occur in patients with and without inhalational injury, particularly when patients are relatively immobile with skin grafts or have significant pain and respiratory splinting. Delirium occurs in up to 30% of patients; although this generally resolves with supportive care only, hypoxia and metabolic disturbances should be ruled out or corrected if necessary.

ADDITIONAL SUGGESTED READING

Ansermino M, Hemsley C. Intensive care management and control of infection. Br Med J 2004;329:220–223.

Hettiaratchy S, Papini R. Initial management of a major burn: I—overview. Br Med J 2004;328:1555–1557.

Hettiaratchy S, Papini R. Initial management of a major burn: II—assessment and resuscitation. Br Med J 2004;329(7457):101–103.

Papini R. Management of burn injuries of various depths. Br Med J 2004;329:158–160.

Abdominal Pain After Motor Vehicle Accident

CC: LUQ pain after MVA.

HPI: Ms. X is a 24-year-old woman who was crossing the street when she was struck on her left side by the side mirror of a car. According to bystanders, she was thrown about 5 feet and lost consciousness for a few minutes. She is brought into the ED on a back board and in C-spine precautions. She is awake and talking, complaining of L-sided abdominal pain. She has had no nausea or vomiting. She recalls the entire incident except for the few minutes during which she was unconscious.

VS: Temp 37.5°C, HR 104, BP 108/75, RR 18, O_2 sat 98% on 4 L NC

PE: *Gen:* WD/WN woman, lying on the gurney in a C-spine collar, tearful; skin is warm and dry with a palpable radial pulse. *Neuro:* Glasgow Coma Scale 14, AO × 3, perseverative questioning, moving all extremities. *Chest:* Breath sounds clear bilaterally, trachea midline, sternum and clavicles stable, tenderness to palpation with abrasions over L lower ribs but no crepitus. *Abdomen:* Soft, nondistended, very tender to palpation over LUQ with contusion over L anterolateral abdomen, no rebound, mild guarding. *Pelvis:* Stable and nontender. *Rectal:* normal tone, heme neg. *HEENT:* PERRL, EOMI, TMs without blood or fluid, R occipitoparietal skull with large hematoma, abrasions over R cheek, no cervical bony tenderness or step-off. *Ext:* Abrasions of R forearm and R hip, R hand with abrasions over palm and tenderness and swelling over R distal forearm/wrist, all neurovascularly intact. *Back:* No bony tenderness or deformity.

THOUGHT QUESTION

- What is your initial assessment of this patient?
- What labs or imaging studies should be obtained in a major trauma patient?

DISCUSSION

The Advanced Trauma Life Support protocol begins with the ABCs: airway, breathing, circulation. This patient is talking (without stridor or respiratory distress) and therefore can be assumed to have a clear airway. If she were nonverbal and unable to protect her airway, or if there was respiratory difficulty or airway obstruction (i.e., due to bleeding or edema), the patient would need to be intubated immediately. She is spontaneously breathing and currently has no evidence of an intrathoracic injury requiring intervention (i.e., chest tube or thoracotomy). She has a palpable radial pulse and an adequate blood pressure. Therefore, after obtaining IV access (i.e., two 14- to 16-gauge IVs), a moderate initial intravenous fluid rate or bolus of 500 to 1000 mL of isotonic fluid (i.e., NS or LR) can be ordered. Once A, B, and C are established, you can proceed with D (disability) and E (exposure). The patient displays no disability (i.e., numbness or paralysis). Exposure requires removal of all the patient's clothing and a thorough examination for other injuries.

"Trauma labs" generally include a hematocrit, blood typing, a chemistry panel, and urinalysis. Additional labs are ordered as indicated by the physical exam (e.g., amylase, blood alcohol, or other toxicology screen). Chest, pelvis, and C-spine plain films are generally performed for all major traumas. Additional imaging studies are ordered in the ED according to suspicion for and mechanism of injury.

CASE CONTINUED

Labs: WBC 12; Hct 44; Plts 214; lytes, amylase, coags WNL; UA neg (no RBCs); Upreg neg

Imaging: *CXR:* No pneumothorax or effusion, nondisplaced fracture L ribs 8, 9, and 10. *Pelvis:* No fracture. *C-spine:* No fractures or dislocations, normal alignment of vertebrae. *R forearm:* Fracture of distal radius and ulnar styloid, slightly displaced but nonangulated.

THOUGHT QUESTION

- What other studies should you consider at this point?

DISCUSSION

This patient has LUQ tenderness with L lower rib fractures. Along with her mode of injury, these are concerning for a splenic injury. This can be evaluated initially in the ED with a "FAST" study (Focused Abdominal Sonography for Trauma) to look for free fluid (i.e., intraperitoneal blood), or if the patient is stable, she can be taken to the CT scanner for imaging of the abdomen and pelvis. If she is unstable or requires immediate craniotomy, a *diagnostic peritoneal lavage* (DPL) can be performed in the ED or operating room to look for intra-abdominal blood or bowel contents.

Given the patient's occipital hematoma and loss of consciousness at the scene, you must be watchful for signs and symptoms of a *closed head injury.* If the patient is to be taken to the operating room, you should consider a preoperative head CT to rule out intracranial bleeding, because you will not be able to monitor for mental status changes while the patient is under general anesthesia.

CASE CONTINUED

An abdomen/pelvis CT shows a grade III splenic injury with a 60% subcapsular hematoma and a 4-cm splenic laceration. In this patient, you elect to take a nonoperative approach, with ICU monitoring and serial hematocrits.

QUESTIONS

42-1. In this case, a positive diagnostic peritoneal lavage result would be which of the following?
- A. 10,000 RBC/mm^3.
- B. 50,000 RBC/mm^3.
- C. 5000 RBC/mm^3.
- D. 100,000 RBC/mm^3.

42-2. Which of the following is a component of the Glasgow Coma Scale?
  A. Eye opening.
  B. Motor strength.
  C. Spinal cord reflexes.
  D. Pupillary response.

42-3. With splenic injury after MVA,
  A. There is a low incidence of other intra-abdominal injury.
  B. No vaccinations are required.
  C. Splenectomy is the treatment of choice.
  D. Bedrest and serial hematocrits are mandatory for nonoperative management.

42-4. Overwhelming postsplenectomy sepsis
  A. Involves gram-positive organisms.
  B. Tends to occur in the immediate postoperative period.
  C. Is very common.
  D. Is more likely after splenectomy for hematologic disorders.

ANSWERS

42-1. D. Needle taps of peritoneal fluid were performed in the 1950s but were abandoned because of a high false-negative rate (and danger of iatrogenic injury if performed inappropriately). Tube paracentesis was then introduced, followed by diagnostic peritoneal lavage in 1965. An NGT and Foley catheter should always be placed before starting a diagnostic peritoneal lavage to decompress the stomach and bladder and to avoid iatrogenic injury to those organs during the procedure. Upon placement of the lavage catheter into the abdomen, an initial aspiration is performed; if this returns 10 to 20 mL of gross blood, the diagnostic peritoneal lavage is considered positive. Feces or bile are also considered positive results. Specific laboratory criteria for a "positive" diagnostic peritoneal lavage differ for blunt and penetrating trauma. In blunt trauma, RBC > 100,000/mm^3 or WBC > 500/mm^3 are considered to be positive for intra-abdominal injury. In penetrating trauma, the parameters vary by hospital (i.e., RBC > 1000 to 50,000/mm^3) depending on the desired threshold of detection. More specifically, a lower detection threshold (e.g., RBC > 1000/mm^3) will result in more false positives, whereas a higher detection threshold (e.g., RBC > 50,000/mm^3) will result in fewer negative laparotomies but a higher false-negative rate with more missed injuries. Comparing CT and diagnostic peritoneal lavage, both have a specificity of 99%, whereas diagnostic peritoneal lavage has a sensitivity of 96% and CT of only 74%. However, diagnostic peritoneal lavage does not identify the specific organ injured and has poor sensitivity for diaphragmatic and retroperitoneal injuries. Therefore, CT and diagnostic peritoneal lavage are often used together as complementary exams.

42-2. A. Table 42-1.

TABLE 42-1 Glasgow Coma Scale (GCS)

Category/Criterion	Patient Response	Score
Eye opening (E):	Spontaneous	4
	To voice	3
	To pain	2
	None	1
Verbal response (V):	Oriented	5
	Confused	4
	Inappropriate words	3
	Incomprehensible	2
	None	1
Motor response (M):	Obeys commands	6
	Purposeful movement	5
	Withdraws to pain	4
	Flexion (to pain)	3
	Extension (to pain)	2
	None	1

The Glasgow Coma Scale (GCS) is used in trauma patients to assess for brain injury. The total GCS points (E V M) = the GCS score: maximum = 15, minimum = 3. The breakdown of points should always be given (e.g., E3, V4, M5 for GCS of 12) to more accurately describe any deficits. A GCS of 15 is normal, 13 to 14 correlates with mild injury, 9 to 12 with moderate injury, and 8 or less with severe brain injury.

42-3. D. Because of the usually significant mechanism of injury, associated *extra*-abdominal injury is also found in 80% to 85% of patients with a splenic injury after an MVA. Management of splenic injury, grade I to II, is generally nonoperative; for grades III or IV, treatment is controversial, with a nonoperative approach being acceptable for those patients who have been hemodynamically stable, require <2 units of blood transfusion, and have no evidence of other intra-abdominal injury. Grade V injury usually requires splenectomy, though splenorrhaphy is preferred when possible to try to preserve the spleen's immunologic function. Thrombocytosis can be present for up to 6 weeks after splenectomy but is not known to occur with splenorrhaphy. Platelet counts rarely exceed 1 million, but if this level is reached, antiplatelet therapy (i.e., aspirin) should be considered to prevent thrombotic complications. In addition to long-term vaccination against encapsulated organisms, penicillin prophylaxis is also recommended for postsplenectomy patients before any invasive procedures.

42-4. D. Overwhelming postsplenectomy sepsis (OPSS) usually involves encapsulated organisms (e.g., pneumococcus, meningococcus, *Escherichia coli*, and *Haemophilus influenza*). It has an incidence of 0.5% to 2% (200 × more than in patients with a normal spleen) and occurs within 2 years of splenectomy in 50% of those patients who develop OPSS. Young children (< 2 years old) seem to be at a much higher risk than older children or adults. This is attributed to the spleen's immunologic function, which may be especially important in young children. Interestingly, this complication seems to be less common after splenectomy for trauma than for other causes. Mortality rates vary between 40% and 70%; therefore, early recognition and treatment is essential.

ADDITIONAL SUGGESTED READING

Brigden ML, Pattullo AL. Prevention and management of overwhelming postsplenectomy infection—an update. Crit Care Med 1999;27:836–842.

Haan JM, Bochicchio GV, Kramer N, et al. Nonoperative management of blunt splenic injury: a 5-year experience. J Trauma 2005;58:492–498.

Richardson JD. Changes in the management of injuries to the liver and spleen. J Am Coll Surg 2005;200:648–669.

Wahl WL, Ahrns KS, Chen S, et al. Blunt splenic injury: operation versus angiographic embolization. Surgery 2004;136:891–899.

CASE **43**

Foot Pain After Motorcycle Accident

CC: R foot pain and numbness ×2 hours.

HPI: Mr. X is a 37-year-old man who was in a motorcycle accident where he suffered a concussion and fractures of the R tibia and fibula. The fractures were reduced and cast in the ED, and the patient was admitted for observation. The following morning, the patient complains of throbbing R foot pain and numbness.

PMHx: None

PSHx: None

Meds: None

All: NKDA

SHx: Noncontributory

VS: Afebrile, HR 73, BP 135/68

PE: *Gen:* WD/WN young man in no acute distress. *R lower leg:* In cast. *R forefoot:* Pink and warm, +edema, palpable pulse. *Neuro:* patient unable to extend R toes, pain with passive flexion of the R toes, R 1st web space between R great toe and 2nd toe insensate to light touch.

THOUGHT QUESTION

- What should you do for this patient?
- What is the cause of his problem?

DISCUSSION

This patient needs to have his cast removed and his leg compartment pressures measured. Simple palpation of the calf in the setting of acute symptoms is unreliable. If the pressures are abnormal or if the symptoms do not resolve with cast removal, the patient has a compartment syndrome and needs a surgical fasciotomy.

Limited by noncompliant fascia and bone, the pressure within an extremity compartment can be elevated by either intramuscular swelling (due to edema or hemorrhage) or by external compression (i.e., tight cast or bandage). With significantly elevated compartment pressure, capillary blood flow can be impaired, leading to tissue ischemia. Generally, the higher the compartment pressure, the greater and more rapid the loss of neuromuscular function. Conversely, mildly elevated compartment pressures can cause dysfunction if the increased pressure is maintained for a long enough time. Without decompression by fasciotomy, muscle and nerve necrosis will occur. The specific neuromuscular deficits will often reflect which compartments are involved (e.g., toe extension and 1st web space deficits result from involvement of the deep peroneal nerve in the anterior leg compartment).

CASE CONTINUED

The cast is removed. Using a Stryker kit, the pressures in each of the four lower leg compartments are measured. His anterior compartment pressure is 37 mm Hg. The rest of his pressures are <20 mm Hg. His symptoms do not improve with cast removal, so he is taken to the operating room for a *fasciotomy*.

THOUGHT QUESTION

■ In addition to trauma, what are other potential causes of an extremity compartment syndrome?

DISCUSSION

In thermal burn injuries, a circumferential full-thickness burn with eschar can compress and restrict the underlying tissues, which are prone to capillary leak and edema from the burn injury itself. In electrical burns, occult tissue injury can cause compartment syndrome even without an eschar. Vascular occlusions can result in tissue reperfusion injury and edema if the arterial ischemia was prolonged (usually >6 to 8 hours) before reperfusion. Unconscious patients (e.g., anesthesia, illicit drug use, stroke) who lie unmoving for long periods can develop compartment syndromes in dependent body parts that have been compressed by the rest of the body (e.g., leg in surgical stirrup, buttocks, arm). Large hematomas (e.g., from bleeding diathesis) within small compartments can also be the source of increased compartment pressure. Even exercise can increase intracompartmental volume and pressure via increased capillary perfusion, interstitial edema, venous congestion, and muscle fiber swelling. This is sufficient to cause an exertional (chronic) compartment syndrome if exercise leads to pain and neurologic dysfunction. Rest usually leads to improvement in symptoms. If exercise is prolonged despite symptoms, however, an acute compartment syndrome can be precipitated.

QUESTIONS

43-1. The "6 Ps" of compartment syndrome are pain, (high) pressure, paresthesia, paresis, and
   A. Purple skin and pulse present.
   B. Pink skin and pulse present.
   C. Purple skin and pulselessness.
   D. Pink skin and pulselessness.

43-2. Which of the following compartments and their respective nerves is correct?
   A. Dorsal forearm and median ulnar nerve.
   B. Anterior leg and superficial peroneal nerve.
   C. Deep posterior leg and tibial nerve.
   D. Superficial posterior leg and saphenous nerve.

43-3. Normal compartment pressure is
   A. 0 to 10 mm Hg.
   B. 10 to 20 mm Hg.
   C. 20 to 30 mm Hg.
   D. <0 mm Hg.

43-4. Which of the following statements is *true*?
A. Muscle ischemia affects the peripheral ends of the muscle belly more than the central portion.
B. Acute ischemia leads to reduced capillary permeability and interstitial edema.
C. Complications of compartment syndrome include infection, amputation, and renal failure.
D. Muscle ischemia can result from prolonged periods of systemic hypertension.

ANSWERS

43-1. B. Contrary to the Ps of an ischemic limb, compartment syndrome involves an intact, distal pulse and pink skin color.

43-2. C. As previously mentioned, the deep peroneal nerve runs in the anterior leg compartment. The fourth compartment of the lower leg is the superficial posterior compartment, and its corresponding nerve is the sural nerve. The two compartments in the arm are also common sites of compartment syndrome (volar compartment more frequently than dorsal). Myoneural necrosis of the volar forearm compartment and the median ulnar nerve leads to *Volkmann's contracture*. The dorsal forearm compartment contains the radial nerve (Fig. 43-1).

43-3. A. A compartment pressure is considered elevated when >30 mm Hg or when it is within 35 to 40 mm Hg of the patient's diastolic blood pressure. A pressure between 10 and 30 mm Hg is abnormal but not always sufficient for a compartment syndrome, unless it satisfies the diastolic blood pressure criteria mentioned above.

43-4. C. Muscle ischemia and compartment syndrome can result from prolonged periods of *hypo*tension. Muscle fibers have collateral circulation at the periphery; therefore, the middle sections are more susceptible to ischemia. The hyperkalemia, acidosis and myoglobinemia produced by myonecrosis can lead to arrhythmia, renal failure and possibly death. Resuscitation with a bicarbonate drip to alkalinize the urine may limit precipitation of myoglobin in the kidneys. Any electrolyte imbalances should be treated aggressively. Ischemic tissue is prone to infection and therefore should be monitored closely.

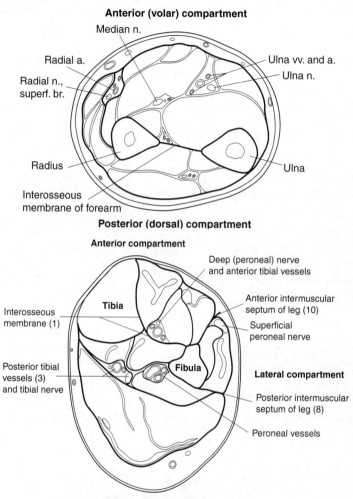

FIGURE 43-1. Compartments of the forearm (A) and lower leg (B). The anterior or volar compartment of the forearm contains the flexors-pronators, which are served primarily by the median nerve. The posterior or dorsal compartment contains the extensors-supinators of the forearm and is innervated by the radial nerve. The exception is the brachioradialis, which is a flexor muscle but is located in the posterior compartment and is supplied by the radial nerve. Forearm fasciotomy requires incisions over each forearm compartment, whereas all four compartments of the calf can be decompressed via just two fasciotomy incisions on the medial and lateral aspects of the lower leg. (*Illustrations by Electronic Illustrators Group.*)

ADDITIONAL SUGGESTED READING

Blaisdell FW. The pathophysiology of skeletal muscle ischemia and
   the reperfusion syndrome: a review. Cardiovasc Surg
   2002;10:620–630.
Kostler W, Strohm PC, Sudkamp NP. Acute compartment
   syndrome of the limb. Injury 2004;35:1221–1227.
Olson SA, Glasgow RR. Acute compartment syndrome in lower
   extremity musculoskeletal trauma. J Am Acad Orthop Surg
   2005;13:436–444.
Velmahos GC, Toutouzas KG. Vascular trauma and compartment
   syndromes. Surg Clin North Am 2002;82:125–41, xxi.

Loss of Consciousness

CC/ID: 38-year-old woman found down by her family.

HPI: Ms. X was in her usual state of good health when she was found on the floor of the bathroom, apparently having tried to use the toilet. There was no witnessed seizure activity. On arrival to the ED, she is alert but confused. Her history is provided by her family.

PMHx: None

PSHx: None

Meds: Birth control pills

VS: Afebrile, BP 150/80, HR 72

PE: *Gen:* Otherwise healthy appearing woman with incoherent speech. Her eyes are closed, but she arouses to pain and loud noises. There are no obvious external signs of trauma. *HEENT:* Difficulty with upward gaze. *Chest:* Clear bilaterally; no rib pain. *Heart:* RRR. *Abdomen:* Soft, nontender, nondistended. *Ext:* Moves all four extremities equally and without difficulty; no deformities noted. *Neuro:* Unable to follow commands but localizes to pain.

THOUGHT QUESTION

- What is the differential diagnosis for this patient's symptoms?
- What tests will you order?

DISCUSSION

The differential in this young, confused, otherwise healthy woman includes seizure of unknown etiology (e.g., due to tumor, toxins, drugs, electrolyte abnormality); subarachnoid hemorrhage (e.g., due to arteriovenous malformation, ruptured aneurysm); or head trauma. Her apparent abducens (cranial nerve VI) palsy may be indicative of hydrocephalus. Important tests to order at this juncture include a full set of labs (assessing for blood loss, electrolyte derangements, coagulopathy), a type specimen to the blood bank, and a head C T.

CASE CONTINUED

Labs: Normal CBC, electrolyte panel, and coags.

Imaging: *Head CT:* Shows diffuse subarachnoid hemorrhage in the basilar cisterns with mild intraventricular hemorrhage, mild hydrocephalus, and effacement of the sulci. The findings are consistent with a ruptured aneurysm (most likely of the anterior communicating artery, basilar tip, or the posterior inferior cerebellar artery—these three account for 75% to 80% of spontaneous subarachnoid hemorrhage).

While the patient is en route from the radiology suite back to the ED, you notice that her monitor is now showing a blood pressure of 185/92 with a heart rate of 53. She is somewhat less arousable than she was previously.

THOUGHT QUESTION

- What is happening in this patient? What do you do next?
- Are there any interventions that may rapidly alter her clinical status?
- What other treatment modalities should you use?

DISCUSSION

The findings of increasing hypertension, decreasing heart rate, and deteriorating mental status are consistent with *Cushing's triad,* which suggests increasing intracranial pressure. This patient should be monitored in an intensive care unit. A ventriculostomy is important in this setting, because it can help to rapidly decompress the elevated intracranial pressure which often ameliorates the Cushing's response. Medications to start at this time would include nimodipine (a calcium channel blocker shown to decrease cerebral vasospasm); a histamine receptor antagonist (there is a high incidence of stress gastritis in this population); an anti-epileptic such as phenytoin (prophylactic in this case, generally recommended when there has been a loss of consciousness or frank seizure activity); and antihypertensives. A four-vessel cerebral angiogram should be ordered. Repair of cerebral aneurysms has classically been accomplished in an open fashion in the operating room, but in recent years endovascular techniques have been successfully used. The decision whether to approach the repair of these lesions in a surgical or endovascular fashion will depend on the location of the aneurysm and the institutional experience and preference.

CASE CONTINUED

After placement of the ventriculostomy, the patient becomes considerably more coherent and is now responding appropriately to questions and commands. When her vitals stabilize, a four-vessel angiogram is performed, revealing an aneurysm of the anterior communicating artery. After discussion with the patient and her family, she undergoes clipping of the aneurysm in the operating room.

QUESTIONS

44-1. On arrival, what Hunt-Hess hemorrhage grade would you have assigned to this patient?

- A. 1
- B. 2
- C. 3
- D. 4
- E. 5

44-2. Which of the following arteries is part of the circle of Willis?
   A. Vertebral.
   B. Ophthalmic.
   C. Middle cerebral.
   D. External carotid.

44-3. What is the most common adult primary brain tumor?
   A. Astrocytoma.
   B. Lymphoma.
   C. Meningioma.
   D. Acoustic neuroma.

44-4. Which of the following tumors commonly metastasize to the brain?
   A. Lung.
   B. Adrenal.
   C. Lymphoma.
   D. Liver.

ANSWERS

44-1. C. The Hunt-Hess grading system is a means of classifying the severity of intracranial hemorrhage based on clinical assessment. The grades range from 1 to 5 (Table 44-1).

TABLE 44-1 The Hunt-Hess Grading System

Grade	Description
1	Mild headache and slight nuchal rigidity
2	Cranial nerve palsy, severe headache, nuchal rigidity
3	Mild focal deficit, lethargy or confusion
4	Stupor, hemiparesis, early decerebrate rigidity
5	Deep coma, decerebrate rigidity, moribund appearance

Based on this patient's confusion/mental status on arrival, she would have been given a grade of 3.

44-2. C. The external carotid artery is an extracranial branch of the common carotid artery that does not contribute to the Circle of Willis. The paired *internal* carotid arteries do (Fig. 44-1).

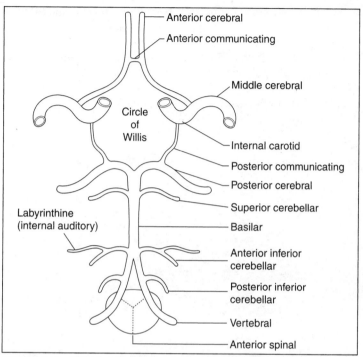

FIGURE 44-1. Arterial contributions to the Circle of Willis. (*Illustrations by Electronic Illustrators Group.*)

44-3. A. Astrocytomas (glial cell tumors) are the most common primary brain tumor in adults.

44-4. A. Melanoma, lung, breast, genitourinary tract, colon/rectum, and sinus tumors are all known to metastasize to the brain; melanoma and lung cancer are the most common. Patients with brain metastases may exhibit a change in affect or may have symptoms of headache, numbness, or motor weakness. A focal neurologic deficit is the most common presenting symptom. Brain MRI or head CT are usually diagnostic.

ADDITIONAL SUGGESTED READING

Black PM, Johnson MD. Surgical resection for patients with solid brain metastases: current status. J Neurooncol 2004;69:119–124.

Keles GE, Berger MS. Advances in neurosurgical technique in the
current management of brain tumors. Semin Oncol
2004;31:659–665.

Liebenberg WA, Worth R, Firth GB, et al. Aneurysmal subarachnoid
haemorrhage: guidance in making the correct diagnosis. Postgrad
Med J 2005;81:470–473.

Tosoni A, Ermani M, Brandes AA. The pathogenesis and treatment
of brain metastases: a comprehensive review. Crit Rev Oncol
Hematol 2004;52:199–215.

Wijdicks EF, Kallmes DF, Manno EM, et al. Subarachnoid
hemorrhage: neurointensive care and aneurysm repair. Mayo
Clin Proc 2005;80:550–559.

Stab Wound

 CC/ID: 19-year-old man with a stab wound to the right lower quadrant

HPI: The paramedics report that the patient was in a knife fight where he was beaten with closed fists to the head before being stabbed in the abdomen. On arrival, he is yelling and agitated. He has alcohol on his breath.

VS: T 36.5°C, BP 145/85, HR 116, O_2 sat 100% 2L NC

PE: *Gen:* WD/WN young man, tattoos across chest, abdomen, and arms. *HEENT:* Pupils dilated but reactive, sclera anicteric. Contusions over R zygomatic arch and periorbital area, no step off. 2-cm superficial laceration transversely across chin. *Chest:* CTA bilaterally, no crepitus, nontender. *Abdomen:* Thin, no scars. No rebound or guarding. Stab wound in RLQ - 1-cm long, not actively bleeding. *Ext:* No clubbing, cyanosis, or edema. Abrasions across knuckles and forearms, small <1-cm lacerations to several fingers.

THOUGHT QUESTION

- Now that you've completed your primary survey (ABCs!), what additional information will assist you in the evaluation of this patient's stab wound?

DISCUSSION

When assessing a stab wound, it is important to try and determine what type of weapon was used (e.g., butcher knife, steak knife, ice pick, broken glass). In combination with the visible skin wound, this information can help you to estimate how deeply the wound

251

might extend and whether or not there might be fragments (e.g., glass, wood, metal) within the wound. It is also helpful to know how long ago the wound was incurred, how much blood was found at the scene, and whether or not the patient has had a tetanus vaccination within the past ten years.

CASE CONTINUED

The patient says that he thinks that the weapon was a small pocket knife. The altercation apparently occurred just before the police and EMS arrived, and you learn that there was minimal blood found at the scene. The patient does not recall ever having received a tetanus shot. He remains belligerent as you proceed.

PMH: "I'm fine, man!"

PSH: unknown

Meds: "I just wanna get outta here!"

All: unknown

Repeat VS remain fairly stable, with a blood pressure of 130/80 and a heart rate of 110.

THOUGHT QUESTION

■ How will you proceed from here?

DISCUSSION

As with any trauma patient, this man should have basic blood tests performed (CBC, electrolytes, type and screen). An upright CXR should be obtained to look for free air under the diaphragm (suggesting viscus injury) and possible rib fractures (although he did not complain of any bony tenderness). A higher wound (i.e., above the level of the umbilicus) might also prompt an evaluation for possible pneumothorax, as the lungs may extend quite inferiorly along the posterior abdomen. Plain films may also help to illustrate the presence of any retained foreign bodies (e.g., knife tip) if this is a concern. Given this patient's evidence of intoxication, a urine toxicology screen and blood alcohol level should be performed. This will help to determine whether or not the patient's sensorium might be altered, which might in turn render his exam more unreliable.

Since the patient is unclear of his tetanus status, a tetanus shot should be administered. Prophylactic antibiotics are also advisable. As long as the patient remains stable and without indications for immediate operative intervention (hemodynamic instability, peritoneal signs), local wound exploration may be performed to assess for depth of injury.

CASE CONTINUED

A trauma lab panel is sent and reveals no abnormal values. The CXR is clear. Urine tox screen shows the presence of both alcohol and amphetamines. Blood alcohol level is 250 (legal limit 80–100). A tetanus shot and 1 gram of cefazolin IV are administered. You go on to perform a local wound exploration and find that the wound grazes only into the subcutaneous fat; the rectus sheath appears to be intact. You continue to observe the patient for sobriety.

THOUGHT QUESTION

- How would your evaluation differ if the patient arrived with a distended, tense abdomen? With "fat" protruding from the stab wound? With the rectus sheath violated on local exploration?
- How would your evaluation differ if the patient arrived obtunded?

DISCUSSION

A distended, tense abdomen with rebound or guarding is consistent with *peritonitis;* in this setting, it is likely caused by blood in the abdomen and requires immediate exploration. Once the patient has had his initial assessment and any additional urgent injuries are ruled out, he should be taken directly to the operating room for a laparotomy. Similarly, "fat" protruding from a stab wound is most likely omentum extending through the wound and is considered *evisceration*. This also requires immediate laparotomy, as the peritoneal cavity has clearly been entered by the stab weapon, and further herniation and strangulation of abdominal contents are possibilities if intervention is delayed. In addition, other injuries behind the herniated tissue may be revealed. The wound should be covered with a warm, moist gauze while waiting for the operating room, and the patient should be started on broad-spectrum antibiotics (i.e., to cover bowel flora). Lastly, if during local wound exploration you discover that the rectus sheath has been penetrated by the stab weapon, this is very concerning for peritoneal penetration as well. If the patient is otherwise stable, laparoscopic or open evaluation of the abdomen may be performed.

In the setting of obtundation and a history of blunt trauma to the head, the patient must also have a thorough neurologic evaluation. If hemodynamically stable, the patient should have an urgent head CT before any definitive treatment for the stab wound. If there is clear evidence of brain injury (i.e., blown pupil, posturing, intracranial hematoma), emergent neurosurgery becomes paramount, and further assessment of the abdominal injury should be performed simultaneously in the operating room. This assessment may be in the form of a diagnostic peritoneal lavage or a definitive laparotomy.

QUESTIONS

45-1. Gunshot wounds to the abdomen:
A. Travel in a straight trajectory.
B. Require operative exploration.
C. Rarely injure organs outside the wound tract.
D. Rarely produce significant intra-abdominal injury.
E. Are usually fatal.

45-2. Stab wounds to the back or flank:
A. Should be treated the same as anterior abdominal stab wounds.
B. Cause visceral injury in >50%.

C. Are best evaluated with laparoscopy.
D. Require CT scan with triple contrast.
E. Are always closed primarily.

45-3. Local wound exploration:
A. Involves local anesthesia and extension of the entrance wound.
B. Begins with digital probing of the wound tract.
C. Should be confirmed with additional studies [i.e., CT or diagnostic peritoneal lavage (DPL)].
D. Reliably rules out injury even if the patient exhibits peritoneal signs.
E. Is a substitute for exploratory laparotomy.

45-4. Abdominal muscle rigidity:
A. Can be caused by bony fractures (ribs, iliac wing, spine).
B. Is an unreliable indicator of peritoneal irritation.
C. Should be confirmed with additional studies (i.e., CT or DPL).
D. Should be assumed to be an abdominal wall hematoma until proven otherwise.
E. Should be treated with narcotics.

ANSWERS

45-1. B. Bullets can expand and fragment and are subject to tumbling and various directional forces. As a result, the bullet path is unpredictable, and blast effects can be significant even outside the bullet trajectory. More than 95% of gunshots to the abdomen result in intra-abdominal injury; therefore all require exploratory laparotomy. Mortality is dependent on the severity of damage incurred and is highly variable.

45-2. D. Triple contrast CT scan (with IV, oral, and rectal contrast) is best in evaluating the retroperitoneum for possible colonic, duodenal, or renal injury. Laparoscopy is unable to visualize the retroperitoneum well, and is more useful for anterior wounds and for ruling out diaphragmatic injury. Back and flank stab wounds result in intra-abdominal injury in <15%, likely related to the extensive musculature that must be traversed in order to reach the peritoneum from the posterolateral direction. After a negative CT scan, most patients are observed for 24–48 hours for possible delayed presentation of a visceral injury. Most stab wounds are left open to heal by secondary intention, although very fresh wounds may be closed primarily.

45-3. A. Digital probing of a stab wound is generally not indicated; a finger may often create its own tract rather than following the actual stab tract, and it may disturb any clot that has formed to temporarily control bleeding. Local wound exploration requires local anesthesia and extension of the entrance wound in order to better expose the wound tract and visualize the anterior abdominal fascia. A negative wound exploration should not be used to disregard a patient's clinical examination; it is always safer to perform a laparotomy if there is any question of visceral injury (i.e., presence of peritoneal signs). Even with evidence of anterior fascial penetration on local exploration, a negative laparotomy occurs in up to 25% and is acceptable because there is a low morbidity associated with negative laparotomy but high morbidity associated with missed visceral injury.

45-4. A. Muscle rigidity can be caused by contiguous bony fractures or contusions. To distinguish this from rigidity related to peritonitis, local anesthesia may be infiltrated into the site of tenderness, which will relieve pain related to abdominal wall injury but not that due to intra-abdominal injury. Abdominal rigidity should be assumed to reflect peritonitis until proven otherwise.

ADDITIONAL SUGGESTED READING

Ahmed N, Whelan J, Brownlee J, et al. The contribution of laparoscopy in evaluation of penetrating abdominal wounds. J Am Coll Surg 2005;201:213–216.

Albrecht RM, Vigil A, Schermer CR, et al. Stab wounds to the back/flank in hemodynamically stable patients: evaluation using triple-contrast computed tomography. Am Surg 1999;65:683–687; discussion 687–688.

DeMaria EJ, Dalton JM, Gore DC, et al. Complementary roles of laparoscopic abdominal exploration and diagnostic peritoneal lavage for evaluating abdominal stab wounds: a prospective study. J Laparoendosc Adv Surg Tech 2000;10:131–136.

Ertekin C, Yanar H, Taviloglu K, et al. Unnecessary laparotomy by using physical examination and different diagnostic modalities for penetrating abdominal stab wounds. Emerg Med J 2005;22:790–794.

Moore EE, Marx JA. Penetrating abdominal wounds. Rationale for exploratory laparotomy. JAMA 1985(10);253:2705–2708.

VII

Perioperative
Period

Preoperative Anesthesia

CC: Preoperative for an inguinal hernia repair.

HPI: Mr. X is a 76-year-old man scheduled for an open bilateral inguinal hernia repair. He is very anxious and is requesting to be "put to sleep" for his operation.

PMHx: HTN, CAD s/p MI 10 years ago, COPD, CRI, BPH

PSHx: Appendectomy as a child

All: Morphine—makes him feel nauseated

Meds: Amlodipine, Nitro-Bid, Combivent inhaler

SHx: Past heavy drinker (none currently), 1 ppd smoker for 40 years, no IV drug use

THOUGHT QUESTION

- What are the options for anesthesia in this case?
- What risk factors in this patient may influence the choice of an anesthetic technique?

DISCUSSION

The possible options are general, regional, or local anesthesia with sedation (called "monitored anesthesia care"). *General anesthesia* is often achieved by inhalational agents, which provide amnesia, analgesia, and some muscle relaxation. Nitrous oxide has minimal cardiovascular effects, but its anesthetic potency is quite weak. The "volatile anesthetics," fluorocarbons such as isoflurane and desflurane, are extremely potent anesthetics, but they are also potent myocardial and respiratory depressants and peripheral vasodilators. Intravenous agents, such as barbiturates, benzodiazepines, propofol, etomidate, and ketamine (all of which provide amnesia), can be used in conjunction with opiates (for analgesia) to achieve general anesthesia. All these IV agents, with the exception of ketamine and etomidate, are potent respiratory depressants. Opiates have no myocardial depressive effects, but they stimulate histamine release and inhibit sympathetic vascular tone; therefore, large doses can cause vasodilation and hypotension. Most patients undergoing general anesthesia require mechanical ventilation, either via an endotracheal tube or a laryngeal mask, and skeletal muscle relaxation using nondepolarizing or depolarizing paralytic agents.

Regional anesthesia can be useful for patients in whom spontaneous ventilation is required or in patients with significant cardiac or respiratory disease where general anesthesia is considered prohibitively risky. Regional anesthesia involves targeted infusion of local anesthetics (i.e., spinal or epidural) and acts by blocking nerve conduction to a body part or dermatomal region. First autonomic, then sensory, and finally motor functions are inhibited. Overdose causes dysrhythmias and seizures. Contraindications for spinal or epidural techniques include anticoagulated patients and those who are preload and afterload dependent, such as patients with aortic stenosis. *Monitored anesthesia care* requires careful and adequate administration of local anesthesia in the surgical field, because although patients are deeply sedated and are likely to be amnestic, they can still respond to both vocal and noxious stimuli.

Because many of the above drugs cause either respiratory or myocardial depression, the risk of adverse events (i.e., respiratory arrest, MI) is not negligible, especially in patients with pre-existing cardiorespiratory disease. This patient has both CAD and COPD and is a current smoker. Therefore, the use of local or regional anesthesia rather than general anesthesia will have fewer cardiac and respiratory effects and risks. His history of alcohol use puts him at risk for liver dysfunction, and so coags should be checked before regional anesthesia is selected. Local anesthesia is associated with the least likelihood of postoperative urinary retention in cases of inguinal hernia repair.

CASE CONTINUED

You counsel this patient to have his inguinal hernias repaired under local anesthesia with sedation. His preoperative labs are notable for normal LFTs, normal coags, and a creatinine of 1.8. His potassium level is 4.7.

THOUGHT QUESTION

■ How does decreased renal clearance affect the perioperative anesthetic considerations?

DISCUSSION

Succinylcholine (a depolarizing muscle relaxant) will raise the plasma potassium by 0.5 to 1.0 mEq/dL. If the patient has borderline hyperkalemia before induction of general anesthesia, then muscle relaxation achieved with succinylcholine could potentially trigger lethal hyperkalemia, especially in the setting of metabolic acidosis. Vecuronium (a nondepolarizing muscle relaxant) and morphine both have active metabolites that are renally cleared. Therefore, they may accumulate in a patient with renal insufficiency. Meperidine, which is often used postoperatively to control shivering, has a nonactive metabolite (normeperidine) that decreases seizure threshold; it is renally cleared and thus can trigger seizures if high amounts are administered to a patient with decreased renal clearance. Because this patient is not undergoing general anesthesia, his renal insufficiency does not alter the anesthetic plan. Postoperative pain control is usually achieved with small doses of morphine or oral narcotics; particular care should be taken if using meperidine.

QUESTIONS

46-1. Which of the following drugs and their reversal agents is *correct*?
   A. Succinylcholine—Narcan.
   B. Sufentanyl—Flumazenil.
   C. Rocuronium—Neostigmine.
   D. Propofol—Edrophonium.

46-2. What is the best local anesthetic agent to use for prolonged postoperative pain control?
   A. Prilocaine.
   B. Lidocaine.
   C. Chlorprocaine.
   D. Bupivacaine.

46-3. Which of the following is associated with increased intracranial and intraocular pressure?
   A. Vecuronium.
   B. Mivacurium.
   C. Succinylcholine.
   D. Rocuronium.

46-4. What is the toxic threshold dose of bupivacaine?
   A. 0.1 mg/kg.
   B. 0.5 mg/kg.
   C. 3.0 mg/kg.
   D. 5.0 mg/kg.

ANSWERS

46-1. C. Narcan is the reversal agent of opiates such as morphine, while flumazenil is the reversal agent for benzodiazepines like versed. Propofol and succinylcholine do not have reversal agents; both are rapidly metabolized and their effects wear off quickly.

46-2. D. The effects of bupivacaine last 2 to 4 hours, whereas those for lidocaine and prilocaine last 30 to 60 and 30 to 90 minutes, respectively. Chlorprocaine is even shorter acting with a duration of 15 to 30 minutes. Prilocaine has the unique side effect of methemoglobinemia. Allergies are more likely to occur to the aminoester drugs (i.e., procaine, tetracaine, chlorprocaine) rather than to the aminoamides (i.e., lidocaine, prilocaine, mepivacaine).

46-3. C. Both atracurium and mivacurium (intermediate and short-acting paralytics, respectively) cause histamine release, whereas succinylcholine does not. Vecuronium and rocuronium have no cardiovascular effects.

46-4. C. Toxicities of local anesthetics are presumed to be additive. These effects are primarily CNS (mental status changes and seizures) or cardiovascular (arrhythmia, myocardial depression). Addition of a small amount of bicarbonate to a solution of local anesthetic results in more rapid onset of and a decrease in the minimum concentration required for nerve conduction blockade. The bicarbonate also acts to buffer the "sting" of infiltrating the (acidic) anesthetic. Addition of vasoconstrictors such as epinephrine can decrease the rate of vascular absorption, thereby allowing more anesthetic to reach the nerve membrane, with a resultant increase in the depth and duration of the anesthesia.

ADDITIONAL SUGGESTED READING

Eger EI 2nd. Characteristics of anesthetic agents used for induction and maintenance of general anesthesia. Am J Health Syst Pharm 2004;61(Suppl 4):S3–10.

Fleisher LA. Anesthetic management and perioperative surveillance. Prog Cardiovasc Dis 1998;40:441–452.

Fredman B, Zohar E, Philipov A, et al. The induction, maintenance, and recovery characteristics of spinal versus general anesthesia in elderly patients. J Clin Anesth 1998;10:623–630.

Golembiewski J. Considerations in selecting an inhaled anesthetic agent: case studies. Am J Health Syst Pharm 200;61(Suppl 4): S10–17.

Mingus ML. Recovery advantages of regional anesthesia compared with general anesthesia: adult patients. J Clin Anesth 1995;7: 628–633.

Postoperative Hypoxia and Pain

CC/ID: 68-year-old man s/p exploratory laparotomy for lysis of adhesions, now with low O_2 sats.

HPI: You are called by the recovery room nurse to see the patient, whose oxygen saturation is 82%. To the best of your knowledge, his case was long and tedious, but otherwise uncomplicated, and he was able to be extubated in the operating room. You instruct the nurse to increase his oxygen delivery and go to the bedside to evaluate.

THOUGHT QUESTION

- What are possible reasons for this patient's desaturation?
- What issues may predispose him to hypoxia?

DISCUSSION

Hypoxia in the postoperative period may be due to a number of causes, including incomplete reversal of neuromuscular blockade, hypoventilation from residual anesthetic agents or narcotics, splinting (from incisional pain) resulting in small tidal volumes and atelectasis, pulmonary edema from excessive intraoperative fluid administration, pulmonary embolism, or primary cardiac failure from a perioperative MI.

A review of the patient's history will be important to look for possible causes of baseline hypoxia, including COPD/tobacco history, obesity, sleep apnea syndrome, pneumonia, or heart failure.

CASE CONTINUED

PMHx: HTN, ex-smoker, quit 2 years ago (60 pyh)

PSHx: Sigmoid colectomy for diverticulitis

Meds: Albuterol MDI, atenolol

VS: Afebrile, BP 125/85, HR 75, RR 24, O_2 sat 82% on 4 L/NC →84% on 100% FM

PE: *Gen:* Agitated, having difficultly speaking. *Chest:* CTA bilaterally, no wheezes or crackles/rales; poor excursions. *Heart:* Regular, no murmur, no gallop. *Neuro:* Unable to lift head off of bed; nerve stimulator: 2 of 4 on train of 4.

THOUGHT QUESTION

- What is the cause of this patient's desaturation?
- What maneuvers will help to improve his oxygen saturation?

DISCUSSION

The patient likely has an element of COPD, suggesting some base-line hypoxia. However, the more notable features in his evaluation are his inability to speak or move his head, and the finding of fewer than four twitches on train-of-4 nerve stimulation. This suggests an incomplete neuromuscular blockade reversal. Although he has probably regained diaphragmatic muscle activity (because it is the muscle most resistant to neuromuscular blockade), he is likely unable to recruit the support of his accessory breathing muscles.

Neuromuscular blockade reversal can be accomplished by adminis-tration of an anticholinesterase such as neostigmine, given in con-junction with an anticholinergic agent such as glycopyrrolate. However, because reversal will not be immediate, it is important to support the patient's airway and breathing. To this end, an oral or nasal airway may be placed, with initiation of bag-mask ventilation. If it appears that the patient is rapidly decompensating or is unable to maintain adequate oxygenation, reintubation may be necessary.

CASE CONTINUED

After the patient is pharmacologically reversed and his breathing supported, his oxygen saturations improve to the mid-90s on oxygen by nasal cannula alone. His vitals are otherwise stable. He now complains of pain.

THOUGHT QUESTION

- What options do you have for ongoing pain management in this patient?

DISCUSSION

Continuous epidural analgesia is an effective means of providing continuous pain control in selected postoperative patients. *Patient-controlled analgesia*, where patients are able to self-deliver intravenous or epidural narcotics by means of a pump, is also useful because it allows patients to receive metered doses of analgesia on demand, without needing to wait for medical staff administration. If pain is expected to be minimal or relatively infrequent, prn (only as needed) intravenous or intramuscular analgesics may be sufficient. Oral pain medications are not initially an option in the NPO postabdominal surgery patient.

QUESTIONS

47-1. Regarding succinylcholine,
A. It is a competitive inhibitor of acetylcholine.
B. It is a long-acting neuromuscular blocker.
C. It cannot be reversed.
D. It is associated with hypokalemia.
E. It is part of a large class of commonly used paralytics.

47-2. Benzodiazepine overdose can be reversed with
A. Acetylcysteine (Mucomyst).
B. Naloxone (Narcan).
C. Metoclopramide.
D. Prochlorperazine.
E. Flumazenil.

47-3. For patients who have had an MI, it is recommended that *elective* surgery be delayed for
   A. There is no need for delay.
   B. 6 weeks.
   C. 3 months.
   D. 6 months.
   E. 12 months.

47-4. The Goldman criteria for evaluating cardiac risk have described which of the following as being independently related to an increase in perioperative cardiac complications?
   A. Age >50 years.
   B. S_3 gallop or jugular venous distension on preoperative examination.
   C. Sinus bradycardia <55 beats per minute.
   D. Neck or extremity surgery.
   E. Mitral regurgitation.

ANSWERS

47-1. C. Neuromuscular blockade is achieved by inhibition of acetylcholine at the neuromuscular junction. Succinylcholine is the only *de*polarizing *non*competitive inhibitor used clinically. Notorious potential side effects of its usage include malignant hyperthermia, dysrhythmias, bradycardia, and *hyper*kalemia. Unlike other (competitive, nondepolarizing) muscle relaxants, succinylcholine cannot be reversed. However, its effects are short-acting (~5 minutes) because it is rapidly hydrolyzed by plasma cholinesterase.

47-2. E. Acetylcysteine (sometimes referred to as *N*-acetylcysteine or Mucomyst) is used to treat acetaminophen toxicity. Naloxone (Narcan) is used to reverse opiate overdose. Prochlorperazine (Compazine) and metoclopramide (Reglan) are used primarily as antiemetics. Reglan is also a promotility agent.

47-3. D. Retrospective studies have shown that the incidence of reinfarction following MI (or acute coronary syndrome, ACS), appears to stabilize after 6 months. The highest rate of reinfarction is within the first 3 months after the cardiac event (Table 47-1).

TABLE 47-1 Rates of Reinfarction

Age of MI (MO)	Rate of Reinfarction (%)
0–3	5.8
3–6	2.3
7–12	1

47-4. B. Analysis of the "Goldman criteria" allows for an assessment of a patient's perioperative cardiac risk. Each of the criteria is assigned a point value; the total number of points a patient has determines his risk. The identified risk factors are listed in Tables 47-2 and 47-3.

TABLE 47-2 The Goldman Criteria

Criterion	Points
S_3 gallop or jugular venous distension on preoperative examination	11
Transmural or subendocardial MI in previous 6 months	10
Premature ventricular contractions, >5 beats/min documented at any time	7
Rhythm other than sinus or premature atrial contractions	5
Age >70 years	4
Emergency operation	3
Intrathoracic, intraperitoneal, or aortic site of surgery	3
Evidence for valvular aortic stenosis	3
Poor general medical condition	3

TABLE 47-3 Patient Risk Based on Goldman Criteria

Total Points	Risk of Cardiac Complications (%)	Risk of Death (%)
0–5	0.7	0.2
6–12	5	2
13–25	11	2
26	22	5

ADDITIONAL SUGGESTED READING

Pedersen T, Dyrlund Pedersen B, Moller AM. Pulse oximetry for perioperative monitoring. Cochrane Database Syst Rev 2003; 3:CD002013.

Watson CB. Respiratory complications associated with anesthesia. Anesthesiol Clin North America 2002;20:513–537.

Postoperative Fever

CC: Postoperative fever.

HPI: A 52-year-old obese woman undergoes a laparoscopic cholecystectomy for acute cholecystitis. Sequential compression devices are placed on her legs preoperatively, per routine. Intraoperatively, there is significant bleeding from the liver bed. The case is converted to an open cholecystectomy, and the bleeding is easily controlled. There are no other events. Postop, she is kept NPO and placed on twice daily heparin injections for DVT prophylaxis. On the evening of postoperative day 1, she develops a fever to 38.6°C.

THOUGHT QUESTION

- What are your thoughts about this fever?
- Do you draw blood cultures?

DISCUSSION

A mild to moderate fever occurring within the first 48 hours postoperatively is generally attributed to atelectasis and should be treated symptomatically. No blood cultures are indicated. However, a patient with very high fever (i.e., ≥39°C) or significant incisional pain should be examined for necrotizing soft tissue infection by checking the wound for erythema, crepitus, or unusual drainage. Such infections acquired in the operative setting tend to assert themselves very quickly and can lead to sepsis and death if unrecognized. The bacteria most commonly involved include *Clostridia*, *Staphylococcus*, and *Streptococcus*.

CASE CONTINUED

PMHx: Diabetes, obesity, and CAD

PSHx: as in HPI

Meds: Insulin, atorvastatin

All: NKDA

SHx: Smokes 1 ppd (30 pyh), no alcohol or other drugs

The patient defervesces, and you continue to await her return of bowel function and overall strength. She complains of abdominal pain and refuses to get out of bed. She makes feeble attempts with her incentive spirometer, taking only shallow breaths. Her wound is clean and dry. Although her initial postoperative fever had resolved by postoperative day 2, on postoperative day 5 she spikes a temperature of 38.7°C and complains of L calf pain and swelling.

THOUGHT QUESTION

- What are your thoughts about this fever?
- Do you draw blood cultures?
- What do you think of her calf pain? How will you evaluate it?

DISCUSSION

The general practice is to perform a workup for any fever that occurs outside of the initial 48-hour postoperative window. This includes urinalysis, blood cultures, CXR, and possibly a CBC if none has been drawn recently. The wound should also be checked for signs of infection. The patient's complaint of calf pain may be an indicator of DVT or of muscle cramps from inactivity or hypokalemia. Calf pain from DVT can often be elicited with passive stretch (*Homan's sign*), although this is not a sensitive or specific finding (~50%). With DVT, the involved lower extremity may be swollen and blanched (*phlegmasia alba dolens*) compared with the contralateral side. After physical examination, evaluation for DVT should continue with a lower extremity *ultrasound* (US). Ultrasound signs of DVT are presence of thrombus, inability to compress the vein, and abnormal blood flow patterns. Duplex US has a 90% sensitivity and specificity compared with the historic and now rarely performed gold standard, contrast phlebography.

CASE CONTINUED

Labs: WBC 12 (no left shift), Hct 38, Plts 234. *Blood cultures:* Pending. *Urinalysis:* 0 to 5 WBC, 0 to 5 RBC, leukocyte esterase neg, nitrite neg.

Imaging: *CXR:* Bibasilar atelectasis, no infiltrates or edema, no effusion. *Lower extremity duplex scan:* L common femoral vein thrombosis.

THOUGHT QUESTION

- How and for how long will you treat these findings? What parameters will you use?

CASE CONTINUED

The patient is started on a heparin drip, her subcutaneous heparin injections are discontinued, and an oral anticoagulant (warfarin) is also begun. The heparin drip should be adjusted so that the PTT is 1.5–2.5 times the normal range within the first 24 hours of treatment. When the INR is therapeutic (goal 2.0–3.0), the heparin drip can be stopped. Subcutaneous low molecular weight heparin injections (i.e. enoxaparin 1 mg/kg BID) can be used in lieu of an unfractionated heparin drip. This may allow the stable patient to be discharged to home prior to reaching an acceptable INR. Anticoagulation therapy is continued for at least 6 weeks.

QUESTIONS

48-1. Which of the following is a risk factor for DVT?
   A. Age <40 years.
   B. Recent weight loss.
   C. Female sex.
   D. Operation >2 hours.
   E. Nulliparity.

48-2. Treatment of DVT in a patient with a contraindication to anticoagulation (e.g., fall risk, hemorrhagic stroke) might include
  A. Vein stripping.
  B. Hyperbaric oxygen.
  C. Placement of vena caval filter.
  D. Venous bypass.
  E. Venous thrombotripsy.

48-3. The most common causes of fever in the postoperative period are UTI, pneumonia, wound infection, DVT, and
  A. Iatrogenic overheating.
  B. Miscalibrated thermometers.
  C. *C. difficile* infection.
  D. Sinusitis.
  E. Drug reaction.

48-4. Regarding pulmonary embolism
  A. Symptoms and signs include dyspnea, anxiety, chest pain, cough, fever, and pleural friction rub.
  B. Findings include decreased central venous and PA pressure and bradycardia.
  C. Most originate from a DVT of the upper extremities.
  D. Lung perfusion scan is the gold standard for diagnosis.
  E. ECG shows inverted T waves.

ANSWERS

48-1. D. Other risk factors for DVT include male sex, age >40 years, obesity, drug use, previous history of DVT or pulmonary embolism, malignancy, use of oral contraceptives, pregnancy, nephrotic syndrome, lupus anticoagulant, inherited coagulation disorders, and smoking. The physiologic explanation for the development of DVT is embodied by *Virchow's triad*—stasis, hypercoagulability, and endothelial injury. Any two of these three are sufficient to cause DVT; the postoperative state involves both stasis and hypercoagulability (because of release of tissue factor during surgery).

DVT prophylaxis should begin in the operating room when thrombus is the most likely to form. It generally consists of sequential compression devices placed on the legs. Concerns for intra- and postoperative bleeding limit the use of heparin in the immediate perioperative period. Postoperatively, the sequential compression devices can be continued, although it is often more productive (and less uncomfortable) for the patient to walk several times a day. Alternatively, subcutaneous heparin injections can be given. Special consideration for using more than one form of DVT prophylaxis should be given to patients at high risk for DVT (age >40 with obesity, malignancy, trauma, or previous DVT/pulmonary embolism) or with more than one of the general risk factors.

48-2. C. Heparin is the initial first choice for treatment of DVT, because it inhibits thrombin and thromboplastin, and prevents further platelet aggregation and granule release. Fibrinolysis can be performed in a catheter-directed fashion, or systemically with an attendant risk of hemorrhagic complications. Surgical thrombectomy is indicated primarily in cases of *phlegmasia cerulea dolens*, where venous hypertension (from severe venous congestion, causing the extremity to appear "bluish") impairs arterial flow, leading to limb ischemia. Venous bypass, vein stripping, hyperbaric oxygen, and thrombotripsy are not options for treatment of DVT. Insertion of a vena caval filter is useful when anticoagulation is contraindicated, results in complications, or fails to prevent recurrent thromboembolism.

48-3. E. The mnemonic used to recall the most common causes of postoperative fevers is the "5 Ws": wind (atelectasis, 24 to 48 hours postoperatively), water (UTI, 3 to 5 days), wound (cellulitis for early fever, 24 to 72 hours; abscess for late fever, 5 to 10 days), walking (DVT, 3 to 5 days), and wonder drugs (drug reaction, seen within 24 hours of drug administration).

48-4. A. Hemoptysis is also a symptom that can be associated with pulmonary embolism, but it is a late finding and generally represents pulmonary infarction. The degree of pulmonary hypertension is usually proportional to the extent of pulmonary vascular occlusion—the result is an *increase* in central venous and PA pressures (RV overload). The most common ECG findings in pulmonary embolism are right bundle branch block and RV strain. The classic description of an S1-Q3-T3 pattern is seen in only 10%. ABG findings reflect hypoxia (Pao_2 <60) and *hypo*carbia ($Paco_2$ <30, secondary to tachypnea). When definitively positive or negative, *lung perfusion scans* can be diagnostic; however, scans are frequently equivocal because small perfusion defects can be seen with atelectasis, chronic lung or cardiac disease (pneumonitis, CHF, etc.), or pneumonia. *Echocardiography* can be performed at the bedside to quickly evaluate for RV overload, but pulmonary arteriography remains the gold standard for diagnostic imaging of pulmonary embolism. Modern *spiral CTs*, which are high speed/high definition scans, are considered very accurate and can usually be performed more safely and expeditiously than an arteriogram. Spiral CT has largely replaced arteriography in the diagnosis of PE. In most cases, the diagnosis is made using a combination of clinical picture and one or more of the previously mentioned studies.

ADDITIONAL SUGGESTED READING

Badillo AT, Sarani B, Evans SR. Optimizing the use of blood cultures in the febrile postoperative patient. J Am Coll Surg 2002;194:477–487.

Vascular Access

CC: Intubated and obtunded in the ICU.

HPI: Mr. X is a 59-year-old man who had a four-vessel CABG performed 3 days ago. Unfortunately, he suffered a massive stroke perioperatively and remains intubated for altered mental status and airway protection. He is on low dose dopamine, an H_2-receptor blocker, amiodarone, and Lasix. Current IV access is via a R internal jugular introducer sheath (i.e., "Cordis" catheter).

PMHx: Stable angina, HTN

PSHx: None

All: NKDA

THOUGHT QUESTION

- What should you think about when assessing a patient's vascular access needs?
- What additional issues are particularly relevant in the ICU setting?

DISCUSSION

Expected needs for monitoring and interventions will determine the type of vascular access a patient should have. Continuous blood pressure monitoring is accomplished with an arterial line, whereas monitoring of central venous or pulmonary artery pressures will require central venous access. Ease of blood draws should not be the sole reason for placement of central venous or arterial lines. Depending on the clinical situation, long-term venous access may be necessary (e.g., chemotherapy, TPN, hemodialysis, long-term antibiotics), and tunneled catheters or peripherally inserted central venous catheters can be placed. Peripheral intravenous lines are a safe, rapid, and common means of obtaining vascular access. In emergency situations, short, large-bore (i.e., 14 to 16 gauge), peripheral IVs are adequate for resuscitation and, in fact, allow a more rapid flow rate than a typical triple lumen central venous line (as predicted by *Poiseuille's law*, where flow is proportional to $1/r^4$).

Gastrointestinal prophylaxis is an additional issue important to consider in critical care patients, because *stress ulceration* is present in 90% of patients by the third day of an ICU admission. Stress ulcers are superficial, often asymptomatic erosions of the gastric mucosa, distinct from peptic ulcers. The primary cause is believed to be impaired blood flow rather than gastric acidity. However, antiulcer medications, which target acid secretion, and sucralfate, which provides a protective coating to the mucosal lining, are standard GI prophylactic measures. Other concerns when managing an ICU patient are DVT prophylaxis, analgesia and sedation (for patient comfort), and nutrition.

 CASE CONTINUED

The central line needs to be removed because, although the patient remains afebrile, erythema is noted at the skin site. You are asked by the cardiologist to replace the central line so that she can continue the IV medications and start *total parenteral nutrition* (TPN).

THOUGHT QUESTION

- What are the different options for nutritional support in this patient who is unable to take POs?
- What are the indications for TPN?
- Do you agree with replacing the central line?

DISCUSSION

In patients with a functional gastrointestinal tract, enteral feeding is the most efficient and safest means of meeting their nutritional needs. It maintains intestinal integrity against bacterial invasion (*translocation*) by preventing intestinal epithelial disruption and atrophy, which occurs when nutrients (particularly *glutamine*) are absent from the bowel lumen. For longer term enteral nutrition, a gastrostomy or jejunostomy can be placed. For short-term nutrition, a temporary feeding tube can be placed through the nose into either the stomach or duodenum. Controversy exists as to whether or not enteral feeding into the duodenum decreases the risk of aspiration compared to gastric feeding.

If the patient requires extended (>7 days) bowel rest or if the patient is in shock, enteral feeding is inappropriate and parenteral nutrition is the only alternative. As with most IVFs, dextrose is the source of carbohydrate in these parenteral formulas. However, high concentrations are required in order to provide adequate calories, resulting in hyperosmolar solutions, referred to as TPN. TPN is always infused into the central veins because these hyperosmolar solutions are strong irritants to small peripheral veins. If central venous access is not possible, *peripheral parenteral nutrition* (PPN) can be given but with limited caloric content. PPN relies on fat emulsion (composed of soy or safflower oil) rather than carbohydrates as the primary caloric source and is considered protein-sparing nutritional support, because it provides just enough calories to avoid protein (i.e., muscle) breakdown but not enough for protein storage. PPN is intended only for short-term support of nonhypercatabolic, nonprotein-depleted patients.

This patient has a functional GI tract and can be given most of his medications enterally. If the dopamine is not being used for blood pressure support, this patient has no absolute indications for a central line. Because central line placement is not risk free, you should consider recommending feeding tube placement instead.

QUESTIONS

49-1. Complications of vascular access procedures include
   A. Radial artery occlusion in up to 75% of radial artery cannulations.
   B. Subclavian vein thrombosis in 20%.
   C. Thoracic duct injury in central line placement.
   D. Carotid artery puncture in 20% to 30% of attempted internal jugular vein cannulations.
   E. Femoral venous thrombosis in 40% of femoral venous lines.

49-2. The nutritional needs and energy requirements of the critically ill patient
   A. Decrease as the severity of illness increases.
   B. Tend to result in a positive nitrogen balance.
   C. Can be altered to affect respiratory function.
   D. Do not impact overall hospital length of stay.
   E. Are met equally by fats, proteins, and carbohydrates.

49-3. Regarding enteral feeding
   A. Hypertonic formulas should be infused into the duodenum.
   B. Small peptides are absorbed more slowly than intact proteins.
   C. Lipid content is usually limited to 50% total calories.
   D. Fiber is added to decrease diarrhea.
   E. Short chain fatty acids are beneficial in patients with hepatic encephalopathy.

49-4. Patients receiving total parenteral nutrition (TPN) need to be monitored for the development of
   A. Acalculous cholecystitis.
   B. Hypocarbia.
   C. Hypoglycemia.
   D. Splenic thrombosis.
   E. Hypercoagulability

ANSWERS

49-1. C. Radial artery occlusion occurs in up to 25% of radial artery cannulations. Carotid artery punctures occur in 2-10% of internal jugular cannulations. Venous thrombosis of the femoral vein occurs in <10% of femoral lines. Subclavian vein thrombosis is even more uncommon (3%) and is treated with catheter removal. Heparin infusion can be initiated. Although pulmonary embolism from upper extremity vein thrombosis is uncommon (10%), anticoagulation should be initiated and continued for 6 weeks to 3 months. Catheter-associated infections tend to occur in lines that have been in place longer than 3 days. Contrary to popular belief, the evidence has *not* shown that infection occurs more often with lines in the femoral position than the subclavian or internal jugular sites.

49-2. C. Proteolysis occurs in skeletal muscle and organs such as the liver and intestine, leading to a net *negative* nitrogen balance. Therefore, nitrogen requirements in catabolic patients are *increased*. Healthy adults tend to maintain a zero nitrogen balance, or nitrogen equilibrium. Metabolic rate can be estimated by calculating the *basal energy expenditure*, or BEE (kcal/day) = 25 × wt (in kg). Depending on the severity of the physiologic stressor, hypermetabolic states require increased energy expenditure (e.g., fever increases BEE by 10% per degree C increase).

Respiratory quotient (RQ) = CO_2 production/O_2 consumption. The *RQ* for each source of energy is as follows: lipid 0.7, protein 0.8, and glucose 1.0. These values reflect a greater production of CO_2 relative to O_2 consumption for carbohydrates as compared with lipids or proteins. Thus, a patient receiving most of her calories in the form of carbohydrates may be more prone to hypercapnia if she has respiratory dysfunction. Actually, excess calories from any source can result in elevated CO_2 production. This knowledge is sometimes manipulated in trying to wean a patient from mechanical ventilation. Protein-depleted patients have longer hospital stays, possibly related to impaired respiratory muscle strength and a resultant increased incidence of postoperative pneumonia.

49-3. D. Hypertonic formulas should be infused into the stomach because the gastric secretions help dilute and decrease the osmolality. In patients with impaired absorption (e.g., inflammatory bowel disease), use of formulas providing small peptides rather than intact protein can facilitate nutrient absorption and water *re*absorption (thus decreasing diarrhea). Formulas enriched with *branched chain amino acids* are useful in trauma patients (to provide an energy source for skeletal muscle and decrease muscle breakdown) and in hepatic encephalopathy (to antagonize uptake of aromatic amino acids, which can be metabolized into false neurotransmitters). Formula lipid content is usually limited to 30% of total calories because excessive fat ingestion can result in a malabsorptive diarrhea. However, in respiratory failure, the fat content can be increased up to 55% to minimize both metabolic CO_2 production (the RQ is 0.7 for lipids) and the potential for CO_2 retention, which is common with pulmonary dysfunction. In addition to reducing both osmotic and watery diarrhea, fiber can act as a supplemental source of nutrition for the colonic mucosa.

49-4. C. TPN administration requires frequent monitoring of electrolytes and other factors to optimize metabolic homeostasis and to detect complications. Glucose *in*tolerance is a common complication of TPN and may require the addition of insulin to the solution. An average of 20% to 30% of the added insulin is adsorbed to the plastic and glassware of the IV infusion apparatus, so the amount of insulin required is usually artificially elevated.

Oxidant-induced cellular injury is associated with lipid infusions and can lead to impaired oxygenation. CO_2 *retention* is common. *Decreased* production of coagulation factors by the liver results from a deficiency of vitamin K, which is normally provided in the diet or produced by intestinal bacteria.

ADDITIONAL SUGGESTED READINGS

Andrews P, Azoulay E, Antonelli M, et al. Year in review in intensive care medicine, 2004. II. Brain injury, hemodynamic monitoring and treatment, pulmonary embolism, gastrointestinal tract, and renal failure. Int Care Med. 2005;31(2):177–88.

De-Souza DA, Greene LJ. Intestinal permeability and systemic infections in critically ill patients: effect of glutamine. Crit Care Med 2005;33(5):1125–35.

Dhaliwal R, Jurewitsch B, Harrietha D, et al. Combination enteral and parenteral nutrition in critically ill patients: harmful or beneficial? A systematic review of the evidence. Intensive Care Med 2004;30(8):1666–1671.

Marik PE, Zaloga GP. Gastric versus post-pyloric feeding: a systematic review. Crit Care 2003;7(3):46–51.

VIII

Miscellaneous
Patient
Presentations

CASE **50**

Skin Lesion

CC/ID: 62-year-old woman with "age spots."

HPI: The patient is referred to you because of an irregular skin lesion on her left forearm. She also has complaints of left arm fatigue. She tells you she does not quite know why she is in your office, because she has spots all over her body and the one on her arm is no different. She is a native Californian and has spent much of her life in the sun, generally without the use of sunscreen. She does not know of any other irregular or suspicious skin spots. She denies any pain or paresthesias in the concerned limb. She has no other systemic complaints.

PMHx: Reflux disease, hyperlipidemia

PSHx: Removal of a benign back mole

Meds: Ranitidine, lovastatin, ASA

THOUGHT QUESTION

- What criteria are used to describe a skin lesion as "irregular"?
- What will you expect to find on examination?
- What steps will you go through to determine this patient's diagnosis?
- Why might she be having arm symptoms?
- Is there anything else you want to know before proceeding?

DISCUSSION

In this patient, it is likely that her skin lesion meets criteria for possible malignancy—the "ABCs" of skin cancer: <u>a</u>symmetry (irregular or raised), <u>b</u>order (dark or inhomogeneous), <u>c</u>olor (i.e., increased), diameter (i.e., >6 mm), and (progressive) enlargement. Other characteristics may include ulcerations, rolled edges, and scaling. Generally, management of extremity lesions is aided by tissue diagnosis. In most cases, a punch or core biopsy (performed in the office) can give the necessary histologic information. For some large or deep lesions, incisional or excisional biopsy may be planned.

The patient's arm fatigue may be from any number of sources, including trauma, overuse, arthritis/arthralgias, or nerve damage resulting from drugs, systemic medical conditions (such as diabetes), or possibly impingement on the brachial plexus by tumor or some other anatomic abnormality. It will be helpful to further characterize these symptoms and to determine whether she has focal/nerve root deficits or paresthesias.

In addition to filling in the history of her arm symptoms and sun exposure, it may be helpful to know about other exposures, possible skin irritants (including new skin care products, detergents, etc.), and family h/o dysplastic nevi or skin cancer. If the patient has awareness of a suspicious skin lesion, a time line regarding size, growth, pain, and so on may be useful to obtain.

CASE CONTINUED

The patient states that her arm just feels "kind of heavy" but that she has not noticed any other specific features. She has no known reason to be immunocompromised. She denies any family h/o melanoma or other skin disorders.

VS: AVSS

PE: *Gen:* Fair-skinned, lively, active-appearing woman appearing her stated age, in no distress. *Neck:* No lymphadenopathy. *Chest:* Clear. *Ext:* Visibly enlarged left arm as compared with the right; measurement of the diameter around the upper arm shows the circumference on the left to be 1.5 cm greater than on the right. All four extremities move without difficulty. She has multiple macular 2- to 4-mm areas of hyperpigmentation over both arms, but has a notably larger irregular macular lesion on the dorsal side of her L forearm, measuring approximately 10 to 12 mm in greatest diameter. It has heterogeneous pigmentation, and is nonulcerated and nontender to palpation. You also notice another smaller (5 mm to 6 mm) unevenly colored lesion on the lateral part of her upper L arm. *Axillae:* No palpable masses on the R;

multiple small nodules on the L, with one large dominant ~1-cm palpable mass. *Neuro:* Minimally decreased strength on the L versus R arm (patient is R-hand dominant); otherwise nonfocal. *Skin:* Multiple "sun spots" with scattered cherry angiomata. No other suspicious lesions.

You biopsy the two suspicious lesions on the patient's L arm and perform an FNA of the palpable axillary lymph node. Both punch biopsies return with a diagnosis of superficial spreading melanoma, Clark level IV/Breslow thickness 2 mm. Cytology on the lymph node returns positive for melanoma.

You diagnose the patient with stage III melanoma. She subsequently undergoes wide excision of the two cutaneous lesions and a left axillary node dissection.

 QUESTIONS

50-1. Regarding melanoma classification,
A. Clark levels refer to absolute depth of tumor invasion, whereas Breslow levels refer to anatomic planes.
B. Tumor depth (thickness) is inversely related to patient survival.
C. Tumors less than 4 mm deep have a >90% cure rate.
D. Tumors greater than 4 mm deep have a 20% chance of having distant disease.
E. Patients with metastatic disease have a 70% chance of survival at 5 years.

50-2. Basal cell carcinoma
A. Is the second most common form of skin cancer.
B. Is predominantly caused by excess UV-A radiation from sunlight.
C. Is divided into three histologic types: noduloulcerative, superficial, and sclerosing.
D. Requires systemic chemotherapy for adequate treatment.
E. Is most prevalent in the Asian population.

50-3. Which of the following exposures is a risk factor for developing squamous cell carcinoma of the skin?
A. Epstein-Barr virus.
B. Human papilloma virus.
C. Cytomegalovirus.
D. Varicella zoster virus.
E. Poliovirus.

50-4. The advantage of standard wide excision over Mohs micrographic surgery is
- A. Better cosmetic outcome.
- B. The ability to excise positive margins in a carefully directed manner.
- C. Decreased need for reoperation.
- D. Applicability to nonmelanoma skin cancers.
- E. Shorter operative time.

ANSWERS

50-1. B. Breslow Thickness Scale values refer to tumor thickness, whereas Clark Levels of Tumor Invasion use anatomic descriptors (Fig. 50-1). The thicker the tumor, the lower the survival rate. Tumors less than 0.76 mm have a greater than 90% cure rate after simple excision; tumors >4.0 mm have a <70% chance of 5-year survival and a greater than 80% risk of having distant disease. Patients with positive lymph nodes have a 13–69% chance of 5-year survival. Ulceration significantly reduces survival at each tumor stage (Table 50-1).

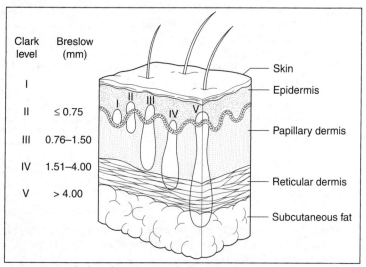

FIGURE 50-1. Clark and Breslow levels for melanoma. Note that Clark levels are based on anatomic planes, whereas Breslow levels are measurement based. A rough correlation between the two is shown. (*Illustration by Electronic Illustrators Group.*)

TABLE 50-1 American Joint Commission on Cancer (AJCC) Staging

Stage	Tnm	Breslow (MM) (Preferred)	Clark's Level	5-year Survival (%)
I	$T_1N_0M_0$	<0.75	II	90
	$T_2N_0M_0$	0.76–1.50	III	
II	$T_3N_0M_0$	1.51–4.0	IV	70
	$T_4N_0M_0$	>4.0	V	
III	Any T, N_1M_0			50
IV	Any T, any N, M_1			20

50-2. C. Basal cell carcinoma is the most common form of skin cancer and is most prevalent in the white population. The predominant etiology is excess exposure to ultraviolet B radiation; as such, tumors tend to arise from sun-exposed skin, especially on the head and neck. The three categories of basal cell carcinoma are noduloulcerative (most common), superficial, and sclerosing. Complete surgical excision is the standard of care for treatment of basal cell carcinoma, although there is evidence to suggest that *topical* chemotherapy with 5-FU, cryosurgery, and cautery/curettage may offer similar cure rates.

50-3. B. Human papilloma virus types 16, 18, 31, 33, and 35 have all been implicated in the development of squamous cell carcinoma. Other risk factors include sunlight exposure, immunosuppression/immunocompromise, chronic ulcers, ionizing radiation, tobacco use, and scars.

50-4. E. Mohs micrographic surgery is usually applied to nonmelanoma skin cancers, though its use in melanoma has been described. The technique involves removal of all gross tumor, followed by excision of a thin layer of tissue 2- to 3-mm deep and with 2- to 3-mm lateral margins. The tissue is carefully mapped, and frozen sections are performed. In this way, precise anatomic location of any residual tumor can be identified and re-excised until all margins are tumor free. Though the Mohs procedure takes longer to perform, it has multiple other benefits (including a low recurrence rate), making it an important operative technique.

📖 *ADDITIONAL SUGGESTED READING*

Abbasi NR, Shaw HM, Rigel DS, et al. Early diagnosis of cutaneous melanoma: revisiting the ABCD criteria. JAMA 2004;292: 2771–2776.

Balch CM, Buzaid AC, Soong SJ, et al. Final version of the American Joint Committee on Cancer staging system for cutaneous melanoma. J Clin Oncol 2001;19:3635–3648.

Lang PG Jr. The role of Mohs' micrographic surgery in the management of skin cancer and a perspective on the management of the surgical defect. Clin Plast Surg 2004;31:5–31.

Thomas JM, Newton-Bishop J, A'Hern R, et al: Excision margins in high-risk malignant melanoma. N Engl J Med 2004;350:757–766.

Bone Pain After Football

CC: Shin pain, fever, and fatigue × 4 days.

HPI: The patient is a healthy 17-year-old man who reports a dull ache in his L shin that has been worsening for the past 4 days. He has also felt feverish and tired. Two weeks ago, he fell and scraped his L leg while playing touch football, but the wound had healed without problems. He recalls no other recent trauma to the area.

PMHx: None

PSHx: None

Meds: None

All: NKDA

SHx: Noncontributory

THOUGHT QUESTION

- What is in your differential diagnosis?
- What imaging studies and lab tests would be useful?

DISCUSSION

Although the association with fever and recent trauma is suggestive of an infectious process (e.g., infected hematoma or bursitis), one must also consider malignancy with inflammation. A CBC, ESR, LFTs (particularly alkaline phosphatase), and blood cultures are important in distinguishing between infectious and noninfectious sources of bony pain. Joint swelling or effusions may prompt evaluation with needle aspiration (*arthrocentesis*). *Plain films* can be an initial screening study for bony destruction (seen as cortical lucencies) and periosteal reaction, though bony changes may not be evident for

14–21 days. Unfortunately, these findings are nonspecific (for infection versus malignancy), and would require further evaluation with either *CT, MRI,* or nuclear *bone scan* to clarify the diagnosis.

CASE CONTINUED

VS: Temp 38.5°C, HR 72, BP 124/64

PE: *Gen:* WD/WN man in no acute distress. *Abdomen:* Soft, NT/ND, no hepatosplenomegaly. *Ext:* L anterior mid-shin with 4 × 7-cm area of erythema and tenderness; no fluctuance or underlying mass; no inguinal lymphadenopathy; L knee with slight swelling, no erythema, nontender, full range of motion; R lower extremity WNL.

Labs:

$$13\text{———}389$$
$$45$$

AST/ALT 41/38
Tbili 0.9
Alk phos 69
ESR 112

Blood cultures and L knee fluid aspiration negative for organisms.

Imaging: *L tib-fib XR:* no sclerosis, no osteolytic lesions, no fracture; possible periosteal elevation in the anterior tibia

Bone scan: focal area of increased activity in the mid tibia

THOUGHT QUESTION

- Given these findings, what is your diagnosis?
- What is your plan for treatment?

DISCUSSION

In this case, the data and physical examination are consistent with osteomyelitis. An elevated sedimentation rate (ESR) is seen in 90% of cases. The WBC is usually normal or slightly elevated. Focal hyperfusion, hyperemia, and increased bony uptake of radiotracer on bone scan are diagnostic findings if there is no evidence of fracture. This is usually a disease of children and adolescents, but it can also occur in immunocompromised patients and diabetics. Trauma is often a precursor, with direct inoculation of bacteria to the bone. However, infection can also occur as a result of hematogenous spread from a remote source. *S. aureus* is the most common organism, though the pathogen may vary depending on the patient's age and mechanism of infection. Treatment involves long-term (>4–6 weeks) IV antibiotics and surgical debridement or drainage if an abscess has formed. If a mass lesion had been found, an incisional biopsy would have been indicated for tissue diagnosis.

QUESTIONS

51-1. Which of the following is a potential complication of acute osteomyelitis?
A. Chronic osteomyelitis.
B. Motor neuropathy.
C. Distal paresthesia.
D. Phantom limb pain.
E. Proprioceptive loss.

51-2. Which of the following disease states predisposes patients to osteomyelitis?
A. Hepatitis.
B. Coronary artery disease.
C. Sickle cell disease.
D. COPD.
E. Acromegaly.

51-3. Paget's disease of the bone involves
A. Femoral bowing.
B. A decrease in hat size.
C. A decrease in alkaline phosphatase levels.
D. Osteoclastic bony destruction.
E. Treatment with cytotoxic agents.

51-4. Current standard treatment of bone tumors includes
A. Hormone therapy.
B. Laser eradication.
C. Radiation therapy.
D. Immunotherapy.
E. Heated limb perfusion.

ANSWERS

51-1. A. Complications of acute osteomyelitis include septic arthritis, growth plate disturbance, pathologic fracture, bone abscess, bacteremia, cellulitis, and chronic osteomyelitis. *Chronic osteomyelitis* results when infection persists in a necrotic nidus of bone, or the sequestrum. A chronic draining sinus tract is often present. To fully treat the infection, the sequestrum must be removed. Free flap placement is often necessary to fill the dead space resulting from bone and soft tissue loss and to increase local blood supply. Neuropathy, distal paresthesias, and proprioceptive loss are not complications of acute osteomyelitis, as nerves are seldom involved. Phantom pain is sometimes seen following amputation.

51-2. C. Patients that seem to be at higher risk for osteomyelitis include those with sickle cell disease, diabetes, AIDS, IV drug abuse, alcoholism, immunosuppression, chronic joint disease, chronic steroid use, orthopedic prostheses, recent surgery, and open fractures. The bacteria seen in osteomyelitis vary according to the underlying disease or source of infection: for instance, osteomyelitis in IV drug abusers most often involves gram-negative organisms such as *Pseudomonas*. Sickle cell disease is frequently associated with *Salmonella* or *S. aureus*. Wounds that occur through an athletic shoe are more likely to be *Pseudomonas* or *S. aureus*. Children less than 4 years of age are more likely to be infected by *H. influenza*, *Enterobacter*, or *Streptococcus*.

51-3. D. Paget's disease of the bone usually involves *tibial* bowing. Sensorineural hearing loss, bone pain, and increased hat size are presenting symptoms. Alkaline phosphatase is markedly elevated due to bone destruction. Mild disease is treated with NSAIDs alone, whereas severe disease can be treated with calcitonin or bisphosphonates. Complications of Paget's disease include pathologic fractures, osteosarcoma, and high-output cardiac failure.

51-4. C. Seventy percent of bony tumors are metastatic. Among primary bone tumors, the most common is *osteosarcoma*. These tend to occur in the distal femur or proximal tibia, or at the metaphyseal ends of the bone. Preoperative (neoadjuvant) chemotherapy increases the number of patients who are able to undergo a limb-sparing operation rather than amputation. Postoperative chemotherapy has been shown to prevent recurrence and improve overall survival (up to 80% at 5 years) in patients with resectable primary tumors. Radiation therapy is useful for local control. There does not seem to be any difference in survival between patients treated with limb-sparing operation versus amputation. Isolated heated limb perfusion is a means of delivering chemotherapeutic drugs directly to an affected extremity, minimizing systemic exposure. It is used primarily in the treatment of melanoma.

ADDITIONAL SUGGESTED READING

Buhne KH, Bohndorf K. Imaging of posttraumatic osteomyelitis. Semin Musculoskelet Radiol 2004;8:199–204.

Gutierrez K. Bone and joint infections in children. Pediatr Clin North Am 2005;52:779–794.

Lazzarini L, Lipsky BA, Mader JT. Antibiotic treatment of osteomyelitis: what have we learned from 30 years of clinical trials? Int J Infect Dis 2005;9:127–138.

Lew DP, Waldvogel FA. Osteomyelitis. Lancet 2004;364:369–379.

Santiago Restrepo C, Gimenez CR, McCarthy K. Imaging of osteomyelitis and musculoskeletal soft tissue infections: current concepts. Rheum Dis Clin North Am 2003;29:89–109.

CASE 52

Incidental Hypercalcemia

CC/ID: 45-year-old woman with hypercalcemia.

HPI: The patient presents to your office following a recent episode of renal colic. She had been seen in the ED with severe flank pain and subsequently passed a kidney stone. Labs drawn were unremarkable except for an elevated serum calcium of 13.5 mg/dL. It was suggested she have this finding followed up on an outpatient basis.

The patient goes on to tell you she has had a few episodes of similar flank pain in the past, but that this had been the worst she could remember. She does sometimes have nonspecific abdominal pain that is usually self-limited, but otherwise describes herself as "perfectly healthy." She has no other complaints.

THOUGHT QUESTION

- What are common causes of hypercalcemia?
- What symptoms are related to hypercalcemia?
- How high or low does the serum calcium need to be in order to experience symptoms?

DISCUSSION

Causes of hypercalcemia include endocrine disorders (hyperparathyroidism, hyperthyroidism, adrenal insufficiency, pheochromocytoma); drug-induced disorders (vitamin D toxicity, thiazide diuretics, lithium toxicity, milk alkali syndrome); malignancy (especially multiple myeloma; solid tumors, which produce parathyroid hormone-related protein; and lymphoma, which causes excess vitamin D production); granulomatous disease (sarcoid, tuberculosis, histoplasmosis, coccidioidomycosis, leprosy); idiopathic disorders such as familial hypocalciuric hypercalcemia; and immobilization. A good history will rule out many of these causes.

The classic constellation of findings in hypercalcemia is "stones, bones, groans, moans, and psychic overtones"—that is, renal calculi, aches and arthralgias, assorted gastrointestinal complaints including nausea and vomiting, and behavioral changes. Because these complaints are so nonspecific, they can be easily missed if not specifically elicited. Any change in calcium homeostasis can lead to symptoms; this explains why hypercalcemic patients who subsequently undergo parathyroidectomy may experience signs of *hypo*calcemia (e.g., Chvostek's or Trousseau's signs) when an elevated calcium drops to normal range. Therefore, there are no absolute calcium values which can predict onset of symptoms.

CASE CONTINUED

PMHx: Prior h/o renal stones

PSHx: appy ~20 years ago

Meds: Occasional antacids for stomach upset

FHx: Negative for multiple endocrine neoplasia, hypercalcemia, or other familial syndromes

ROS: No bone pain, no emotional changes

VS: AVSS

PE: *Gen:* WD/WN woman in no distress. *HEENT:* Anicteric, EOMI, PERRLA. *Neck:* No masses, no enlarged lymph nodes. *Chest:* Clear bilaterally. *Abdomen:* Soft, nontender, nondistended, no masses; well-healed RLQ scar. *Ext:* No clubbing, cyanosis, or edema. No pain or deformity. *Neuro:* Nonfocal.

THOUGHT QUESTION

■ What will be the next step in your evaluation?

DISCUSSION

It is important to look for any correctable causes of hypercalcemia. The patient has no overt signs of tumor (e.g., neck mass, wasting), but this cannot be entirely ruled out. It is possible she has effectively overdosed on her antacids, and a trial of cessation of these may be useful. However, it is necessary to evaluate her parathyroid function. A parathyroid hormone assay and a calcium to phosphate ratio can assist in the diagnosis.

CASE CONTINUED

You order a panel of endocrine function tests and find that her parathyroid hormone (parathormone) level is indeed elevated. In addition, her calcium to phosphate ratio is >33, suggestive of primary hyperparathyroidism. You suspect the patient has a parathyroid adenoma, and because she has had no prior neck surgery, you opt not to do any preoperative localization studies. She undergoes a four-gland parathyroid neck exploration with the finding of a single enlarged gland that is excised. Her postoperative calcium drops to 9, and on subsequent follow-up she notes a marked improvement in her symptoms.

QUESTIONS

52-1. Besides hyperparathyroidism (or parathyroid hyperplasia), what other findings are associated with multiple endocrine neoplasia type 1 (MEN-1)?

    A. Pituitary adenoma and pancreaticoduodenal (neuroendocrine) tumors.

    B. Hyperthyroidism and mucosal neuromas.

    C. Pancreatic tumors and medullary thyroid cancer

    D. Adrenal insufficiency and acromegaly.

    E. Pheochromocytoma and pituitary adenoma.

52-2. Arterial supply to the parathyroid glands is from the left and right

    A. Superior and inferior parathyroid arteries.

    B. Superior thyroid arteries.

    C. Inferior thyroid arteries.

    D. Middle thyroid arteries.

52-3. Which of the following parathyroid localization techniques is most sensitive for detecting parathyroid tumor?
A. Palpation.
B. Ultrasound.
C. Computed tomography (CT) scan.
D. Magnetic resonance imaging (MRI).
E. Nuclear medicine (sestamibi) scan.

52-4. Secondary hyperparathyroidism is seen in patients with
A. Liver disease.
B. Renal disease.
C. Lung disease.
D. Pituitary disease.
E. Pancreatic disease.

ANSWERS

52-1. A. MEN-1 is characterized by parathyroid hyperplasia, pituitary adenomas, and pancreatic (and duodenal) tumors. MEN-2a is characterized by medullary thyroid cancer, parathyroid hyperplasia, and pheochromocytoma. MEN-2b is characterized by medullary thyroid cancer, pheochromocytoma, and mucosal neuromas. Treatment for the hyperparathyroid component of these syndromes involves subtotal (3 1/2-gland) parathyroidectomy, or total (4-gland) parathyroidectomy with autotransplantation. Autotransplantation typically involves placement of 10 to 20 small (1-mm) suture-tagged segments of parathyroid tissue into the sternocleidomastoid or forearm muscles. This allows for continued postoperative calcium homeostasis.

52-2. C. Arterial supply to the parathyroid glands is via the right and left inferior thyroid arteries. Venous drainage is via the inferior thyroid veins. The superior thyroid and esophageal arteries are uninvolved. There is no such thing as a parathyroid or middle thyroid artery.

52-3. E. Sestamibi scan is the best noninvasive localization study for abnormal glands, with a sensitivity of 70% to 90% for solid tumors and a specificity of 77% to 100% (Fig. 52-1). Ultrasound has a 60% sensitivity for finding an ectopic gland at reoperation, with a slightly higher sensitivity at the time of the initial operation. Its utility is very operator-dependent. Selective venous sampling is generally used only when other techniques have failed (including angiography) and has a sensitivity and specificity that varies markedly according to the center performing the study. Other imaging modalities include CT (70% sensitivity initially, 50% to 60% sensitivity at reoperation) and MRI (57% to 90% sensitivity at reoperation). Parathyroid glands are usually NOT palpable, making this method generally unhelpful for localization purposes. The most likely site for an ectopic parathyroid gland is in the thymus.

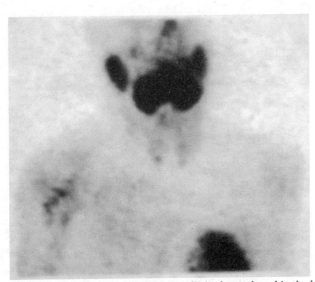

FIGURE 52-1. Note the technetium-99m uptake in the neck and in the heart. Later images should be expected to show some clearing of the tracer from the thyroid, making it easier to identify the increased uptake in the parathyroid adenoma. (*Image provided by Department of Radiology, University of California, San Francisco.*)

52-4. B. *Secondary* hyperparathyroidism is seen in patients with renal failure, where there is calcium wasting and chronic (appropriate) elevations of parathyroid hormone. *Tertiary* hyperparathyroidism is a state of autonomous parathyroid hyperplasia (inappropriate), most commonly described in patients who have undergone renal transplantation but who continue to elaborate excessive amounts of parathyroid hormone.

ADDITIONAL SUGGESTED READING

Inzucchi SE. Management of hypercalcemia. Diagnostic workup, therapeutic options for hyperparathyroidism, and other common causes. Postgrad Med 2004;115:27–36.

Kearns AE, Thompson GB. Medical and surgical management of hyperparathyroidism. Mayo Clin Proc 2002;77:87–91.

Udelsman R. Primary hyperparathyroidism. Curr Treat Options Oncol 2001;2:365–372.

Testicular Pain

 CC/ID: 14-year-old boy with acute onset of testicle pain.

HPI: The patient presents to the ED with an approximately 1-hour history of sharp severe pain in his left testicle. The pain radiates into his lower left abdomen, and he believes the affected testicle is getting larger. He reports that he had a similar pain ~1 year ago, but it was short-lived. He has had no fevers/chills/sweats, nausea, or vomiting. He has not voided since the onset of his symptoms, and so is unable to tell you of any urinary complaints. He denies any h/o trauma and has been feeling otherwise well. He is not sexually active.

PMHx/
PSHx: Negative

Meds: None

All: NKDA

THOUGHT QUESTION

- What is your differential diagnosis for this patient? What will you look for on exam?
- What is your timeframe for coming to a diagnosis?

DISCUSSION

The differential diagnosis of acute scrotum includes testicular torsion, torsion of the testicular appendages, acute epididymo-orchitis, tense hydrocele, and acute incarcerated inguinal hernia. On exam, a torsed testicle will present as a swollen, exquisitely tender, elevated (high-riding) mass in the scrotum. Torsion of the testicular appendages (vestigial remnants of the Müllerian ducts) will present as a tender pea-shaped mass at the head of the epididymis.

Incarcerated hernias may be reducible or may be associated with gastrointestinal symptoms but are often easily confused with testicular pathology.

If testicular torsion is suspected, there is a 6-hour window for correction before strangulation of the blood supply renders the testicle unsalvageable.

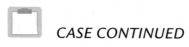

CASE CONTINUED

VS: AVSS

PE: *Gen:* Very uncomfortable young man in considerable distress. *Abdomen:* normal active bowel sounds; soft, nontender, nondistended. *Groin:* No masses. *Genitals:* Very tender swollen left testicle, resting high in the scrotal sac.

Labs: Urinalysis is normal

THOUGHT QUESTION

- The patient's mother is fearful of surgery and wants to know how you can be sure of the diagnosis without having performed any "tests." What do you tell her?

DISCUSSION

It is important to emphasize the need for expediency in this setting. The testicular salvage rate if detorsion is performed within 6 hours of symptoms is up to 97%, versus <10% if performed later than 24 hours. If the diagnosis of testicular torsion is in doubt, color-flow Doppler ultrasound could be obtained to evaluate for (lack of) blood flow to the testicle. A radionuclide testicular scan would give similar information. If after appropriate evaluation the diagnosis remains unclear, surgical exploration for diagnosis (and treatment) is warranted. Remember, if testicular torsion is clinically suggested, immediate surgical exploration should be performed regardless of laboratory studies because a negative finding upon exploration of the scrotum is more acceptable than the loss of a salvageable testis.

CASE CONTINUED

Ultrasound examination confirms testicular torsion. The patient undergoes surgical exploration with detorsion of the left testicle and orchiopexy. Orchiopexy is performed on the right testicle as well, because there is a high incidence of bilaterality of the anatomic condition that predisposes to torsion. Fortunately, the left testicle appeared viable and there was no indication for orchiectomy.

QUESTIONS

53-1. Testicular torsion is caused by the spontaneous twisting of
A. The testicular pedicle.
B. A patent processus vaginalis.
C. A scrotal hydrocele.
D. The scrotal sac.
E. The vas deferens.

53-2. Cryptorchidism is usually corrected when diagnosed because of
A. Increased risk of impotence.
B. Increased risk of testicular cancer.
C. Inability to secrete androgens.
D. Growth retardation.
E. Paradoxical estrogen secretion.

53-3. More than 90% of all testicular cancers are
A. Germ cell tumors.
B. Leydig cell tumors.
C. Sertoli cell tumors.
D. Gonadoblastomas.
E. Sarcomas.

53-4. Epididymo-orchitis is associated with
A. Hematuria.
B. Sexually transmitted organisms.
C. Leukopenia.
D. Bilateral painful, swollen testicles.
E. Need for emergent orchiectomy.

ANSWERS

53-1. A. Testicular torsion is the twisting of a testicle on its vascular supply. A patent processus vaginalis leads to an indirect inguinal hernia. Scrotal hydroceles are related to incomplete obliteration of the processus vaginalis during testicular descent.

53-2. B. Poor spermatogenesis and increased risk of cancer (~30 times higher than in the normal population) are sequelae of cryptorchidism (undescended testicle). Because of these, surgical intervention is required. The abdominal testis remains capable of androgen secretion.

53-3. A. Ninety to ninety-five percent of all primary testicular tumors are germ cell tumors. Seminomas account for ~35% of these; nonseminomas account for the rest (20% embryonal cell, 5% teratoma, <1% choriocarcinoma, and 40% mixed cell).

53-4. B. Pyuria and leukocytosis with a left shift are frequent findings. Younger men who are sexually active will frequently have *Chlamydia* or *Neisseria gonorrhea* infections. Older men tend to have urinary tract obstruction with associated infection (*E. coli*, *Proteus*, *Klebsiella*, *Enterobacter*, *Pseudomonas*). Epididymo-orchitis generally affects only one testicle, with the other testis being normal. Treatment is with antibiotics.

ADDITIONAL SUGGESTED READING

Dogra V, Bhatt S. Acute painful scrotum. Radiol Clin North Am 2004;42:349–363.

Eaton SH, Cendron MA, Estrada CR, et al. Intermittent testicular torsion: diagnostic features and management outcomes. J Urol 2005;174(4 Pt 2):1532–1535, discussion 1535.

Garner MJ, Turner MC, Ghadirian P, et al. Epidemiology of testicular cancer: an overview. Int J Cancer 2005;116:331–339. Review.

Kolon TF, Patel RP, Huff DS. Cryptorchidism: diagnosis, treatment, and long-term prognosis. Urol Clin North Am 2004;31:469–480, viii–ix. Review.

Urinary Hesitancy

CC/ID: 70-year-old man with difficulty voiding.

HPI: The patient presents with a 3- to 4-month h/o progressive difficulty initiating urination. He reports no burning, frequency, or pain. He has been in generally good health and as a result has not seen a physician in several years. He asks you if he would benefit from one of those "roto-rooter jobs" friends of his have had.

PMHx: Mild HTN (not requiring medications), arthritis

PSHx: Knee surgery ~20 years ago; vasectomy

Meds: Daily aspirin, anti-inflammatories prn

All: Penicillin, meperidine (Demerol)

SHx: Retired welder; smoker, formerly ~1 ppd × 40 years, now about 1/2 ppd; social drinker; no h/o illicit drugs

FHx: Orphaned, family history unknown

VS: AVSS

PE: *Gen:* Vigorous African-American man, appearing younger than stated age, in no distress. *Abdomen:* No scars; normal active bowel sounds; soft, nontender/nondistended; no masses, no palpable bladder. *Ext:* Some swelling of the left leg as compared with the right; prominent inguinal lymph nodes. *Genitals:* No gross external lesions or anatomic irregularities. *Rectal:* normal tone; firm/indurated, moderately enlarged prostate, left >right; no other masses; guaiac heme negative.

THOUGHT QUESTION

- What do you believe is the cause of this patient's symptoms?
- Are there any features in his history that may be contributory?
- Why might he have leg swelling?
- What tests will you order to assist in the diagnosis?

DISCUSSION

Complaints of bladder outlet obstruction (here, presenting as hesitancy) in an elderly man are frequently due to enlargement of the prostate. This patient has not had any routine physical or screening exams in some time, so evaluation of both benign and malignant causes should be undertaken. Risk factors for cancer of the prostate include age, African-American race, positive family history, high dietary fat intake, and cadmium exposure (found in cigarettes, batteries, the welding industry). Prior vasectomy is an inconclusive contributor to risk. The patient's leg swelling and asymmetrically enlarged gland could be indicative of malignancy with local bulky lymphadenopathy causing lymphedema of the ipsilateral leg.

Tests to include in evaluation are a urinalysis, serum BUN and creatinine, liver function test including alkaline phosphatase, a postvoid residual, and a PSA level. Transrectal ultrasound and/or a transrectal ultrasound-guided biopsy is useful in the setting of an irregular prostate on exam or an elevated PSA. It is worth noting that PSA alone may be elevated in BPH, urethral instrumentation, infection, or prostatic infarction. Tissue diagnosis is therefore important to exclude malignancy.

CASE CONTINUED

The patient is found to have an elevated PSA. Biopsy reveals prostate cancer and is assigned a Gleason score of 6 (3 + 3). Metastatic workup/imaging studies show some enlarged lymph nodes in the left groin. There is no other evidence of disease extension. He is started on a course of neoadjuvant hormonal therapy (LHRH agonists, to induce androgen deprivation, i.e., medical castration) to be followed by external-beam radiotherapy.

QUESTIONS

54-1. The maximum Gleason score is
   A.   4.
   B.   6.
   C.   8.
   D.   10.
   E.   12.

54-2. The 10-year disease-free survival in patients with organ-confined cancer of the prostate who undergo radical resection (of the prostate) is
   A.   <5%.
   B.   10% to 20%.
   C.   30% to 40%.
   D.   50% to 60%.
   E.   >70%.

54-3. Prior to the increase in incidental diagnosis of renal lesions (based on noninvasive imaging studies), the historic clinical presentation of *renal cell cancer* included
   A.   Epigastric pain, dysuria, hepatic dysfunction.
   B.   Suprapubic pain, hematuria, hypertension.
   C.   Flank pain, hematuria, abdominal mass.
   D.   Bone pain, pyuria, hematuria.
   E.   Back pain, oliguria, early satiety.

54-4. Regarding bladder cancers:
   A.   Greater than 90% are adenocarcinoma.
   B.   Women are more frequently affected than men.
   C.   Hematuria is a common presentation.
   D.   Locally advanced disease is treated by transurethral resection alone.
   E.   All stages of disease are treated with adjuvant radiation.

ANSWERS

54-1. D. The Gleason grading system is based on the microscopic glandular architecture of cancerous prostatic tissue seen under a low-power field. The tissue is given two grades, each ranging from 1 to 5, which represent the two patterns of cancer most commonly observed (1 being the most well differentiated, 5 being the least). If only one pattern is seen, then the same value is given twice. The Gleason score is the sum of these two grades and there-fore the value will range from 2 to 10.

54-2. E. Radical resection of the prostate involves removal of the entire prostate, the seminal vesicles, and the ampullae of the vas deferens. Patients with organ-confined disease have a 10-year disease-free survival of 70% to 85% in several series. Patients with focal extracapsular invasion have a 10-year disease-free survival of ~75%. Patients with more extensive extracapsular extension have a 10-year disease-free survival of ~40%. Higher Gleason score (≥7) is associated with an increased risk of progression.

54-3. C. Sixty percent of patients will have hematuria. Flank pain or abdominal masses are seen in 30%. About 40% of patients have hypertension. Bone pain is a sign of advanced disease and has been reported in 20% to 30% of patients.

54-4. C. Ninety percent of bladder malignancies are *transitional cell* tumors. Men are more frequently affected by a ratio of ~3:1. Hematuria is a presenting symptom in 85% to 90% of patients with bladder cancer. UTI and bladder irritability (frequency, dysuria) are other presentations. Local disease can be treated by transurethral resection and chemotherapy. Locally advanced disease requires radical cystectomy and chemoradiation.

ADDITIONAL SUGGESTED READING

Prostate Cancer Trialists' Collaborative Group: Maximum androgen blockade in advanced prostate cancer: an overview of the randomised trials. Lancet 2000;355:1491–1498.

Routh JC, Leibovich BC. Adenocarcinoma of the prostate: epidemiological trends, screening, diagnosis, and surgical management of localized disease. Mayo Clin Proc 2005;80: 899–907.

Earache

CC: 9-year-old boy with right ear pain.

HPI: The patient presents with a recent h/o cough, congestion, and runny nose. His parents tell you that he seemed to be
recovering from his "flu" when he started to complain of right ear
pain. The boy tells you his ear "feels funny", like when he dives to
the bottom of the deep end of the pool. He has had fevers as high as
101°F, and his parents believe he is having trouble hearing.

**PMHx/
PSHx:**   Asthma, hay fever

Meds: prn inhalers

VS: Temp 38°C, BP 100/60, HR 100

PE: *Gen:* WD/WN boy in no distress, occasionally fidgeting
with his right ear. *HEENT:* Remarkable for an erythematous,
inflamed, bulging R TM; L TM is normal. *Neck:* Several 1- to 2-cm
nontender, mobile, cervical lymph nodes on the R. *Chest:* CTA
bilaterally.

THOUGHT QUESTION

- What is the differential for ear pain?
- What is this patient's diagnosis? What are the most
  common organisms? What are predisposing factors to
  this illness?
- How will you treat this? What happens if treatment is
  incomplete or delayed?

DISCUSSION

The many sources of ear pain include trauma, sudden changes in pressure (e.g., while flying or swimming), blockage of the ear canal (such as with a foreign object), otitis externa or media, mastoiditis, allergies, ruptured eardrum, sinusitis, tooth abscess, referred pain from a sore throat, ear tumors, and temporomandibular joint syndrome.

This patient has *acute otitis media*, an infection of the middle ear. The most common causative organisms are upper respiratory tract in origin, the top three of which are *Streptococcus pneumoniae*, *Haemophilus influenzae*, and *Moraxella catarrhalis*. These organisms reach the middle ear because of reflux of nasopharyngeal bacteria and fluids or because of dysfunctional eustachian tube drainage, often secondary to obstruction related to inflammation, allergy, large adenoids, or neoplasm. Standard treatment is with antibiotics, though there is some evidence that, depending on the clinical situation, watchful waiting may be appropriate, with antibiotics started only if symptoms fail to improve. However, incomplete/delayed treatment may result in early recurrence, TM perforation, mastoiditis, meningitis, or hearing loss.

CASE CONTINUED

You treat the boy with a 10-day course of antibiotics and recommend NSAIDs for pain. He does well, although you end up seeing him three or four more times over the next couple of years for recurrent episodes. When the patient is 12 years old, he returns to see you several weeks after one of his treatment courses, saying that he feels better but there is still something wrong with his hearing.

On examination, you note that his TMs are grayish in color, retracted, and with air-fluid levels behind them. Pharyngeal exam reveals slightly enlarged adenoids.

THOUGHT QUESTION

■ What is this condition?
■ What is the likely cause?

DISCUSSION

The patient has otitis media with an effusion, or *serous otitis media*. This condition does not imply infection, so antibiotics are not warranted. Among the most common precursors to serous otitis media is thick residual fluid from prior acute otitis media. In small children (aged 1 to 3 years), the length or angle of the eustachian tubes is often inadequate to offer proper middle ear drainage. In older patients, nasopharyngeal obstruction (e.g., adenoids, polyps, or other tumors) is a frequent culprit.

 CASE CONTINUED

The patient is put on decongestants and antihistamines, but the effusion fails to completely clear after several weeks. You decide to observe the patient, but he returns with persistent difficulty hearing.

 THOUGHT QUESTION

■ What surgical option might be entertained at this point?

 DISCUSSION

Myringotomy (or middle ear ventilation) tubes offer what are effectively artificial eustachian tubes. These are placed in the anteroinferior TM, allowing fluids to drain and air to enter. In most cases, these tubes are extruded within 1 year. Ideally, they will allow for complete drainage of the offending fluid until better anatomic drainage is established. Sometimes tubes will need to be replaced if they are prematurely extruded. Adenoidectomy might also be considered.

 QUESTIONS

55-1. Otitis externa is commonly associated with
   A. An inflamed tympanic membrane.
   B. Sore throat with swallowing.
   C. History of swimming.
   D. Need for oral antibiotics.
   E. Runny nose and nasal congestion.

55-2. Regarding TM perforations,
  A. Central perforations are more easily treated than marginal ones.
  B. Central perforations are more likely than marginal ones to develop into cholesteatoma.
  C. Otitis media is seldom involved.
  D. They rarely occur in the setting of ear infections.
  E. They never heal spontaneously.

55-3. Treatment of cholesteatoma
  A. Requires mastoidectomy.
  B. Is necessary to avoid ear deformity.
  C. Is medical.
  D. May result in injury to the basilar artery.
  E. Can be accomplished in the office.

55-4. The Rinne test is used to assess hearing. Normally,
  A. Air conduction is greater than bone conduction.
  B. Bone conduction is greater than air conduction.
  C. Air conduction equals bone conduction.
  D. Conduction depends on the age of the patient.
  E. This test evaluates for sensorineural (rather than conductive) deficits.

ANSWERS

55-1. C. Otitis externa, or "swimmer's ear," is a relatively common presentation. Patients may complain of pain, itching, or hearing loss. There is frequently a history of swimming, other water sports, or ear trauma (i.e., sticking objects such as cotton-tipped swabs into the external ear canal). Examination reveals auricle pain and redness. The mainstay of treatment is eardrops, which usually contain some combination of an acid (to acidify the canal, thereby discouraging bacterial growth), a drying agent, antibiotics, and steroids. Oral antibiotics are *not* generally required. A wick may be placed in the ear canal if it is swollen shut, allowing for improved drainage of desquamated cells and debris.

55-2. A., 55-3. A. Perforations commonly occur during an acute bout of otitis media. Central perforations, which do not extend to the outer rim of the TM (i.e., the annulus), often heal spontaneously or else can be simply closed surgically. Marginal perforations, on the other hand, carry the risk of growth of external auditory canal epithelium into the middle ear, forming a sac that ultimately becomes a cholesteatoma. Cholesteatomas are basically epidermal inclusion cysts that tend to grow posteriorly into the mastoid cavity, putting them into close proximity with the cochlea, vestibular labyrinth and semicircular canals, carotid artery, facial nerve, sigmoid sinus, jugular bulb, middle cranial fossa, and posterior cranial fossa. Because these cysts/tumors can erode into any of these nearby structures, severe complications can ensue. Potential sequelae include meningitis, brain abscess, total hearing loss, facial nerve paralysis, carotid artery blowout, and sigmoid sinus thrombosis. Removal of a cholesteatoma requires mastoidectomy.

55-4. A. Sound is usually transmitted through the external and middle ear to the inner ear. This conduction pathway can be short-circuited by placing a vibrating tuning fork on the mastoid bone directly behind the ear, effectively bypassing the external and middle ears. This is the basis for the Rinne hearing test. Normally, air conduction is greater than bone conduction. If bone conduction is greater (i.e., perceived as louder by the patient), it implies a *conductive* (rather than sensorineural) hearing deficit, because sound is not being conducted as expected through.

ADDITIONAL SUGGESTED READING

American Academy of Pediatrics: Diagnosis and management of acute otitis media. Pediatrics 2004;113:1451–1465.

Kenna MA. Otitis media and the new guidelines. J Otolaryngol 2005;34(Suppl 1):S24–32.

Louis J, Burton MJ, Felding JU, et al. Grommets (ventilation tubes) for hearing loss associated with otitis media with effusion in children. Cochrane Database Syst Rev 2005;(1):CD001801.

Sore Throat

CC: 15-year-old girl with 3-day h/o sore throat and difficulty swallowing.

HPI: The patient presents with an intensely painful sore throat that has failed to improve despite throat lozenges, saline gargling, drinking cool liquids, and avoiding solid foods. She thought that she might have a cold, though she has been without cough or runny nose. She says she is pretty sure she has had fevers (she has not specifically measured her temperature). She mentions some difficulty sleeping, but the onset of this trouble preceded her current symptoms.

PMHx: Ear infections in early childhood

PSHx: None

Meds: Recent Tylenol for fever and discomfort

All: To cats and pollen; NKDA

SHx: Not sexually active; denies smoking

VS: Temp 39°C, BP 100/50, HR 100

PE: *Gen:* Ill-appearing teenager in moderate distress. *HEENT:* TMs clear; oropharynx—bilaterally enlarged tonsils covered with whitish exudate; posterior pharynx, nasopharynx, nose, and larynx appear normal. *Neck:* Bilateral anterior cervical lymphadenopathy. *Chest:* Clear to auscultation bilaterally.

Labs: Mononucleosis spot test—negative

THOUGHT QUESTION

- What are causes of sore throat?
- What would you like to do for this patient?

315

DISCUSSION

The differential for sore throat is fairly extensive and includes viral, gonococcal, or allergic pharyngitis, (streptococcal) tonsillitis, mononucleosis, peritonsillar abscess, alcohol or tobacco damage, pharyngitis sicca (dry throat), and oral cavity or oral pharyngeal cancers. The most common of these is viral pharyngitis.

This patient appears to have a bacterial tonsillitis, a common occurrence in children and young adults. Some would obtain a throat culture for verification, although this practice is not routine in immunocompetent patients. In sick patients, it is generally appropriate to treat empirically with antibiotics directed against oropharyngeal bacteria (most commonly *Streptococcus*).

CASE CONTINUED

You prescribe a 10-day course of penicillin-based antibiotics and instruct the patient to take the entire course even though it is likely she will feel better within 3 or 4 days. She agrees to be compliant. However, you end up seeing the patient 8 or 10 times over the next 3 years for recurrent episodes of tonsillitis. Before her leaving for college, she asks if maybe she should just have her tonsils removed.

THOUGHT QUESTION

- What are the indications for tonsillectomy and/or adenoidectomy (T&A)?
- What are the risks of this procedure?

DISCUSSION

There is some controversy over the absolute indications for T&A, and this is reflected in the decreasing frequency of this procedure as compared with 10 or 20 years ago. Still, it remains one of the most common surgical procedures performed today. The clearest indications are carcinoma of the tonsil, peritonsillar abscess, congestive heart failure (cor pulmonale, related to constant upper airway obstruction), and tonsillitis causing respiratory difficulties, dysphagia, or requiring hospitalization. Less clear indications include recurrent tonsillitis, sleep disturbances, and recurrent otitis media. Recent reviews suggest there is a benefit to performing T&A in children with severe recurrent tonsillitis (variably defined as four to five episodes a year for 2 years or three episodes a year for 3 + years), but good randomized controlled data are limited. There are no good studies on indication for T&A in adults.

Risks of this procedure range from postoperative throat discomfort to minor bleeding to death. Among the most frightening complications is catastrophic hemorrhage requiring carotid artery ligation. Other potential complications include nasopharyngeal stenosis, acute cervical adenitis +/– abscess formation, airway obstruction secondary to subglottic edema, aspiration of foreign bodies or blood clots, mediastinal emphysema, otalgia, palatal incompetence, and food, fluids, and air escaping from the nose. Serious complications are rare, with a reported overall complication rate of 2% to 15%.

 ## QUESTIONS

56-1. Peritonsillar abscesses occur in the space between the tonsil and
   A. The posterior pharynx.
   B. The adenoids.
   C. The opposite tonsil.
   D. The lateral pharyngeal wall.

56-2. The risk of developing a recurrent peritonsillar abscess after drainage is approximately
   A. <1%.
   B. 10%.
   C. 25%.
   D. 50%.
   E. >90%.

56-3. Regarding acute viral laryngitis,
   A. Antibiotics are not effective.
   B. Exercising vocal cords prevents scarring.
   C. It is an inflammatory swelling of the epiglottis.
   D. Hoarseness is rare.
   E. It usually follows episodes of cigarette smoking.

56-4. Enlargement of pharyngeal structures may lead to obstructive sleep apnea. Patients with this problem are sometimes referred for uvulopalatopharyngoplasty. This procedure involves resection of the

A. Uvula, epiglottis, and hard palate.
B. Uvula, base of tongue, and lingula.
C. Uvula, hard palate, and posterior pharynx.
D. Uvula, hard palate, and nasal septum.
E. Uvula, portion of the soft palate, and tonsils.

ANSWERS

56-1. D., 56-2. B. Peritonsillar abscesses are generally mixed anaerobic infections of the space between the tonsil and the lateral pharyngeal wall. Patients present with intense pain that is usually unilateral. Diagnosis is made clinically and treatment involves aspiration and antibiotics. Because the peritonsillar space is obliterated by the first infection, recurrent abscesses will involve the *parapharyngeal* space. As a result, infection can quickly involve the carotid artery and jugular vein or can spread inferiorly and involve the superior mediastinum. Because there is a 10% risk of developing a recurrent abscess, many advocate tonsillectomy once a patient has presented with peritonsillar abscess.

56-3. A. Acute viral laryngitis is an inflammatory swelling of the vocal cords, usually associated with either an acute upper respiratory tract infection or with a recent h/o yelling, such as at a sports event. Patients present with hoarseness. Antibiotics are not effective. Patients should be cautioned to use their voices softly and sparingly, because abuse may cause scarring and permanent hoarseness.

56-4. E. Uvulopalatopharyngoplasty involves resection of the tonsils and adjoining lateral pharyngeal wall tissues, the uvula, and a portion of the soft palate. When the pharyngeal and palatal wounds are closed, the pharynx is tightened and the nasopharyngeal opening into the oropharynx is enlarged. In principle, this decreases oropharyngeal collapse and inspiratory obstruction during sleep.

ADDITIONAL SUGGESTED READING

Burton MJ, Towler B, Glasziou P. Tonsillectomy versus nonsurgical treatment for chronic / recurrent acute tonsillitis. Cochrane Database Syst Rev 2000;(2):CD001802.

Darrow DH, Siemens C. Indications for tonsillectomy and
    adenoidectomy. Laryngoscope 2002;112(Pt 2 Suppl 100):6–10.
Johnson BC, Alvi A. Cost-effective workup for tonsillitis: Testing,
    treatment, and potential complications. Postgrad Med 2003;113,
    115–118, 121.
Raut VV, Yung MW. Peritonsillar abscess: the rationale for interval
    tonsillectomy. Ear Nose Throat J 2000;79:206–209.
Tewfik TL, Al Garni M. Tonsillopharyngitis: clinical highlights.
    J Otolaryngol. 2005;34 Suppl 1:S45-49.

CASE **57**

Refractory Hypotension

CC/ID: Dizziness and chest pain on deep inspiration

HPI: The patient is a 34-year-old woman who reports a one day history of sore throat and "feeling hot and cold." She had a restless night and woke this morning with right-sided chest pain on taking deep breaths, slight shortness of breath (particularly when lying on her right side), and dizziness. She has an occasional productive cough and feels quite thirsty.

PMH: none

PSH: none

Meds: none

All: NKDA

SH: one glass of wine with dinner

FH: none

VS: T 38.3°C, BP 65/35, HR 99, O2 sat 96% RA

PE: *Gen:* WD/WN woman, mild tachypnea. *HEENT:* Eyes anicteric, mucus membranes dry. *Chest:* CTA L side, decreased BS R upper 1/2 with expiratory wheeze but no crackles. *Abdomen:* No scars; nondistended. No rebound or guarding. *Ext:* No clubbing, cyanosis, or edema. Cool but not notably diaphoretic.

THOUGHT QUESTION

- What is your assessment at this point? What treatment would you administer? What other studies would you want?
- How would your assessment change if this patient were three days post-operative from an abdominal procedure?

320

DISCUSSION

Given the patient's relative hypotension, dry mucus membranes, and complaints of dizziness and thirst, the clinical picture is one of dehydration or intravascular volume depletion. Intravenous fluids are indicated. Other initial studies that would help in evaluating this patient are a CXR and bloodwork, particularly a CBC and electrolytes to assess for infection and dehydration.

Post-operative respiratory symptoms, particularly pleuritic chest pain and shortness of breath, are concerning for aspiration pneumonia and pulmonary embolism. The same basic blood tests should be sent, and you should consider an ABG as well, particularly if the patient has had an acute change in oxygen saturation or oxygen requirement. A spiral chest CT, rather than a CXR, would likely provide the most information in the post-op setting (i.e., pleural effusion, consolidation, embolism). Low blood pressure may be due to third-spacing, but cardiac dysfunction (i.e., MI or failure) should also be considered, especially in older patients.

You order a two liter bolus of lactated Ringers solution, and the patient's blood pressure improves slightly to 80/40. Two albuterol nebulizer treatments are also administered. The CXR shows RUL consolidation but no effusion or pneumothorax. Unfortunately over the next hour or so, the patient becomes progressively more hypoxic (O_2 sat 86% on 100% nonrebreather mask). Despite L lateral decubitus positioning, she becomes more tachypneic and her cough more frequent and productive.

THOUGHT QUESTION

- What are the indications for intubation?
- What is the definition of shock? What are the types of shock and how are they distinguished and treated? What kind of shock could be occurring in this patient? How will you confirm this?

DISCUSSION

The general indications for intubation are inability to oxygenate or ventilate, airway patency or protection, pulmonary toilet (management of excessive secretions), and increased work of breathing with insufficient physiologic reserve. Timely recognition of the need for intubation is preferred, as delayed intervention may lead to cardiopulmonary collapse. Quantitative measures that are often used to indicate impending respiratory failure include RR >30, PaO_2 <70 mmHg, and $PaCO_2$ >55mmHg.

Shock is defined as a physiologic derangement that results in inadequate end organ perfusion. Shock can be classified as septic, neurogenic, cardiogenic, hypovolemic, or traumatic, depending on the etiology. Infection associated with hypotension is indicative of sepsis, or *septic* shock. A systemic inflammatory response to the bacteria and related endo/exotoxins is often a contributing factor to the systemic vasodilation. *Neurogenic* shock can occur following cervical or thoracic spinal cord injury. It is characterized by loss of sympathetic tone with unopposed vagal tone below the level of injury, leading to peripheral arteriolar and venous dilation (warm, pink extremities). *Cardiogenic* shock occurs with severe heart failure and is exemplified by hypotension in the setting of adequate or even excess intravascular volume. A unique type of cardiogenic shock results from extrinsic compression, as with pericardial tamponade or tension pneumothorax; here diastolic filling is limited and should be treated with volume infusion and immediate relief of the increased intrathoracic pressure. *Hypovolemic* shock is the most common type of shock and can be secondary to hemorrhage (following total blood volume loss of at least 30%) or to loss of plasma volume, either through extravascular fluid shifts ("third-spacing", i.e., pancreatitis, SBO) or through excessive GI, urinary, or insensible losses. In the case of trauma, there is often both a hemorrhagic, or hypovolemic, component and a direct tissue injury component, which can provoke a systemic inflammatory response; this combination may be referred to as *traumatic* shock (Table 57-1).

TABLE 57-1 Finding and Treatment of Subcategories of Shock

Type	HR	CO	SVR	Treatment
Septic	↑	↑	↓	IVF, vasoconstrictor (if fluid inadequate), treatment of infection
Neurogenic	↑↓	↑↓	↓	IVF, vasoconstrictor
Cardiogenic	↑↓	↓	↑	Diuresis, inotropy, antiarrhythmic, vasodilator, intra-aortic balloon pump
Hypovolemic	↑	↓	↑	IVF, control of ongoing losses

This patient appears to have a pneumonia with hypotension, suggesting septic shock. She is otherwise healthy and has had no recent trauma. When the etiology of shock is unclear or multifactorial, the procedure of choice is placement of a pulmonary artery catheter. Also known as a Swan-Ganz catheter, it is an invasive means of measuring pulmonary artery pressures and cardiac output and of estimating systemic vascular resistance. An alternative study would be an echocardiogram, although this would give you limited information regarding cardiac contractility and ventricular filling. This would be most useful in cardiogenic shock to clarify a particular cardiac pathology.

CASE CONTINUED

Because of her limited ability to oxygenate, the patient is intubated and taken to the ICU, where she remains hypotensive. Her initial labs sent from the ED are notable for a WBC of 1.3, Cr 0.9, total bili 3.3. Blood cultures eventually show gram-positive cocci in pairs and chains.

Broad-spectrum antibiotics are started. With aggressive fluid resuscitation (25 L of IVF over 6 hrs) and phenylephrine, dopamine, and norepinephrine drips, the patient's BP is maintained at 80/35, but she becomes progressively more difficult to oxygenate and ventilate. A repeat CXR now shows bilateral infiltrates. Her ABG is pH 7.19/$PaCO_2$ 55/PaO_2 50/HCO_3 15/sat 78% on FiO_2 of 1.0, PEEP 15, PIPs in the 50s. A pulmonary artery catheter is placed and shows a PCWP of 14 mmHg. Moreover, her abdomen has become tense, urine output has fallen off, and creatinine has increased to 1.7. A bladder pressure is measured and is 54 mmHg.

THOUGHT QUESTION

- What respiratory syndrome may be developing? How is this diagnosed? How is it treated?
- What abdominal syndrome may be developing? How is this diagnosed? How is it treated?

DISCUSSION

Acute respiratory distress syndrome (ARDS) is a diffuse inflammatory process involving both lungs. The most common predisposing condition is sepsis (ARDS develops in up to 40%); mortality rates vary from 35–70% (higher when age >60 years) and are related primarily to multisystem organ failure. Clinical criteria for ARDS are diffuse bilateral pulmonary infiltrates, refractory hypoxemia (PaO_2/FiO_2 <200), presence of a predisposing condition, and pulmonary wedge pressure <18 mmHg (i.e., no left-heart failure). Management is supportive and attempts to minimize ventilator barotrauma and oxygen toxicity, reduce lung water, and maintain tissue oxygenation.

Abdominal compartment syndrome (ACS) is defined by increased intra-abdominal pressure (IAP) leading to multiorgan compromise. ACS results from the aggressive fluid resuscitation and altered microvascular permeability of a shock state, which together can lead to marked visceral edema and reduced abdominal wall compliance (due to soft tissue edema). ACS is most commonly seen in the trauma setting, but may become evident in any patient who requires large volume resuscitation (as in pancreatitis, laparotomy, or other types of shock). Decreased cardiac output occurs from caval compression and mechanical compression of capillary beds (leading to increased SVR). Lung compliance is reduced such that high airway pressures are required for ventilation. Renal dysfunction results from decreased glomerular filtration rate due to a combination of decreased cardiac output and renal vein compression. Other effects of increased IAP include visceral mucosal ischemia, as well as increased intracranial pressure due to impaired cerebral venous outflow. Treatment requires a decompressive laparotomy with delayed abdominal closure when the acute shock process is resolved.

QUESTIONS

57-1. Vasodilation in sepsis affects the:
- A. Arterial system.
- B. Venous system.
- C. Arterial and venous systems.
- D. Lymphatic system.
- E. Portal venous system.

57-2. The most common cause of shock in patients with acute spinal cord injury is
    A. Cardiogenic.
    B. Hemorrhage.
    C. Neurogenic.
    D. Sepsis.
    E. Hypoadrenal.

57-3. Normal bladder pressure is:
    A. <5 mmHg.
    B. <15 mmHg.
    C. <25 mmHg.
    D. <35 mmHg.
    E. <50 mmHg.

57-4. For ARDS, the recommended ventilatory tidal volume is:
    A. 3 cc/kg.
    B. 6 cc/kg.
    C. 9 cc/kg.
    D. 12 cc/kg.
    E. There is no recommended tidal volume.

ANSWERS

57-1. C. In sepsis, vasomotor tone is affected in both the arterial and venous systems. Reduced venous tone leads to blood pooling and effective blood volume loss, while reduced arterial tone (due primarily to dilatation of the small arterioles in skeletal muscles) leads to decreased systemic vascular resistance. The combined decrease in arterial and venous vasomotor tone is the main cause of hypotension in sepsis, although bacteria-induced release of proinflammatory cytokines (TNF-α and IL-1) may also lead to myocardial depression.

57-2. B. Hemorrhage is the most common cause of hypotension, even in a traumatic spinal cord injury patient and must be ruled out before neurogenic shock is diagnosed. Look for intra-abdominal and intrathoracic sources. *Hypoadrenal* shock is rare and usually occurs in the setting of a separate and distinct critical illness. In the United States, the most common cause of hypoadrenal shock is severe stress (major infection, operation, trauma) in the setting of chronic corticosteroid administration, which suppresses the normal adrenal output and limits the ability to respond to the stressor. Occasionally, adrenal infarction due to hypotension or adrenal hemorrhage due to coagulopathy may occur and lead to acute adrenal insufficiency. Diagnosis requires a high degree of suspicion. Refractory shock is often the only finding; other signs include hyponatremia, hypochloremia, hyperkalemia (due to decreased mineralocorticoid activity), fever, and acute abdomen. Plasma cortisol and corticotrophin levels should be obtained and a cosyntropin stimulation test performed. Treatment consists of high-dose intravenous steroids.

57-3. B. Transurethral bladder pressure measurement is used to estimate intra-abdominal pressure in the evaluation of abdominal compartment syndrome. Normal bladder pressure is <10–15 mmHg. Decompressive laparotomy is recommended when bladder pressure is >30 mmHg, although the clinical condition of the patient must also be used to assess the need for and timing of operation.

57-4. B. Traditional ventilator management utilizes tidal volumes of 10–12 cc/kg. However, in patients with ARDS, lower tidal volume (6 cc/kg) has been shown to decrease both mortality and number of days requiring ventilator use.

ADDITIONAL SUGGESTED READING

Brower RG, Ware LB, Berthiaume Y, et al. Treatment of ARDS. Chest 2001;120:1347–1367.

Malbrain ML, Chiumello D, Pelosi P, et al. Incidence and prognosis of intraabdominal hypertension in a mixed population of critically ill patients: a multiple-center epidemiological study. Crit Care Med 2005;33:315–322.

Moore AF, Hargest R, Martin M, et al. Intra-abdominal hypertension and the abdominal compartment syndrome. Br J Surg 2004;91:1102–1110.

Sugrue M. Abdominal compartment syndrome. Curr Opin Crit Care 2005;11:333–338.

Ventilation with lower tidal volumes as compared with traditional tidal volumes for acute lung injury and the acute respiratory distress syndrome. The Acute Respiratory Distress Syndrome Network. N Engl J Med 2000;342:1301–1308.

Ware LB, Matthay MA. The acute respiratory distress syndrome. N Engl J Med 200;342:1334–1349.

Headache

 CC/ID: 38-year-old man with chronic headaches, post-nasal drip, and cough.

HPI: The patient is a schoolteacher who presents with a nearly one year history of persistent frontal headaches and nasal congestion. He says that he seems constantly to be experiencing mucus-type secretions in the back of his throat, which makes the coughing worse. He has on several occasions been treated with antibiotics, but the symptoms keep returning. He is anxious to know whether anything else can be done.

THOUGHT QUESTION

- What is this patient's likely diagnosis? How would you confirm this? What criteria are important?

- What antibiotics would be (or should have been) appropriate? What other therapies are indicated?

DISCUSSION

The patient's history and symptom complex is consistent with sinusitis (or rhinosinusitis), a common disease that affects some 30 million people in the United States. The most common symptoms reported by patients are nasal congestion, pain, pressure, and postnasal discharge. The diagnosis of sinusitis, as defined by the Rhinosinusitis Task Force (RTF) of the American Academy of Otolaryngology-Head and Neck Surgery, is primarily a clinical one, and requires the presence of 2 major or 1 major and 2 minor criteria (Table 58-1). The diagnosis of chronic sinusitis requires the presence of these same criteria for ≥12 weeks, in addition to one other sign of inflammation: discolored nasal discharge; nasal polyps; polypoid swelling; edema or erythema of the middle meatus or ethmoid bulla; or granulation tissue seen on rhinoscopy.

TABLE 58-1 Criteria for Diagnosis of Sinusitis

Major Criteria	Minor Criteria
Facial pain or pressure	Headache
Nasal obstruction or blockage	Halitosis
Nasal discharge or purulence or discolored postnasal discharge	Fatigue Dental pain
Hyposmia or anosmia	Cough
Purulence in the nasal cavity	Ear pain, pressure, or fullness
Fever (for acute sinusitis)	Fever (for chronic sinusitis)

The pathogenesis of sinusitis is related to a change in sinus ostia patency, ciliary function, or quality of secretions. Typically, obstructed ostia result in stagnant secretions in the sinus, which in turn lead to a decrease in pH, lower oxygen tension, bacterial overgrowth, and mucosal inflammation.

Other diagnoses with similar presentations include allergic fungal sinusitis, allergic rhinitis, cystic fibrosis, foreign bodies in the airway, malignant nasopharyngeal, nasal cavity, or sinus tumors, turbinate dysfunction, nasal polyposis, dental abscess, NSAID sensitivity, or chronic headache of other etiology.

Culprit bacteria include gram positive organisms, gram negative organisms, and anaerobes. Anaerobes are a more significant pathogen in adults than children. It is common to initiate treatment with amoxicillin +/- clavulanate, progressing to clarithromycin or other antibiotic such as a second generation cephalosporin or quinolone if initial treatment fails. As in all cases of antibiotic use, selection of medication must be tailored to information provided by local antiobiograms and patient allergy histories. Neither cultures nor blood work are routinely obtained at this stage but may be helpful if symptoms persist.

CASE CONTINUED

The patient goes on to tell you that he has been treated on four different occasions with antibiotics. The treatment courses have each been of 3–6 weeks' duration, with only temporary relief of symptoms. He has also tried decongestants, antihistamines, and nasal saline washes to variable effect. He was given a prescription for a steroid inhaler, but was afraid to use it given all the negative things he has heard about steroid use.

PMHx: environmental allergies

PSHx: arthroscopic knee surgery in his 20s

MEDs: Allegra prn

All: NKDA

SHx: denies smoking, alcohol, or other drug use

EXAM: *Gen*—healthy appearing man in no distress, sniffling and coughing occasionally. *HEENT*—watery eyes, slightly reddened; TMs clear; nares red and irritated—examination with nasal speculum reveals turbinate swelling with purulent exudates; oropharynx slightly red; no significant cervical lymphadenopathy; percussion tenderness over the forehead. *Chest*—clear bilaterally.

THOUGHT QUESTION

- The patient tells you he had a bad experience with his knee operation and is "a little wary of going under the knife again." What could you offer the patient as a next step in his management?

DISCUSSION

The patient has chronic sinusitis based on history, exam, and duration of symptoms. It is possible to continue treatment with antibiotics, but it is likely that his symptoms will recur, as antibiotics alone will not address the underlying mechanical problem of poor sinus fluid clearance. Decongestants may continue to be helpful in reducing tissue edema and facilitating drainage, although tolerance to nasal preparations may develop if used for longer than 3–5 days at a time. Steroids have been shown to be a useful adjunct in treatment, as they can significantly decrease local inflammation. The patient should be counseled that the rate of systemic absorption of inhaled corticosteroids is relatively low and that they can be taken safely. Other nonoperative interventions include the use of mucolytics/steam inhalation, nasal irrigations, and treatment of underlying causes (e.g., allergy). Anecdotally, garlic and horseradish root may be effective homeopathic decongestants. To avoid further intervention, the patient should try to maximize symptom control with these described methods.

CASE CONTINUED

The patient continues with nasal irrigations and occasional steroid nasal sprays. He seems to respond favorably, and you don't see him for some time. He returns several months later stating that he does not think he's making enough progress and that he's now willing to consider more aggressive intervention.

THOUGHT QUESTION

- Now what? How will you plan for an operation? What imaging studies will you obtain?
- In what anatomic area would you expect to find pathology?

DISCUSSION

The typical operation for chronic sinusitis (or recurrent acute sinusitis, defined as >3–4 infections/year) is *functional endoscopic sinus surgery* (FESS), which is performed transnasally (no incisions). Open trephination approaches are less frequently performed. The goal of therapy in either case is to unclog and open the ostia through which the sinuses drain. This results in up to 90% long-term patency and symptom improvement. Knowing which sinuses are affected will help direct the procedure. *Sinus CT* is the imaging modality of choice, as the diagnosis can be confirmed and detailed anatomic information can be obtained. Plain XR films are not generally recommended in the evaluation of chronic sinusitis, as visualization is often inadequate. MRI is not recommended as a first-line imaging study.

The patient's history of frontal headaches, purulent exudates at the middle meatus, and forehead tenderness to percussion suggest pathology in the frontal sinus.

QUESTIONS

58-1. In adults with sinusitis, the most commonly affected sinuses are the
  A. Ethmoid.
  B. Frontal.
  C. Maxillary.
  D. Sphenoid.
  E. Temporal.

58-2. A patient with ethmoid sinusitis might be expected to have symptoms of pain or pressure
A. Behind the ears.
B. In the forehead.
C. Above the upper lip.
D. At the angle of the jaw.
E. Along the inferior orbit/medial canthus.

58-3. Which of the following is a common causative organism in acute sinusitis?
A. *H. influenzae.*
B. *E. coli.*
C. *B. Fragilis.*
D. *P. Aeruginosa.*
E. *C. albicans.*

58-4. Potential complications of FESS for chronic sinusitis include
A. Meningitis.
B. Tonsillitis.
C. Otitis.
D. Mastoiditis.
E. Pharyngitis.

ANSWERS

58-1. C. The maxillary sinuses are most commonly affected in adults.

58-2. E. Classically, sinus pain and pressure occur over the offending anatomic location. Thus, *ethmoid* sinusitises may present with tenderness over the medial canthus and inferior orbit. *Maxillary* sinusitis will typically cause cheek discomfort or pain in the upper teeth. *Frontal* sinusitis is usually experienced in the forehead. *Sphenoid* sinusitis is retroorbital, but radiates to the occiput and vertex.

58-3. A. *Haemophilus influenzae* and *Streptococcus pneumoniae* are the organisms most commonly found in acute sinusitis in adults. In children, the organisms are the same, with the addition of *Moraxella catarrhalis*. In older children, *Staphylococcus aureus* may also be seen. The infecting organisms in *chronic* sinusitis are more variable and more likely to be polymicrobial, with a higher incidence of anaerobic organisms (such as *Bacteroides*). In systemically impaired patients, such as those with diabetes, cancer, renal failure, or immuno-suppression, *Candida*, *Aspergillus*, and *Phycomycetes* may be found.

58-4. A. Meningitis and brain abscess resulting from CSF leak are among the potential complications of FESS for chronic sinusitis. Other complications include orbital and periorbital injuries (hematoma/hemorrhage, emphysema), blindness, diplopia, dental pain, adhesions, stenosis, hyposmia/anosmia, nasolacrimal duct injury, epistaxis, skull base injury, and intracranial injury.

ADDITIONAL SUGGESTED READING

Benninger MS, Ferguson BJ, Hadley JA. Adult chronic rhinosinusitis: definitions, diagnosis, epidemiology, and pathophysiology. Otolaryngol Head Neck Surg 2003;129 (3Suppl):S1–32.

Bhattacharyya N, Fried MP. The accuracy of computed tomography in the diagnosis of chronic rhinosinusitis. Laryngoscope 2003;113:125–129.

Damm M, Quante G, Jungehuelsing M. Impact of functional endoscopic sinus surgery on symptoms and quality of life in chronic rhinosinusitis. Laryngoscope 2002;112:310–315.

Metson RB, Gliklich RE. Clinical outcomes in patients with chronic sinusitis. Laryngoscope 2000;110:24–28.

Hip Pain

CC/ID: persistent R hip pain

HPI: The patient is a fairly active, 65 year-old woman who for the last several years has had progressive R > L hip "tightness" and pain. The pain seems to be worse in the area of her groin, but is occasionally present in her buttock. She notices the pain most with activity or weight-bearing. She especially finds it difficult to put on her socks or to get out of her car. Most of the time, she takes ibuprofen, with variable relief of her symptoms. She denies any history of trauma, though she believes she may have had "problems" with her right hip in childhood.

PMHx: mild asthma, hypothyroidism

PSHx: cataract surgery, breast surgery ~5 years ago

MEDs: multivitamin, calcium supplement, levothyroxine, prn ibuprofen, and inhalers

All: NKDA

SHx: denies smoking, alcohol, or other drug use. Retired legal secretary.

THOUGHT QUESTION

- How will you evaluate this patient's symptoms?
- Are there any other issues in the history that might be useful?
- What are the causes of hip pain? What are the most likely?
- What provocative tests may be used in the evaluation of hip pain?

DISCUSSION

The normal hip functions as a "ball and socket" joint, with the femoral head acting as the "ball" and the acetabulum acting as the "socket." This configuration normally allows for smooth range of motion in multiple planes. Any condition that affects either of these structures can lead to deterioration of the joint; deterioration of the joint leads to pain or loss of function. Hip pain can thus result from a number of factors, including trauma, degenerative disease, inflammation, developmental dysplasia, childhood hip disorders, cancer, or necrosis. The most common cause of ball-socket disruption is osteoarthritis. In addition, back or spine problems may lead to a radiculopathy that is appreciated as hip pain. Buttock claudication may also be described as hip pain.

In this case, the patient has already informed you that she has no history of trauma. It may be worth investigating the nature of her childhood hip "problem," but it is unlikely to change your management. A history of cancer as the reason for her breast operation may prompt an evaluation for bony metastases. The relationship of the pain to walking or other exercise should be clarified to assess for the possibility of peripheral vascular disease.

Physical evaluation will include examination of the hip joint, gait, previous incisions, abnormal swelling of the hip or limb, abrasions or other signs of trauma, and limb length discrepancy (which is important for operative planning). Femoral and pedal pulses should be documented. Provocative tests include: *straight leg raise* (when done against resistance, will elicit groin pain in joint pathology; if back or posterior hip pain is elicited, radicular pathology is suggested) and *Trendelenburg's sign* (when standing on the affected leg, the opposite hip normally rises; if it drops, this signifies weak hip abductors and is considered a positive test for joint dysfunction).

CASE CONTINUED

On specific questioning, the patient denies any history of back pain. She reports that her breast operation was a lumpectomy for benign disease. The hip pain occurs on initiating activity such as walking or getting up from sitting. It actually seems to lessen as she continues to move or as the day progresses. She does not experience buttock, thigh or calf pain, or cramping with walking.

Exam: *Gen*—overweight woman in no distress. *Lower extremities*—no gross deformity, contractures, or scars. Moderately decreased range of motion (passive and active) on the right >left. Motor strength diminished but equal. 2+ femoral/pedal pulses bilaterally. Sensation and reflexes intact. Right limb slightly shorter than left. Positive Trendelenburg's sign.

Labs: CBC, coags, and ECG are WNL.

Imaging: Plain films of the pelvis and hip reveal no significant bony deformity, with the exception of degenerative changes in the right > left hip.

You diagnose the patient with severe degenerative osteoarthritis. As a first line of treatment, you prescribe a weight reduction plan and physical therapy. In addition, you have her continue to take NSAIDs, adding glucosamine and chondroitin sulfate to her regimen.

THOUGHT QUESTION

- What are the indications for hip arthroplasty?
- What risks should the patient (and you) be aware of before recommending surgery?

DISCUSSION

Hip arthroplasty is typically reserved for patients who have a deteriorated hip joint and who have failed conservative management (persistent debilitating pain, significant deformity, and/or a significant decrease in the activities of daily living). Many believe that it is preferable to delay this procedure for as long as possible, because of the risk of eventual joint failure. However, some studies have suggested that better outcomes and fewer complications may be achieved if surgery is performed *before* the development of significant deformity, joint instability, contractures, functional loss, or muscle atrophy.

In addition to the usual perioperative and anesthetic risks, the potential complications specifically associated with the procedure include fracture, nerve or vascular injury, cement-related hypotension, infection, dislocation, implant failure/fracture, thromboembolism, osteolysis, and leg length discrepancy.

If proceeding to surgery, this patient should be advised to stop taking ibuprofen and aspirin for at least one week prior to surgery, as continuation of NSAIDs has been shown to increase perioperative bleeding up to twofold.

QUESTIONS

59-1. Patients who undergo total hip arthroplasty should be instructed to:
- A. Avoid all activity.
- B. Avoid impact activities, manual labor, heavy lifting, and high intensity sports.
- C. Increase activity significantly to prevent premature failure of the replaced joint.
- D. Avoid hip abduction and adduction as much as possible; hip flexion and extension should be encouraged.
- E. Avoid hip flexion and extension as much as possible; hip abduction and adduction should be encouraged.

59-2. Which of the following patients is the best candidate for placement of a prosthetic hip?
- A. 6-year-old with slipped capital femoral epiphysis.
- B. 40-year-old with paraplegia.
- C. 50-year-old with rheumatoid arthritis and an acute urinary tract infection.
- D. 70-year-old with spondyloarthropathy and h/o CHF, COPD, HTN, and chronic DVT.
- E. 85-year-old man with osteoarthritis and no major comorbidities.

59-3. Surgical alternatives to total hip arthroplasty include
- A. Dislocation and debridement.
- B. Amputation.
- C. Femoral osteotomy.
- D. Knee arthroscopy.
- E. Femoral-femoral artery bypass graft.

59-4. Patients with lateral femoral cutaneous nerve entrapment (meralgia paresthetica) have hyperesthesia or hyperthesia of the
- A. Anterolateral thigh.
- B. Posterolateral thigh.
- C. Lateral knee.
- D. Inguinal ligament.
- E. Superior buttock.

ANSWERS

59-1. B. Particularly in the young and active, patients need to be made aware that premature failure of the replaced joint may occur if activity levels are not reduced. High impact activities and sports should be avoided. There is no reason to limit regular activity or range of motion, as the prosthetic joint is designed to function in multiple planes.

59-2. E. Hip arthroplasty should not be performed in cases of active infection (it is always unwise to implant prosthetic material in the setting of potential bacteremia and bacterial seeding), significant medical comorbidity, skeletal immaturity, paraplegia or quadriplegia, or permanent muscle weakness. Age is not a contraindication if the patient is an otherwise good operative candidate.

59-3. A. Many intracapsular hip disorders may be treated with surgical dislocation and debridement of the joint space. Other less radical surgical options include intertrochanteric or periacetabular osteotomy to improve anatomic deformity and biomechanics, core decompression to remove necrotic debris from the femoral head, resection arthroplasty (a salvage procedure that creates an articulation between the proximal femur and the iliac bone), hip arthroscopy, and hip arthrodesis (fusion), which is rarely performed. Amputation is not necessary. Fem-fem bypass is a procedure for arterial insufficiency and is not indicated in this setting.

59-4. A. *Meralgia paresthetica* refers to the dysesthetic syndrome that results from entrapment of the lateral femoral cutaneous nerve. This nerve provides sensation to the anterolateral thigh, and entrapment of the nerve can lead to either heightened or decreased sensation along its distribution.

ADDITIONAL SUGGESTED READING

Fortin PR, Penrod JR, Clarke AE, et al. Timing of total joint replacement affects clinical outcomes among patients with osteoarthritis of the hip or knee. Arthritis Rheum 2002;46:3327–3330.

Lyman S, Sherman S, Dunn WR, et al. Advancements in the surgical and alternative treatment of arthritis. Curr Opin Rheumatol 2005;17:129–133.

Strickland JP, Berry DJ. Total joint arthroplasty in patients with
  osteopetrosis: a report of 5 cases and review of the literature.
  J Arthroplasty 2005;20:815–820.
Wenz JF, Gurkan I, Jibodh SR. Mini-incision total hip-arthroplasty:
  a comparative assessment of perioperative outcomes.
  Orthopedics 2002;25:1031–1043.

Obesity

CC/ID: Three women inquiring about surgical options for weight loss.

HPI: The patients are three sisters, ages 35, 38, and 43. They explain to you that they have spent their entire adult lives worrying about "weight problems." The eldest tells you that she has "never been able to lose the weight" since the birth of her second child. The youngest reports that she has been a "chronic dieter" all her life. They all express frustration at being unable to lose weight and keep it off. While home together over the holidays, they decided to make a group effort to slim down. After much consideration, they have determined that surgical intervention might be the best option for reaching their goals.

You scan their intake chart and note that they are each 5′6″ tall. Their weights (in pounds) are 235, 195, and 285, respectively.

THOUGHT QUESTION

- How is obesity defined? What comorbidities have been associated with obesity?

- How do you determine a body mass index (BMI)? What is the BMI of your patients and in what weight status does this place them?

DISCUSSION

Obesity affects more than 31% of Americans, at an estimated cost of more than $80 billion for the treatment of medically-related diseases and services. The Centers for Disease Control and Prevention have defined obesity as a BMI of >30. BMI is calculated as weight (in kg) divided by height (in m^2).

Severe obesity is associated with a number of health problems, including noninsulin dependent diabetes, hypertension, cardiovascular disease, pulmonary dysfunction, gallbladder disease, obstructive sleep apnea, gastroesophageal reflux, and osteoarthritis. There may also be an association with cancers of the breast and colon. It is important to look for such comorbidities in the obese patient, as many of them can be reversed or prevented with significant and sustained weight loss.

Regarding your patients, they have BMIs of 37.9, 31.5, and 46, respectively. This places all of them into the category of obese (Table 60-1).

TABLE **60-1** Weight Classification by Body Mass Index

BMI	Weight Status
Below 18.5	Underweight
18.5–24.9	Normal
25.0–29.9	Overweight
30.0 and above	Obese

CASE CONTINUED

You learn that the youngest woman (BMI 37.9) has had problems with hypertension and high sugars, both of which are controlled medically. She underwent laparoscopic cholecystectomy last year for symptomatic gallstones. She most recently was on the Zone diet but found it difficult to consistently eliminate carbohydrates from her meals. She initially lost almost 20 lbs but has since put most of it back on. She tries to walk for about 15 to 20 minutes two or three times a week, but admits that she often misses sessions.

The middle sister (BMI 31.5) has not had any major medical problems, but she often suffers from aching joints. She has no set exercise or diet program, but says that she is on her feet a lot during the workday. Her weight hasn't changed much in the past few years.

The eldest sister (BMI 46) has also had problems with hypertension, but attributes it to raising her kids. She had a brief scare with a "possible heart attack" a couple of years ago, but she has had no episodes since. She is on medications for her blood pressure and heart. She reports that she really doesn't eat very much, and that she is always running around after her kids. She tells you that she would like to eat healthier, but that it is difficult when the kids only seem to want fast food.

THOUGHT QUESTION

- Are these patients candidates for obesity surgery?

DISCUSSION

The criteria for weight-loss surgery was described in a 1991 NIH consensus statement. To be considered a candidate, a patient must be morbidly obese, with a BMI >40 (usually equivalent to about 100 lbs or more over ideal body weight). Alternatively, a patient with a BMI between 35 and 40 AND an obesity-associated morbidity (as discussed above) may also be eligible. Generally speaking, patients should have failed previous attempts at medically-supervised weight reduction programs and should be deemed to have an acceptable medical risk for surgery. Patients who are not able to comply with postoperative follow up, who have alcohol or other substance-abuse problems, or who have active, uncontrolled psychiatric disease are NOT good candidates. It is important to stress that the goal for patients should be an improvement in over-all health, as opposed to only a change in cosmetic appearance.

Assuming that the sisters have documented attempts at weight loss, have no known psychoses or addictions (patients are often screened by a psychiatrist before being considered for bariatric procedures), have realistic expectations for outcomes, are committed to long-term follow up, and are otherwise good surgical risks, then the youngest and oldest might be considered as operative candidates, using the NIH criteria.

CASE CONTINUED

The two eligible sisters are scheduled for surgery. They both undergo uncomplicated laparoscopic procedures: one a restrictive type and the other both restrictive and malabsorptive. Postoperatively, they follow the nutritionist's instructions for eating habits and quickly lose weight. The middle sister, inspired by her siblings, is also able to improve her dietary and exercise habits. Each of the women loses approximately 30–50% of her excess body weight at one year after surgery, with marked improvements in their various other medical problems.

QUESTIONS

60-1. Which of the following procedures is purely restrictive?
A. Gastric bypass.
B. Vertical banded gastroplasty (VBG).
C. Biliopancreatic diversion (BPD).
D. Duodenal switch.
E. Abdominal colectomy.

60-2. Which of the following patients (all with a BMI >40) is least likely to be offered bariatric surgery?
A. Active 65-year-old.
B. 16-year-old student.
C. 35-year-old with a history of exploratory laparotomy following a motor vehicle accident.
D. 42-year-old with a history of a previous (failed) obesity operation.
E. 30-year-old alcoholic with a recent DUI conviction.

60-3. What percentage of patients undergoing weight-loss surgery may be expected to achieve weight loss >50% of excess body weight?
A. <10%.
B. 10–40%.
C. 40–60%.
D. 60–80%.
E. 80–90%.

60-4. Possible complications of weight loss surgery include:
A. Vitamin C deficiency.
B. Steatohepatitis.
C. Diabetes.
D. Anastamotic leak.
E. Esophageal reflux.

ANSWERS

60-1. B. *Restrictive* procedures encourage a reduction in caloric intake via the creation of a small gastric reservoir. This is a mechanical restriction, where patients are intended to feel "full" with less volume consumed. *Malabsorptive* procedures bypass variable lengths of small bowel, such that caloric intake is reduced by limiting systemic enteric absorption. This is largely a functional restriction.

Operations for weight loss capitalize on one or both of these strategies. In appropriate patients, the outcomes are comparable.

The procedures most commonly performed (laparoscopic or open):

- Gastric bypass—restrictive and malabsorptive (small gastric reservoir, gastrojejunostomy with roux-en-y limb).
- Biliopancreatic diversion (BPD)—mostly malabsorptive, with a restrictive component (distal gastrectomy with jejuno-ileal bypass).
- Duodenal switch—mostly malabsorptive, with a restrictive component (like BPD, but with a pylorus-preserving gastrectomy and gastro-ileal bypass).
- Vertical banded gastroplasty (VBG)—restrictive (small gastric pouch, with distal/remainder of stomach stapled off; band at pouch narrows outlet).
- Laparoscopic adjustable gastric band—restrictive (similar to VBG, with an adjustable band placed at the proximal stomach, creating a narrow outlet; no staple line).

60-2. E. Age, previous abdominal surgery, and previous failed bariatric procedures are not necessarily contraindications to weight-loss surgery. Adolescent patients with medically-complicated obesity are being offered these procedures with increasing frequency, although this practice still remains somewhat controversial. Older patients may also benefit from surgery, but the impact on obesity-related comorbidities may not be as great as for younger patients. As discussed in the case, patients with active substance abuse problems or psychoses are not considered surgical candidates.

60-3. E. Unfortunately, medical management for obesity has a poor success rate, with only 5–10% of patients able to achieve long-lasting, significant weight reduction. Surgical procedures have been effective in achieving weight loss of ≥50% of excess body weight in 80–90% of patients.

60-4. D. Major complications of bariatric surgery are primarily seen in the perioperative period. Mortality is usually less than 1% and morbidity is approximately 15%. Complications include wound infections, anastomotic leak (for procedures involving an anastomosis), pulmonary emboli, vitamin B12 and iron deficiency, and bowel obstruction. Obesity-related diseases including steatohepatitis, diabetes, and reflux are typically improved following surgery.

ADDITIONAL SUGGESTED READING

Ali MR, Fuller WD, Choi MP, et al. Bariatric surgical outcomes. Surg Clin North Am 2005;85:835–852, vii.

Buchwald H; Consensus Conference Panel. Bariatric surgery for morbid obesity: health implications for patients, health professionals, and third-party payers. J Am Coll Surg 2005:200:593–604.

Buchwald H, Avidor Y, Braunwald E, et al. Bariatric surgery: a systematic review and meta-analysis. JAMA 2004;292: 1724–1737.

Colquitt J, Clegg A, Loveman E, et al. Surgery for morbid obesity. Cochrane Database Syst Rev 2005;4:CD003641.

Inge TH, Krebs NF, Garcia VF, et al. Bariatric surgery for severely overweight adolescents: concerns and recommendations. Pediatrics 2004;114:217–223.

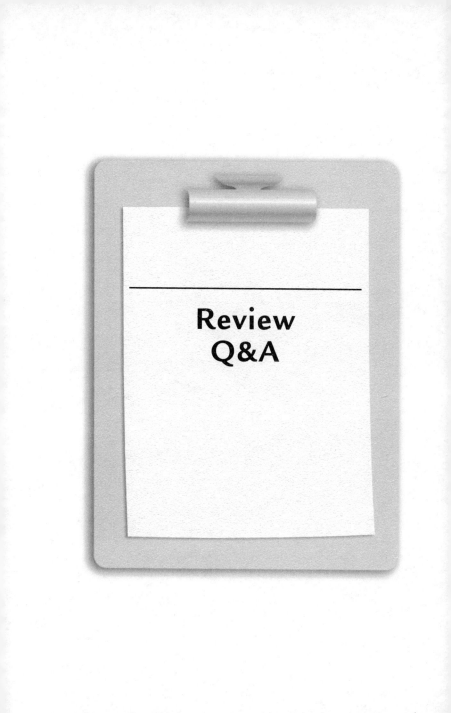

Review
Q&A

Questions

1. A 60-year-old man with a several-month history of hoarseness and a neck mass presents to your office. At this point, the single most effective method of diagnosis is:
- A. Incisional biopsy of the neck mass
- B. Excisional biopsy of the neck mass
- C. Fine-needle aspiration (FNA) of the neck mass
- D. CT scan of the head, neck, and chest
- E. Laryngoscopy with biopsy
- F. Flexible bronchoscopy

2. Prophylactic mastectomy in women who are at moderate to high risk for developing breast cancer:
- A. Reduces that risk by 90%
- B. Involves removal of all of the breast glandular tissue
- C. Should be offered to all women with diffuse ductal carcinoma in situ (DCIS)
- D. Can be avoided by placing the patient on tamoxifen therapy
- E. Has no role in the modern management of breast disease

3. A 60-year-old woman comes to you with stereotactic breast biopsy findings of ductal carcinoma in situ (DCIS) in two quadrants. You recommend that she undergo:
- A. Observation with repeat mammography in 1 year
- B. Sentinel lymph node biopsy
- C. Two-quadrant lumpectomy
- D. Simple mastectomy with an option for immediate reconstruction
- E. Modified radical mastectomy

4. A young woman presents to your office with a mammogram showing a nodular density in the left breast. Since it is nonpalpable, you send her for stereotactic core needle biopsy. A finding of atypical ductal hyperplasia:

    A. Requires surgical referral for excision
    B. Is benign and can be followed expectantly
    C. Warrants administration of tamoxifen chemotherapy
    D. Is commonly found in women who are lactating
    E. Predicts future inflammatory breast cancer

5. A 50-year-old woman comes to you with a palpable breast mass discovered on self-exam. You perform a fine needle aspiration (FNA) that reveals adenocarcinoma. When she asks you about preoperative versus postoperative chemotherapy, you tell her that preoperative (neoadjuvant) therapy is associated with:

    A. An increase in overall survival
    B. Increased rates of breast conservation
    C. Improved locoregional control
    D. Improved disease-free survival
    E. Fewer side effects

6. You are asked to evaluate a healthy, nonlactating 42-year-old woman with a tender, fluctuant subareolar mass with surrounding erythema. Regarding this condition:

    A. Recurrences are uncommon
    B. The most likely causative organism is *Staphylococcus*
    C. Percutaneous aspiration should not be attempted
    D. Antibiotics are not necessary
    E. Mammography is the diagnostic study of choice

7. Which of the following features is associated with the best prognosis for a patient with breast cancer?

    A. Estrogen receptor positive tumor
    B. Pregnant patient
    C. Tumor with overexpression of HER-2/neu
    D. Male sex
    E. Patient age <35

8. You have been asked to evaluate a 40-year-old man for breast cancer. Which of the following features would constitute a positive risk factor?

    A. BRCA1 gene mutation
    B. BRCA2 gene mutation
    C. Gynecomastia
    D. Asian heritage
    E. Anabolic steroid use

9. A 50-year-old man is found to have an isolated 2-cm gastric ulcer along the mid-lesser curve of his stomach. This lesion is classified as:

    A. Type I, and is associated with normal or decreased acid secretion

    B. Type II, and is associated with NSAID use

    C. Type III, and is associated with malignancy

    D. Type IV, and is associated with lesions at the GE junction

    E. Type V, and is associated with atrophic gastritis

10. Appropriate treatment of *Helicobacter pylori* typically involves:

    A. Antibiotics alone

    B. Proton pump inhibitors alone

    C. A combination of antibiotics and a proton pump inhibitor

    D. Acid neutralization with sucralfate

    E. A combination of sucralfate and a proton pump inhibitor

11. A 52-year-old patient presents to you with a several month history of dysphagia, regurgitation, and bad breath. A barium swallow reveals a blind pouch coming off of the cervical portion of the esophagus. Appropriate treatment for this patient should include:

    A. Behavioral modification

    B. Botulinum toxin injections

    C. Diverticulectomy alone

    D. Cricopharyngeal myotomy

    E. Esophagectomy

12. A 40-year-old woman with a long history of gastroesophageal reflux undergoes screening endoscopy, with findings of a small hiatal hernia. She recalls that her uncle had a similar hernia that required operation and wants to know if she will require that as well. Presence of which of the following features is most likely to lead to a need for surgical intervention?

    A. Gastroesophageal junction (GEJ) located at the hiatus

    B. GEJ located in the abdomen

    C. GEJ located in the chest

    D. Gastric fundus in the abdomen

    E. Gastric fundus in the chest

    F. Presence of a true hernia sac

13. Regarding Barrett's esophagitis:
    A. Most patients who progress to carcinoma are men aged 55–60 years
    B. Patients with low-grade dypslasia should undergo esophagectomy
    C. High-grade dysplasia should be treated with antacids and an antireflux procedure
    D. Endoscopic surveillance is not necessary if symptoms are controlled
    E. It may be seen in up to 50% of patients with symptoms of reflux

14. The enterocutaneous fistula that is most likely to close spontaneously is:
    A. Ileal
    B. Jejunal
    C. Gastric
    D. Radiation-induced
    E. Tract <2 cm
    F. 24-hour output >500 ml

15. A patient requires major small bowel resection for ischemia, leaving him with <100 cm of small bowel. Which of the following would you expect postoperatively?
    A. Preservation of the ileocecal valve will decrease the likelihood that parenteral nutrition will be required
    B. Preservation of the jejunum will be more important to adaptation/increase in absorption than will preservation of the ileum
    C. Decrease in gastrin levels
    D. Increased risk for kidney stones due to elevated increased urinary calcium
    E. Intestinal adaptation will be complete within 1 year of resection

16. A 45-year-old woman has been on proton pump inhibitors for treatment of her gastroesophageal reflux disease (GERD). With regards to follow-up endoscopy, which of the following is expected?
    A. Inhibited progression of dysplasia
    B. Reversal of intestinal metaplasia
    C. Effects of treatment only seen if gastric acidity is normalized
    D. Regression of Barrett's changes
    E. Increased squamous islands in Barrett's segments

17. An 80-year-old nursing home resident has a 3-day history of abdominal pain and progressive abdominal distension. Her laboratory studies are normal, and her abdominal x-ray shows a sigmoid volvulus. Appropriate initial management is:

- A. Immediate laparotomy
- B. Neostigmine
- C. Promotility agents
- D. Rigid or flexible sigmoidoscopy
- E. Percutaneous decompression

18. A 76-year-old woman who recently underwent total hip replacement presents with a 4-day history of abdominal distension. Laboratory tests reveal some minor electrolyte abnormalities, and radiography shows a distended colon with no transition point, no evidence of mass, and a cecum that is 12 cm in diameter. Initial treatment of this condition:

- A. Definitely includes surgical intervention
- B. Is with a cholinesterase inhibitor
- C. Does not require correction of any electrolyte abnormalities
- D. May be associated with tachycardia
- E. Should include encouragement of an oral diet

19. An otherwise healthy 58-year-old woman presents with fecal and urinary incontinence. On examination, concentric rings of mucosa are seen prolapsing through the anus. Management of this condition:

- A. Will require a hysterectomy
- B. Can only be performed from an abdominal approach
- C. Will require a diverting colostomy
- D. Does not necessarily include a bowel resection
- E. Can effectively be accomplished with strengthening exercises alone

20. *Helicobacter pylori* infection is believed to have a pathogenic role in:

- A. Reflux esophagitis
- B. Gastric adenocarcinoma
- C. Pancreatitis
- D. Mallory-Weiss gastric tears
- E. Gallstone formation

21. You are asked to evaluate an elderly ICU patient with abdominal pain. You note that he is 4 days status post CABG, and that he has intermittently required pressors for blood pressure support. On examination, he is somewhat somnolent but seems to respond to palpation of his abdomen, particularly on the left side. Colonoscopy shows patchy areas of mucosal ischemia. With regards to this patient's abdominal process:

    A. It is confined to the sigmoid colon
    B. It is more common in young patients
    C. Angiography is required for diagnosis
    D. It will usually resolve with antibiotics and other supportive care
    E. Continued use of vasopressors will help reverse the problem

22. A 66-year-old man undergoes upper endoscopy for evaluation of peptic ulcer disease. About 8 hours after the procedure, he presents to the ED reporting pain and swelling in his neck. On examination, he has subcutaneous emphysema and hemodynamic signs of sepsis. Which of the following would be contraindicated?

    A. Gastrografin swallow study
    B. CT scan of the neck
    C. Immediate surgical exploration
    D. Lateral cervical spine films
    E. Nasogastric intubation

23. A 30-year-old woman presents to the ED with a 5 to 6 hour history of vague, persistent abdominal pain and nausea. She tells you that just prior to arrival, she passed a stool containing mucus and blood. You obtain a CT scan that the on-call radiologist tells you looks most consistent with intussusception. At this point you:

    A. Administer neostigmine
    B. Take the patient urgently to the operating room for exploration and bowel resection
    C. Ask the radiologist to perform a barium enema
    D. Admit the patient for bowel rest, NGT decompression, and intravenous fluids
    E. Perform colonoscopy
    F. Discharge the patient with analgesics and instructions to return if the symptoms do not improve in 12–24 hours

24. An obese 50-year-old woman with a longstanding history of postprandial epigastric pain presents with a 36-hour history of progressive abdominal distension, nausea, and vomiting. On examination, she has a tympanitic abdomen with minimal diffuse tenderness to palpation. An abdominal series shows distended loops of bowel, a few air fluid levels, calcification in the right lower quadrant, and pneumobilia. Appropriate management will require resuscitation followed by:

    A. Esophagogastroduodenoscopy (EGD)
    B. Colonoscopy
    C. Endoscopic retrograde cholangiopancreatography (ERCP)
    D. Angiography
    E. Operative intervention

25. A 44-year-old alcoholic was admitted five days ago to the ICU with a diagnosis of acute pancreatitis. He continues to be febrile, leukocytotic, and somewhat hemodynamically labile. The need for surgical intervention is most accurately determined by:

    A. Computed tomography (CT) of the abdomen
    B. Percutaneous needle aspiration
    C. Abdominal ultrasound
    D. Indium WBC scan
    E. Lipase level

26. A healthy 42-year-old man who is involved in a motor vehicle accident comes in complaining of vague abdominal pain. You obtain an abdominal CT scan, which is unremarkable except for a 2.5 cm mass in the right adrenal gland. Prior to the accident, he had been asymptomatic. Prior to discharging the patient, you advise that he:

    A. Undergo adrenalectomy
    B. Complete tests to determine whether the tumor is functional
    C. Obtain a follow-up CT scan in 5 years
    D. Ignore this incidental finding
    E. Get a fine needle aspiration biopsy of the tumor

27. You suspect that a TPN-dependent, obtunded ICU patient may have acalculous cholecystitis. After obtaining a right upper quadrant ultrasound that shows gallbladder sludge without pericholecystic fluid, gallbladder wall thickening, or ductal dilatation, the best test to obtain would be:

    A. HIDA (cholescintigraphy) scan
    B. Abdominal CT scan
    C. Endoscopic retrograde cholangiopancreatography (ERCP)
    D. Magnetic resonance cholangiography (MRC)
    E. Gastrograffin swallow

28. Budd-Chiari syndrome is a disorder produced by occlusion of the hepatic veins. It is associated with a history of hepatitis, pregnancy, tumor, abscess, trauma, or hematologic or hypercoagulable derangements. The classic triad of clinical findings is:
  A. Hepatomegaly, spider angiomata, and melena
  B. Right upper quadrant pain, early satiety, and encephalopathy
  C. Ascites, abdominal pain, and esophageal varices
  D. Jaundice, right upper quadrant pain, and fever
  E. Right upper quadrant pain, hepatomegaly, rapid development of ascites

29. A 50-year-old alcoholic presents to the emergency department with his third episode of significant variceal bleeding. He has in the past been successfully treated with transfusion, sclerotherapy, and banding. He is a Child's A cirrhotic. After resuscitation and stabilization, appropriate surgical options for him at this juncture should include:
  A. Esophagectomy
  B. Liver transplant
  C. Portosystemic shunt
  D. Paracentesis
  E. His Child's class precludes any viable surgical interventions

30. Three weeks following her first admission for acute pancreatitis, a 37-year-old woman presents in follow-up with a slight fullness in her left upper quadrant. She is nontender to palpation and is otherwise asymptomatic. You obtain an abdominal CT scan, which reveals an 8-cm, low-density collection in the tail of the pancreas. At this point, you recommend that the patient undergo:
  A. Observation and follow-up CT scan
  B. Percutaneous drainage
  C. Operative exploration, debridement, and drainage
  D. Endoscopic retrograde cholangiopancreatography (ERCP)
  E. A 2-week course of antibiotic therapy

31. The finding of pneumatosis intestinalis in a patient with abdominal pain:
  A. Is a normal variant
  B. Cannot be seen on plain x-rays
  C. Signifies intravascular dehydration
  D. Usually mandates surgical intervention
  E. Should be followed by an enteroclysis study to further evaluate

32. A 67-year-old woman undergoes esophagectomy for Barrett's esophagus. She does well following her operation, and is started eventually on an oral diet. She seems to be tolerating this well, but as you are considering pulling her chest tube, she begins to drain a milky white fluid. Laboratory analysis confirms a high triglyceride content. The next step in management should be:
  A. Surgical closure of the fistula
  B. Bowel rest and total parenteral nutrition
  C. Pleuroperitoneal shunt
  D. Dietary supplementation with medium-chain triglycerides
  E. Pleurodesis

33. A 30-year-old G_2P_1, 18-weeks-pregnant woman presents to your office with right upper quadrant pain, nausea, and vomiting. Her vital signs are stable, exam confirms RUQ tenderness to palpation, and her WBC is moderately elevated. Ultrasound confirms the presence of gallstones, without pericholecystic fluid or gallbladder wall thickening. You admit her to the hospital for intravenous antibiotics, but her symptoms worsen over the course of the next 12–24 hours. You recommend:
  A. Changing to a different antibiotic
  B. Percutaneous cholecystostomy
  C. Termination of the pregnancy
  D. Induction of labor
  E. Laparoscopic cholecystectomy

34. The most likely causative organism in biliary tract sepsis is:
  A. *Enterobacter*
  B. *Bacteroides fragilis*
  C. *Escherichia coli*
  D. *Enterococcus*
  E. *Clostridium perfringens*

35. Which of the following is pathognomonic of obturator hernia?
  A. Pain in the ipsilateral hip, medial thigh, and knee that is exacerbated by extension and relieved by flexion of the thigh (Howship-Romberg sign)
  B. Pain in the ipsilateral lower quadrant with extension of the hip (psoas sign)
  C. Pain in the contralateral lower abdomen with palpation (Rovsing's sign)
  D. Pain in the calf with ankle flexion (Homan's sign)
  E. Pain in the leg with walking that is relieved by rest

36. Early (<72 hours from onset of symptoms) versus late chole-cystectomy for acute cholecystitis is associated with:

A. Increased operative time
B. Increased rate of conversion to open procedure
C. No change in complication rate
D. Increased hospital stay
E. Increased operative blood loss

37. Botulinum toxin has been safely and routinely used as treatment for:

A. Hypertrophic scars
B. Osteoarthritis
C. Gastroesophageal reflux
D. Anal fissures
E. Hyperhidrosis

38. A 55-year-old woman with a history of multiple abdominal operations presents with a wound separation. On examination, you note that she has exposed prosthetic mesh in her midline wound. The next step in her management should now include:

A. Total parenteral nutrition
B. Excision of only the exposed section of mesh
C. Covering the exposed mesh with new, sterile mesh
D. Diverting ileostomy, away from the mesh
E. Computed tomography (CT) of the abdomen

39. You are called to evaluate a 58-year-old man with an umbilical hernia and ascites. Which of the following would be cause for immediate operative intervention?

A. Worsening ascites
B. Plans for the patient to undergo transjugular intrahepatic portosystemic shunt (TIPS) this admission
C. Incarcercation and skin ulceration
D. Leaking from the hernia
E. Hernia larger than 3 cm

40. You suspect a diagnosis of small bowel obstruction in a patient with intermittent abdominal pain and bloating. Applicable imaging studies to consider, from most to least sensitive are:

A. Plain abdominal x-ray > abdominal computed tomography (CT) scan > enteroclysis
B. Plain abdominal x-ray > enteroclysis > abdominal CT scan
C. Abdominal CT scan > plain abdominal x-ray > enteroclysis
D. Abdominal CT scan > enteroclysis > plain abdominal x-ray
E. Enteroclysis > plain abdominal x-ray > abdominal CT scan
F. Enteroclysis > abdominal CT scan > plain abdominal x-ray

41. A patient with a neuroendocrine tumor of the beta cells of the islets of Langerhans would be expected to have symptoms of:
A. Hyponatremia
B. Hypoglycemia
C. Hypocalcemia
D. Hypokalemia
E. Diarrhea

42. A 48-year-old woman has a known parathyroid adenoma that was diagnosed after an incidental finding of hypercalcemia. She has been asymptomatic, and has not wanted to undergo parathyroidectomy. She presents to the emergency department with symptoms of anorexia, vomiting, and dehydration. Her laboratory tests are remarkable for a contraction alkalosis and a calcium level of 18 mg/dl. EKG shows a shortened QT interval. Appropriate management in this patient may include:
A. Normal saline hydration, thiazide diuretics, oral phosphate
B. Normal saline hydration, loop diuretic, bisphosphonate
C. Colloid volume replacement, thiazide diuretics, calcitonin
D. Colloid volume replacement, loop diuretic, vitamin D
E. Cagnesium, thiazide diuretics, gallium

43. Regarding the finding of a solitary thyroid nodule in a child younger than 5 years of age:
A. No intervention is indicated, as there is no risk of malignancy
B. It is only seen in patients who have a family history of hereditary thyroid cancer
C. There is an increased prevalence of cancer now that fewer children are exposed to neck irradiation
D. The incidence of malignancy is higher than in adults
E. It is only seen in geographic areas of iodine deficiency

44. A 46-year-old woman with a recent diagnosis of metastatic thyroid cancer comes to your office for a second opinion. She understands that thyroidectomy is recommended, and wants to hear your views on adjuvant therapy with radioactive iodine (^{131}I). You explain to her that her response would depend on the tumor type, with the most avid iodine concentration seen in:
A. Papillary thyroid cancer
B. Medullary thyroid cancer
C. Anaplastic thyroid cancer
D. Other cancers metastatic to the thyroid
E. Lymphoma

45. A young model is diagnosed with a parathyroid adenoma, which she is anxious to have removed. However, she is worried about the cosmetic impact. You inform her that
  A. An 8–10 cm collar incision is hardly noticeable.
  B. Focused parathyroidectomy through a small incision will be more painful because of increased wound manipulation.
  C. The success of focused parathyroidectomy in locating and removing the hyperactive adenoma (as compared with a standard 4-gland exploration) is clearly inferior.
  D. The risk of injury to the vocal cords is much higher with focused parathyroidectomy.
  E. The success of focused parathyroidectomy in the identification and removal of the involved gland is >90%–95% if there is agreement between the relevant perioperative studies.

46. Normal rate of expansion for AAA is estimated to be
  A. 0.1 cm per year
  B. 0.2–0.4 cm per year
  C. 0.5–0.7 cm per year
  D. 0.7–1.0 cm per year
  E. >1.0 cm per year

47. In comparing breast conservation therapy (BCT) for invasive ductal carcinoma to modified radical mastectomy (MRM):
  A. The survival rate is better for BCT
  B. The survival rate is better for MRM
  C. The local recurrence rate is higher for BCT, but the survival is equivalent
  D. The local recurrence rate is higher for MRM, but the survival is equivalent
  E. There are no differences between BCT and MRM in terms of local recurrence or survival

48. The most common histology of male breast cancers is:
  A. Ductal carcinoma in situ (DCIS)
  B. Lobular carcinoma in situ (LCIS)
  C. Invasive ductal carcinoma (IDC)
  D. Invasive lobular carcinoma
  E. Medullary carcinoma
  F. Inflammatory carcinoma

49. As compared to conventional open techniques for inguinal hernia repair, laparoscopic hernia repair is associated with
A. Shorter operative time
B. Fewer vascular injuries
C. Fewer visceral injuries
D. No difference in time to return of usual activity
E. A similar rate of hernia recurrence when compared to open repairs with mesh

50. Routine administration of prophylactic preoperative antibiotics has been clearly shown to decrease infection rates in which of the following elective procedures?
A. Inguinal hernia repair with mesh
B. Laparoscopic cholecystectomy for biliary colic
C. Excisional breast biopsy for a suspicious breast mass
D. Sigmoid colectomy for large villous adenoma
E. Thyroidectomy for cancer

51. A surgical margin of 5 mm is appropriate for primary melanoma that is
A. In situ.
B. Up to 1 mm in depth.
C. Up to 2 mm in depth.
D. Up to 4 mm in depth.
E. It is not appropriate to have such a small margin in melanoma.

52. A 57-year-old woman comes into the ED with complaints of upper leg pain and fever. The triage nurse orders an x-ray that shows the presence of periosteal elevation in the mid-femur. Diagnosis may be confirmed by:
A. Evidence of fracture on X-ray.
B. A history of arthritis.
C. The finding of rosettes on bone biopsy.
D. An elevated WBC.
E. Positive blood culture.

53. The estimated lifetime risk of a man developing prostate cancer is
A. 1 in 5.
B. 1 in 10.
C. 1 in 20.
D. 1 in 50.
E. 1 in 100.

54. The most common site of a visceral arterial aneurysm is:
   A. Renal artery
   B. Superior mesenteric artery
   C. Splenic artery
   D. Celiac artery
   E. Hepatic artery

55. Energy required for walking is highest after:
   A. Above knee amputation (AKA)
   B. Below knee amputation (BKA)
   C. Transmetatarsal amputation (TMA)
   D. Symes amputation
   E. Knee disarticulation

56. A 75-year-old man presents to the emergency room after being found on the floor by his wife. He is unable to speak or move his right arm and leg. The next step in his management should be:
   A. Start heparin immediately
   B. Obtain a carotid duplex ultrasound
   C. Take him emergently to the operating room
   D. Obtain a head CT
   E. Start aspirin immediately

57. A 56-year-old woman is found on an abdominal ultrasound for gallstones to have a 3.5-cm infrarenal abdominal aortic aneurysm. You advise her that she should:
   A. Have the aneurysm fixed as soon as possible
   B. Forget about it
   C. Have a surveillance ultrasound every year
   D. Eat more fruits and vegetables
   E. Start an exercise regimen

58. A 63-year-old man is referred to you for bilateral calf cramping after walking four blocks. He is a busy, slightly overweight executive, who eats fast food, smokes two packs a day, and has chronic insomnia. What is the most important lifestyle change that may affect the progression of his disease?
   A. Start taking a lipid-lowering drug
   B. Stop smoking
   C. Exercise regularly
   D. Eat healthier
   E. Reduce stress

59. An ankle-brachial index (ABI) is:
  A. The diameter of the ankle divided by the diameter of the arm
  B. A measure of the degree of stenosis in the superficial femoral artery
  C. The diastolic blood pressure at the ankle divided by that at the arm
  D. Abnormal if <0.9
  E. Useless for following patients over time

60. Sepsis, vasopressors, and digitalis are all factors that may be associated with:
  A. Nonocclusive mesenteric ischemia
  B. Abdominal aortic aneurysm rupture
  C. Deep venous thrombosis
  D. Acute cerebral ischemia
  E. Hypercoagulable syndrome

61. A 55-year-old patient is scheduled for sigmoid colectomy for recurrent diverticulitis. His past medical history includes diabetes, hypercholesterolism, anemia, and atrial fibrillation. Which of his regular medications should he be advised to take on the morning of his operation?
  A. Insulin
  B. Oral hypoglycemics
  C. Statin therapy
  D. Iron
  E. Coumadin

62. A 64-year-old woman presents with a long-standing history of atrial fibrillation, for which she has been on anticoagulation therapy. Surgical management of this problem:
  A. Is not possible, as this is a primarily medical problem
  B. May involve replacement of the aortic valve
  C. Disrupts aberrant pathways through multiple incisions in the heart muscle
  D. Replaces the natural cardiac pacemaker
  E. Requires transplant

63. A 52-year-old man is found on routine CXR to have a chest mass. Lateral views suggest a posterior mediastinal lesion. No previous CXR is available for comparison. The most likely etiology is:
  A. Thymoma
  B. Substernal goiter
  C. Esophageal leiomyoma
  D. Brachiocephalic aneurysm
  E. Ganglioma

64. A 71-year-old patient is referred to you for evaluation of a lung nodule seen on x-ray. You learn that the patient was treated for lung cancer ~3 years prior. He tells you that he underwent chemotherapy and radiation, and that his course was complicated by "low salt levels and something about holding on to too much water." On examination, you see radiation port site tattoos but no chest scars. The most likely histology of his prior cancer is:
  A. Small-cell lung cancer
  B. Squamous cell cancer
  C. Adenocarcinoma
  D. Bronchioalveolar carcinoma
  E. Large cell carcinoma

65. Two years following resection of a node-positive colon cancer, your patient is found to have a solitary mass on a routine screening chest x-ray. The mass was not present on previous preoperative imaging studies. Regarding this lesion:
  A. If isolated, resection is indicated
  B. Primary treatment is radiation
  C. Positive emission tomography (PET) is not helpful
  D. A normal serum carcinoembryonic antigen (CEA) level excludes metastatic disease
  E. Percutaneous biopsy should be avoided

66. A 56-year-old man with a history of pancreatic cancer presents with shortness of breath and a new pleural effusion. The most appropriate treatment for him at this time is
  A. Arrangement of hospice care
  B. Plan for repeated periodic outpatient thoracentesis
  C. Placement of chest tube thoracostomy
  D. Fluid drainage and pleurodesis
  E. Open drainage via thoracotomy

67. Surgical treatment for patients with myasthenia gravis
  A. Is more likely to result in complete remission if the patient is over 60
  B. Is most likely to result in complete remission if performed within 3 years of diagnosis
  C. Results in complete remission in up to approximately 40% of patients
  D. Has a prognosis that is most reliably predicted by the histologic features of the thymus
  E. Is more successful in women

68. A patient with a history of jejuno-ileal bypass presents with renal calculi. The stones are most likely composed of:
A. Uric acid
B. Bilirubin
C. Cholesterol
D. Calcium oxalate
E. Cystine

69. Initial management of a hemodynamically stable trauma patient with a nonextravasating renal laceration extending through the renal cortex and medulla should include:
A. Immediate laparotomy and nephrectomy
B. Laparotomy and partial nephrectomy
C. Laparotomy and primary renal repair
D. Angiography and renal artery embolization
E. Observation and serial hematocrits

70. Prostate cancer
A. Has no causal relationship with benign prostatic hypertrophy (BPH)
B. Is the leading cause of cancer death among men in the United States
C. Can specifically be identified by an elevation in prostate specific antigen (PSA) levels
D. Decreases in incidence with age
E. Frequently metastasizes to the kidneys

71. A 42-year-old woman presents with a large abdominal mass. Imaging and eventual laparotomy suggest that the mass emanates from the bowel. The resected specimen stains positive for c-kit. The patient should be informed that:
A. Her expected survival is less than 1 year
B. Recurrent disease is common
C. She will need to be started on hormone therapy
D. There is no available adjuvant therapy for her tumor
E. Radiation therapy offers her a good chance for cure

72. Following a low anterior resection (LAR) for rectal cancer, a 65-year-old patient with a T3N0M0 adenocarcinoma should undergo
A. Close follow-up
B. Adjuvant chemotherapy
C. Adjuvant radiotherapy
D. Adjuvant chemoradiation
E. Reoperation for abdominoperineal resection (APR)

73. Which of the following associations between genetic marker and disease is correct?

- A. Adenomatous polyposis coli (APC)—familial adenomatous polyposis (FAP)
- B. BRCA1—esophageal cancer
- C. k-ras—breast cancer
- D. RET—pancreatic cancer
- E. p-53—lymphoma

74. A 66-year-old man with a history of abdominal pain and weight loss is explored for bowel obstruction. At operation, she is found to have an "apple-core" tumor in the proximal jejunum. Regarding this lesion:

- A. It will likely be responsive to radiation
- B. Chemotherapy is effective in prolonging survival
- C. It is less likely to be seen in patients with Crohn's disease
- D. It is most likely to be a carcinoid tumor
- E. 5 year survival is 15%–20%

75. A 56-year-old woman who presents with crampy abdominal pain, diarrhea, and flushing is found to have elevated urinary 5-HIAA levels. The most likely primary site of the source of her symptoms is the:

- A. Stomach
- B. Small bowel
- C. Appendix
- D. Colon
- E. Rectum

76. Keloids

- A. Result from scar overgrowth of the original wound edges
- B. Differ from hypertrophic scar by staying within the boundaries of the original wound
- C. Tend to regress spontaneously with time
- D. Occur most commonly on the limbs
- E. Are most commonly observed in patients aged 40–60 years.

77. You recommend that your patient have an epidural anesthetic placed for postoperative pain management. Your discussion of potential complications would include

- A. Hypertension
- B. Bradycardia
- C. Intracranial hematoma
- D. Prolonged postoperative ileus
- E. Need for absolute bedrest

78. You are scheduling a 76-year-old patient for a lower limb revascularization procedure. You remember that perioperative beta-blockade:

A. Is ideally started as soon as the patient is awake after surgery

B. Can also be effected using calcium-channel blockers

C. Should be targeted to a goal heart rate of 80–100 beats per minute

D. Has been shown to reduce cardiac morbidity and mortality for up to 2 years after operation

E. Commonly leads to problems with intraoperative hypotension

79. A 30-year-old woman complains of a one week history of L arm swelling and heaviness. She is a former college swimmer and continues to work-out at the gym three times a week. She does not recall any trauma or other injury to her arm. There is no numbness or tingling. After diagnostic imaging studies, which of the following is the most common initial treatment?

A. Exploration and first rib resection

B. Thrombolysis and stenting

C. Anticoagulation

D. Aspirin

E. Warm compresses and arm elevation

80. A 20-year-old man has recently noted cramping in his R calf with walking more than three blocks. He is not a smoker and has no family history of atherosclerosis. On examination, he has palpable pedal pulses when his foot is in a neutral position but no pulses when the foot is plantarflexed. Which of the following is the most likely diagnosis?

A. Early arterial occlusive disease

B. Popliteal adventitial cystic disease

C. Buerger's disease

D. Acute embolism

E. Popliteal artery entrapment

81. A patient is being considered for femoral-tibial bypass. Which of the following options is the most desirable conduit?

A. Cephalic vein

B. Expanded polytetrafluoroethylene (ePTFE)

C. Superficial femoral vein

D. Greater saphenous vein

E. Internal iliac artery

82. The most common cause of superior vena cava syndrome is:
   A. Chronic in-dwelling dialysis catheter
   B. Apical pulmonary tumor
   C. Chemotherapy infusion
   D. Thoracic outlet syndrome
   E. Lymphoma

83. Which of the following is the most common causative organism of primary arterial infections?
   A. *Candida*
   B. *Staphylococcus*
   C. *Streptococcus*
   D. *Salmonella*
   E. *Escherichia*

84. Which of the following is an example of a selective portosystemic shunt?
   A. Portocaval
   B. Mesocaval
   C. Proximal splenorenal
   D. Distal splenorenal
   E. Transjugular intrahepatic portosystemic

85. A 48-year-old man presents with a swollen, painful, and pale left leg. Evaluation reveals an occlusive left iliofemoral deep venous thrombosis. May-Thurner syndrome involves which of the following anatomic relationships?
   A. Left iliac vein runs over the left iliac artery
   B. Left iliac vein runs under the left iliac artery
   C. Left iliac vein runs over the right iliac artery
   D. Left iliac vein runs under the right iliac artery

86. You perform an open appendectomy on a 77-year-old woman for ruptured appendicitis. In the OR, you found a necrotic appendix with a localized pocket of pus. After closing the fascia, you decide to leave the skin open to avoid wound infection. Which of the following is true regarding delayed primary closure (DPC)?
   A. Less effective at preventing wound infection than healing by secondary intention
   B. Faster healing time than secondary intention
   C. Should be performed on POD #5 after wound contraction has begun
   D. Should be performed even if signs of infection are present
   E. Requires general anesthesia

87. Wound healing involves the phases of inflammation, epithelialization, fibroplasia, and
   A. Collagenization
   B. Homogenization
   C. Maturation
   D. Hemostasis
   E. Angiogenesis

88. A patient with rectal cancer undergoes preoperative radiation therapy to improve resectability prior to abdominoperineal resection. Which of the following wound healing complications is more likely after radiation?
   A. Infection
   B. Keloid formation
   C. Nerve compression
   D. Seroma
   E. Hematoma

89. The same patient has an uncomplicated procedure, but on postoperative day 8, his bandages become saturated with copious pinkish fluid draining from the inferior aspect of his abdominal incision. There is no erythema or fever. Which of the following is the most likely diagnosis?
   A. Superficial wound infection
   B. Seroma
   C. Necrotizing fasciitis
   D. Anastomotic leak
   E. Dehiscence

90. You are called to evaluate a newborn who developed tachypnea, cough, and excessive secretions after her first feeding. The neonatal team was unable to pass a nasogastric tube into the stomach, and the CXR shows the NGT curled in the mediastinum with air seen in the stomach. The baby is being kept in a head up position with the NGT to suction. What is the most likely diagnosis?
   A. Esophageal atresia (EA) with distal tracheoesophageal fistula (TEF)
   B. EA with proximal TEF
   C. EA with both proximal and distal TEF
   D. EA without fistula
   E. TEF without EA ("H-type")

91. Which of the following is associated with omphalocele but not with gastroschisis?
- A. Bowel
- B. Peritoneal sac
- C. Nonrotation of bowel
- D. Amniotic peritonitis
- E. Urgent repair

92. You are called urgently to a delivery. The baby is tachypneic, grunting, and cyanotic. He has decreased breath sounds on the left and distant heart sounds. His abdomen is scaphoid. You intubate the baby, and on his initial CXR, you see air-filled loops of bowel in the left chest. Your next step is to:
- A. Take the baby emergently to the operating room
- B. Place a sump gastric tube to low suction
- C. Maintain peak inspiratory pressures >35 mmHg
- D. Begin extracorporeal membrane oxygenation (ECMO)
- E. Place a left-sided chest tube

93. A neonate on day of life three begins to have bilious emesis. You question the mother and find that she has had very few stools. She has a distended but soft abdomen. Gentle rectal examination reveals a forceful release of air and liquid stool. A plain x-ray shows dilated loops of bowel but no discrete transition point. You suspect Hirschsprung's disease and order a contrast enema, which shows proximal colonic dilation and distal narrowing. What is the definitive way to make this diagnosis?
- A. Contrast enema
- B. Anorectal manometry
- C. CT pelvis
- D. Colonoscopy
- E. Rectal biopsy

94. Which of the following is the recommended initial bolus for a pediatric trauma patient?
- A. 5 cc/kg lactated Ringer's
- B. 10 cc/kg lactated Ringer's
- C. 20 cc/kg lactated Ringer's
- D. 50 cc/kg lactated Ringer's

95. What is the Glasgow Coma Scale score for a patient who opens his eyes only to painful stimuli, speaks inappropriate words, and withdraws his arms and legs to painful stimuli?

    A. 3
    B. 6
    C. 9
    D. 12
    E. 15

96. A patient has been stabbed in the neck. He is brought into the emergency department awake and alert, speaking in full sentences in a normal voice, and without any reported dysphagia. You examine his neck and find a wound posterior to the sternocleidomastoid muscle, just below the angle of the jaw. Which anatomic zone is involved?

    A. Zone I
    B. Zone II
    C. Zone III
    D. None of the above

97. A tall, thin, 32-year-old man presents to the emergency department with shortness of breath. He experienced similar symptoms a year ago, at which time he was diagnosed with a primary spontaneous pneumothorax and was able to be treated with observation alone. An upright CXR today reveals a recurrent spontaneous pneumothorax with near total lung collapse. After placing a chest tube and reexpanding the lung, you counsel the man that:

    A. The risk of recurrence is now 50%
    B. Smoking will be protective against further incidents
    C. Pleurodesis is the gold standard for prevention of recurrence
    D. Surgical resection of the underlying blebs requires thoracotomy
    E. He should avoid air travel for the rest of his life

98. Which of the following types of transplant rejection is reversible?
    A. Hyperacute
    B. Acute
    C. Chronic
    D. All of the above
    E. None of the above

99. Daclizumab (Zenapax) belongs to which of the following immunosuppression drug categories?
- A. Corticosteroid
- B. Antiproliferative
- C. Calcineurin inhibitor
- D. Antilymphocyte
- E. Anti-IL-2 receptor

100. A young woman presents to your office with a pulsatile mass in her neck, just below her jaw. She reports a "funny feeling" when swallowing. An ultrasound of the neck ordered by her primary care physician reveals a vascular mass between the internal and external carotid arteries. Carotid body tumors:
- A. Are typically painful
- B. Get their blood supply from the external carotid
- C. Are found in the medial layer at the carotid bifurcation
- D. Are generally malignant
- E. Should be observed

Answers and Explanations

1. C	26. B	51. A	76. A
2. A	27. A	52. E	77. B
3. D	28. E	53. B	78. D
4. A	29. C	54. C	79. C
5. B	30. A	55. A	80. E
6. B	31. B	56. D	81. D
7. A	32. B	57. C	82. A
8. B	33. E	58. B	83. B
9. A	34. C	59. D	84. D
10. C	35. A	60. A	85. D
11. D	36. C	61. C	86. B
12. F	37. D	62. C	87. C
13. A	38. E	63. E	88. A
14. B	39. C	64. A	89. E
15. A	40. F	65. A	90. A
16. E	41. B	66. D	91. B
17. D	42. B	67. C	92. B
18. B	43. D	68. D	93. E
19. D	44. A	69. E	94. C
20. B	45. E	70. A	95. C
21. D	46. B	71. B	96. B
22. E	47. C	72. D	97. A
23. B	48. C	73. A	98. B
24. E	49. E	74. E	99. E
25. B	50. D	75. C	100. B

1. C. The most efficient workup of a palpable neck mass is by FNA, because it will direct subsequent workup, diagnosis, staging, and treatment. FNA can identify squamous cell cancer (SCC) and adenocarcinoma with a fairly high degree of sensitivity and specificity, which in turn can direct the need for further interventions.

Because the differences between reactive lymphadenopathy and lymphoma cannot be reliably distinguished by FNA, those findings usually require open biopsy for diagnosis. In those cases, a limited (incisional or excisional) operative procedure may be planned. Outpatient laryngoscopy may be useful, but it will generally need to be done in conjunction with bronchoscopy and esophagoscopy (EGD) to fully evaluate for SCC, and is less appropriate as a first step. CT scan is indicated later in the workup, depending upon the results of the FNA and panendoscopy.

2. A. For women who are at moderate to high risk (by family or individual history, or by genetic markers such as BRCA1, BRCA2, or HNPCC), prophylactic mastectomy reduces the risk of breast cancer by approximately 90%. It does not, however, protect all patients from the disease.

Prophylactic mastectomy typically removes most but not all breast tissue. Its practice in patients with diffuse ductal carcinoma in situ (DCIS) is controversial, and should not be uniformly offered in the absence of other risk factors. Tamoxifen therapy does not confer nearly the same prophylactic benefit, as many patients with the BRCA1 mutation tend to develop ER/PR negative tumors.

3. D. Proven ductal carcinoma in situ (DCIS) in multiple quadrants is considered multicentric disease. Simple mastectomy with the option of immediate reconstruction constitutes optimal management. Notably, most DCIS is not multicentric, and breast conservation therapy can usually be achieved.

Sentinel lymph node biopsy for DCIS is controversial and would certainly not be performed without removal of the primary tumor. It may be indicated in some instances of high-grade DCIS or needle biopsy findings of microinvasion. Lumpectomy alone would be insufficient for the reasons mentioned above.

4. A. The finding of *atypical ductal hyperplasia* on a core needle biopsy should be followed with excisional biopsy. Up to 40% of patients will have the diagnosis upgraded to DCIS or invasive cancer upon more complete tissue sampling. A confirmed diagnosis of atypical ductal hyperplasia on excisional biopsy can be followed expectantly. There are no current indications for tamoxifen in this setting.

5. B. The major role for neoadjuvant chemotherapy in breast cancer is in downstaging disease and allowing more patients to be treated with breast-conservation therapy. Thus, it is primarily recommended as initial management for tumors deemed too large for lumpectomy. Large studies have shown no difference in terms of overall survival, progression-free survival, or locoregional recurrence. The side effect profile is similar regardless of perioperative timing. Notably, clinical objective response to chemotherapy is not a significant prognostic factor.

6. B. *Staphylococcus aureus* is the most commonly isolated organism in breast abscesses. Alpha-hemolytic streptococci and anaerobic bacteria can also be found. However, antibiotic therapy should initially be directed at gram-positive organisms. Subareolar abscesses typically occur in young, healthy, nonlactating women. They are thought to result from damaged ducts that become obstructed with accumulated debris. Recurrence is common if the underlying ductal pathology is not addressed surgically. Percutaneous aspiration is successful in up to 85% of patients. Ultrasound examination may be helpful to define the anatomy.

7. A. The most powerful predictor of prognosis is axillary node status, followed by tumor size and receptor status. Patients with estrogen-receptor positive tumors have a 10% increase in 5-year disease-free survival over those with estrogen-receptor negative tumors. On the other hand, HER-2/neu overexpression is associated with decreased disease-free survival.

Women who are pregnant or <35 years old at diagnosis have a worse prognosis. Breast cancer in males tends to be diagnosed at more advanced stages, accounting for its poorer prognosis. However, when controlled for stage, there is no survival difference as compared with women.

8. B. Although the risk of breast cancer in women is increased in carriers of either the BRCA1 or BRCA2 mutations, only mutations in BRCA2 is known to confer an increased risk in men.

Male breast cancer constitutes less than 1% of all male cancers and about 0.5% of all cases of breast cancer. Risk factors include Klinefelter's syndrome (47, XXY), African-American or Jewish heritage, obesity, cirrhosis, and family history. Gynecomastia is the most common form of male breast enlargement and is not a risk factor for male breast cancer. Although use of anabolic steroids has been associated with hepatocellular, prostate, and renal cell cancers, it has not been shown to increase male breast cancer risk.

9. A. An isolated lesion found in the body of the stomach (most commonly along the lesser curve) is a Type I ulcer and is associated with low to normal gastric acid levels. These are the most common gastric ulcers, comprising 50%–60% (Table 1).

TABLE 1 Classification of Gastric Ulcers

Type	% of gastric ulcers	Location	Acid secretion	Recommended operation
I	50–60	Body, usually lesser curve	nl/↓	Antrectomy
II	25	Body, associated with duodenal ulcers	↑	Vagotomy & antrectomy (V&A)
III	15	Prepyloric	↑	V&A
IV	<5	Near GE junction	nl/↓	Resection if possible (may require gastrectomy)
V		Any		Discontinue aspirin/NSAIDs

Type II gastric ulcers are also found in the body of the stomach but are associated with a concomitant duodenal ulcer. Gastric acid hypersecretion is present. These ulcers represent approximately 25% of all gastric ulcers.

Type III gastric ulcers are prepyloric and are also associated with acid hypersecretion.

Type IV gastric ulcers are similar to Type I ulcers, except that they occur high on the lesser curve, close to the gastroesophageal (GE) junction. These are associated with low to normal acid secretion.

Type V gastric ulcers are by definition associated with NSAID use and can occur throughout the stomach.

All gastric ulcers are at risk for malignant changes, so biopsies are always indicated during endoscopic evaluation. Larger lesions (3 cm) have a greater risk for malignancy than smaller ones.

Superficial gastritis and atrophic gastritis are commonly associated with gastric ulcer and may be linked to *H. pylori* infection. All types of gastric ulcer are associated with *H. pylori*, so eradication is always appropriate first-line therapy. Moreover, ulcers may recur with *H. pylori* reinfection.

10. **C.** Eradication of *H. pylori* typically includes at least 2 antibiotics in conjunction with a proton pump inhibitor (PPI). Cessation of NSAIDs is also recommended. Omeprazole is the most commonly used PPI. Most antibiotic regimens are administered for 14 days, and include:

Clarithromycin + amoxicillin
or Tetracycline + metronidazole

11. **D.** Treatment of a Zenker's diverticulum typically involves both diverticulectomy and cricopharyngeal myotomy. As with most epiphrenic diverticula, the pathophysiology involves an increase in intraluminal pressure, leading to pulsion-type herniation. Myotomy addresses the muscle hypertonicity and is always required to avoid recurrence.

In cases where the diverticulum is small, diverticulectomy may be omitted. In older or high risk patients, diverticulopexy, leaving the mouth of the diverticulum facing downward, may be appropriate. Diverticulectomy alone does not address the primary pathophysiologic problem. Esophagectomy is not required. Behavioral modifications will not change this primary neuromuscular problem. Botulinum toxin injections have been used in achalasia, but have no described role in treatment of Zenker's diverticulum.

12. **F.** Hiatal hernias that involve a hernia sac are commonly referred to as paraesophageal hernias and are most likely to require surgical intervention.

Type I hiatal hernias, also referred to as "sliding hernias," are the most common, and involve displacement of the gastroesophageal junction (GEJ) into the chest. Because the longitudinal axis of the stomach stays in line with the esophagus, the risk of incarceration or volvulus is low. These hernias do not have a true hernia sac.

Type II and III hernias are the paraesophageal hernias. In type II ("rolling") hernias, the GEJ is in a normal position, and a sac containing the gastric fundus and body develops alongside the esophagus. In type III ("mixed") hernias, the GEJ is displaced into the chest along with the sac containing part of the stomach. In these types of hernias, the stomach can rotate on a separate axis, leading to incarceration, volvulus, ischemia, and perforation. Because of these risks, elective surgical intervention is frequently recommended upon diagnosis. Paraesophageal hernias are increasingly common with advancing age.

13. A. Barrett's esophagitis is a premaligant lesion in which columnar epithelium replaces normal squamous epithelium (metaplasia). Most patients who go on to develop carcinoma in the setting of Barrett's esophagitis are men aged 55–60. Esophagectomy is recommended in patients with high grade dyplasia, because high grade dysplasia is pathologically difficult to distinguish from carcinoma in situ, leading to possible sampling error and missed diagnoses. Patients who undergo regular endoscopic surveillance (usually every two years) are more likely to present with lower-stage cancers than patients who do not participate in surveillance programs. Antireflux procedures may be appropriate in patients with no or low-grade dysplasia. In patients with symptoms of gastroesophageal reflux disease (GERD), 10%–15% will be diagnosed with Barrett's.

14. B. Jejunal, esophageal, pancreatic, and colonic fistulas are more likely to close than those arising in the stomach or ileum. Postoperative, diverticular, or post-appendicitis fistulas will generally close spontaneously, whereas those due to Crohn's disease, foreign bodies, or radiation exposure are less likely to do so. Long fistula tracts have increased resistance and a decreased likelihood of epithelialization, making them more likely to close than short ones. Low-output fistulas (<500 ml/24 hours) are 3 times more likely to close spontaneously than high output fistulas.

The mnemonic FRIEND can help to remember features which tend to keep fistulas open:
  F—foreign body
  R—radiation
  I—infection
  E—epithelialization
  N—neoplasm
  D—distal obstruction

15. A. Patients who have <120 cm of small bowel will have features of short gut syndrome, including diarrhea, fluid and electrolyte deficiencies, malnutrition, and increased risk of gallstones. Patients with <60–80 cm of small bowel are dependent on parenteral nutrition for survival. Preservation of the ileocecal valve improves bowel function, such that an intact ileocecal valve can allow patients with very little remaining small bowel to not require TPN. Proximal resections are generally better tolerated than distal ones, because the ileum can increase its absorptive capacity more effectively than the jejunum. Patients typically have hypergastrinemia. The increased risk of kidney stones is due to increased urinary oxalate that results from increased colonic oxalate absorption. The structural and functional changes associated with adaptation may continue for years.

16. E. Proton pump inhibitors (PPIs) are effective in decreasing symptoms of chronic GERD and in healing esophagitis. This is true even if gastric acidity is not normalized. Endoscopic follow-up in patients on PPIs shows an increase in the number of squamous epithelial islands within Barrett's segments, but biopsies from these islands often show continued underlying intestinal metaplasia. This suggests that PPI treatment may not result in clinically significant regression of Barrett's epithelium. There is no evidence that these medications inhibit progression to high-grade dysplasia.

17. D. Sigmoid volvulus commonly occurs in bedridden, institutionalized patients. Every attempt should be made to reduce the obstruction nonoperatively. This may include rigid or flexible sigmoidoscopy, barium enema, and/or insertion of a rectal tube. Success may be achieved in 70%–80% of cases using these techniques. Spontaneous reduction has been reported. Immediate laparotomy is not a first option unless there is peritonitis and concern for perforation, because of the increased morbidity and mortality of an operation in these patients. Neostigmine is used in colonic pseudo-obstruction and would not be appropriate here. There is no role for promotility agents in the face of a mechanical obstruction. Percutaneous decompression has been described for cecal volvulus, but not for sigmoid volvulus.

18. B. Ogilivie's syndrome (colonic pseudo-obstruction) is a massive dilation of the colon without mechanical obstruction. It may develop after operation, injury, or severe illness. Treatment with the cholinesterase inhibitor *neostigmine* increases acetylcholine activity and induces coordinated colonic propulsion. As such, neostigmine is a common first-line agent in the treatment of this disorder. Because of its pharmacologic action, bradycardia may result, so administration should be done in a monitored setting, with atropine available as needed.

If the obstruction fails to resolve, colonoscopic decompression or surgical intervention may be required to prevent ischemia and perforation. Primary causes such as electrolyte abnormalities should always be corrected.

19. D. Rectal prolapse (procidentia) is distinguished from hemorrhoids by the finding of concentric rings of mucosa (with or without associated underlying bowel wall) protruding through the anus. Hemorrhoidal prolapse, on the other hand, classically has radial grooves, which mark the separation between individual piles.

The management of rectal prolapse is surgical, with both perineal and abdominal approaches described. The approach depends on the overall health of the patient (perineal approaches are somewhat more easily tolerated, but may be less durable), the degree of prolapse, and the experience of the surgeon. In some instances, it may be appropriate to suspend the rectum from the sacrum without resection (rectopexy). Other abdominal surgical options include sigmoidectomy, sigmoidectomy with rectopexy, and variations involving mesh. Perineal options include reinforcement of the anus with a constrictive band (Thiersch operation), perineal proctosigmoidectomy (Altemeier procedure), and mucosal stripping and plication of the rectal circular muscle (Delorme procedure).

Hysterectomy will not fix a rectal prolapse. Colostomy can help with incontinence, but will not affect the prolapsing tissue. Strengthening exercises for the perineal muscles (e.g., Kegel exercises) may be a useful adjunct, but alone will not treat the prolapse.

20. B. The discovery of *H. pylori* has dramatically changed the way that diseases of the foregut are assessed, diagnosed, and treated. *H. pylori* infection has been implicated in the pathogenesis of duodenal and gastric ulcers. Furthermore, *H. pylori* has been classified as a definite carcinogen in the development of both adenocarcinoma and gastric lymphoma, specifically mucosa-associated lymphoid tumors (MALTomas).

21. D. Ischemic colitis is the most common form of bowel ischemia. It results from a number of different etiologies, including drugs, abdominal aortic or mesenteric vascular procedures, low flow states due to cardiac failure or other types of shock, and a variety of vasculitides and coagulopathies. Often, no specific etiology is found. In most cases, ischemic colitis can be treated with antibiotics and supportive care, although a small number of patients will progress to full-thickness necrosis or develop a subsequent stricture.

Although ischemic colitis can occur anywhere in the colon, it is most commonly seen in the splenic flexure and descending and sigmoid colon. Approximately 90% of cases occur in patients older than 60 years of age. Colonoscopy is the preferred diagnostic modality, as angiography often does not show a specific lesion. Vasopressors often preferentially cause vasoconstriction of the peripheral and mesenteric vessels and may actually exacerbate the problem.

22. E. This patient's presentation is highly suspicious for (cervical) esophageal perforation. Placement of a (blind) nasogastric tube is discouraged, as it may exacerbate the problem. The diagnosis may be confirmed by extravasation on gastrografin (a water-soluble contrast agent) swallow or CT scan, or by subcutaneous air seen on lateral cervical spine films. Neck exploration based on clinical grounds is appropriate. Whether or not the perforation can be identified or repaired, the most important aspect of surgical management in this case is *drainage* of the affected area.

23. B. The most appropriate treatment for intussusception in adults is operative exploration and (usually) bowel resection. Although intussusception most commonly occurs in early childhood, adult cases account for about 5%. In adults, the lead point is typically a mass such as a polyp, tumor, focus of endometriosis or Meckel's diverticulum. Operative intervention is required because of the high risk that a pathologic lead point is present (tumor until proven otherwise!). Although contrast enema is typically the best diagnostic (and potentially therapeutic) study in children, abdominal CT seems to be more accurate in adults.

24. E. The patient has a "gallstone ileus" that is best treated with operative intervention. It is a condition that occurs in patients with cholelithiasis, who have recurrent episodes of cholecystitis with eventual adhesion formation between the gallbladder and the gastrointestinal tract. With progressive bouts of inflammation, the gallstones can then erode into the bowel, where they may become impacted and cause a mechanical obstruction. The distal ileum/ileocecal valve is the most frequent site of obstruction. Air in the biliary tree may give a clue to this diagnosis, as it is consistent with the presence of a cholecystoenteric fistula. Operative treatment involves enterotomy and stone retrieval. Cholecystectomy and fistula closure is often delayed, sometimes indefinitely, because of the difficulty with operating in this inflamed area.

25. B. The inflammatory process that is seen in necrotizing pancreatitis may be sterile or infected. Several studies have suggested that patients with sterile necrosis may be managed nonoperatively with bowel rest, total parenteral nutrition, and analgesics. The use of antibiotics in this instance remains somewhat controversial. On the other hand, if infected pancreatic necrosis is identified, the most appropriate management is intravenous antibiotics and operative debridement. The most accurate method for determining whether necrotizing pancreatitis is infected is by aspiration, gram stain, and culture of the pancreatic phlegmon.

CT, ultrasound, and nuclear medicine studies do not indicate whether the inflammatory process is infected, but can give an indication as to the extent of inflammation and necrosis. Lipase and amylase levels do not reflect bacterial infection.

26. B. All patients with adrenal incidentalomas should undergo studies to determine whether the tumor is functional. The studies should include determination of fractionated urinary and/or plasma metanephrines (to detect subclinical pheochromocytoma), serum potassium (and aldosterone, if the patient is hypertensive) to detect aldosteronoma, and cortisol levels and/or dexamethasone suppression test to look for Cushing's syndrome. Patients who have a functional tumor should undergo resection. If the tumor is nonfunctional, then follow-up imaging is indicated. The follow-up scan should be done in 6–12 months. For tumors that are greater than 6 cm at diagnosis, then removal is indicated, as the risk of malignancy is higher. Since the advent of laparoscopic adrenalectomy, many surgeons have lowered the size limit to 4 cm for universal recommendation of removal. Patients who have a known history of prior malignancy AND who do not have evidence of a functional adrenal tumor may be candidates for fine needle aspiration (FNA) to confirm the presence of metastatic disease. FNA is otherwise avoided because of the risk of track seeding or stimulation of potential pheochromocytoma.

27. A. The most sensitive test for acute acalculous cholecystitis is cholescintigraphy (HIDA scan). The test is often performed with morphine, which causes contraction of the sphincter of Oddi, increasing pressure in the common bile duct. Failure of the cystic duct and gallbladder to fill is diagnostic. Acalculous cholecystitis is most commonly seen in critically ill patients, and is often difficult to diagnose because of the patients' altered mental status, unreliable physical exam, and difficult to interpret laboratory tests. Morphine cholescintigraphy in acute cholecystitis has a sensitivity of 65%–90% in critically ill patients versus 50%–75% for ultrasound.

28. E. The classic clinical triad associated with Budd-Chiari syndrome is rapidly developing ascites, right upper quadrant pain, and hepatomegaly, with ascites being the most common presenting sign. In fulminant Budd-Chiari syndrome, liver failure can progress rapidly to profound coma or death. Milder forms may be associated with jaundice, bleeding esophageal varices, and encepthalopathy. Option "d" is the triad associated with acute cholangitis.

In Western countries, the major causes of obstruction are hematologic disorders, such as polycythemia vera or factor V (Leiden) mutation. Veno-occlusive disease (VOD) of the liver is a related disorder, but differs in its occlusion of small central or sublobular veins rather than in the hepatic veins themselves. Treatment is geared toward relief of hepatic engorgement and prevention of recurrence. The most effective therapy for a patient with completely thrombosed hepatic veins and a patent inferior vena cava is portosystemic shunt.

29. C. Initial treatment of variceal bleeding is supportive, and should include volume resuscitation with blood products, somatostatin, and lactulose as needed to decrease encephalopathy. Endoscopic treatment successfully stops bleeding in up to 90% of patients. First-line prevention of rebleeding is generally accomplished with endoscopic obliteration of varices with sclerotherapy or band ligation. When first line management is unsuccessful, portal decompression or devascularization should be considered. Transjugular intrahepatic portosystemic shunt (TIPS) has largely replaced open procedures, as it has a lower perioperative morbidity and does not disrupt future options for transplant. However, patency rates for open portosystemic shunts are significantly better, and may be appropriate in patients in whom follow-up will be difficult. Several types of operative (open) portosystemic shunts have been described, and the choice of which to use depends largely on the condition of the patient and the institutional preference/experience.

Esophagectomy is not an appropriate surgical option. Liver transplant is reserved for the patient who fails decompressive therapy, and is usually contraindicated in a patient who is still drinking. Paracentesis may temporarily relieve symptoms related to ascites (if present), but does nothing to prevent recurrence. This patient's Child's class is relatively favorable.

30. A. The patient has a pancreatic pseudocyst, with no signs or symptoms to suggest superinfection. Asymptomatic patients may be safely observed, and should be followed-up with serial abdominal CT scans. At least 25% of pseudocysts will resolve spontaneously, with spontaneous resolution more likely in the setting of acute rather than chronic pancreatitis. Indications for intervention would include free rupture, hemorrhage, or an increase in size. In those instances, percutaneous approaches have a lower initial success rate than endoscopic or operative techniques.

31. B. Pneumatosis intestinalis is a relatively rare finding of air in the bowel wall, and is most commonly associated with intestinal ischemia and transmural infarction. Patients who also have portomesenteric venous gas are more likely to have transmural infarction than are those with pneumatosis alone. The overall presentation and condition of the patient will guide this assessment, and any patient in whom dead bowel is suspected will require immediate operative intervention. Other (nonoperative) conditions in which pneumatosis has been described include inflammatory bowel disease and pancreatitis. It is possible to see pneumatosis on plain x-rays, although it is usually easier to see on CT. There is no role for a contrast study such as enteroclysis in this setting.

32. B. Chylothorax and chylous ascites may occur following mediastinal or retroperitoneal operations. The incidence of postoperative chylothorax ranges from 0.2%–0.5%, and symptoms usually appear at 2–10 days postop. Diagnosis is confirmed by the finding of chylomicrons, a fat content higher than that of the plasma, or a triglyceride level of >100 mg/dl in the fluid. The output is usually 500 to 1000 mL/day. The mainstay of treatment is drainage of the fluid, total parenteral nutrition (TPN), and bowel rest. In addition, somatostatin therapy has been shown to help with closure of lymphatic fistulas. The majority of these leaks will close with conservative management. Surgical closure is only considered when noninvasive approaches have failed. Dietary supplementation with medium-chain triglycerides (MCT) is not effective. Pleurodesis is used in cases of intractable pleural effusions (usually malignant), but has no role in the treatment of chylothorax.

33. E. The optimal time to perform operative biliary procedures in pregnancy is during the second trimester. During the first trimester, operative intervention (open or laparoscopic) is associated with an increased risk of spontaneous abortion and possible teratogenicity. During the third trimester, there is an increased risk of injury to the uterus and induction of premature labor. Acute cholecystitis must be judiciously managed, as progression of the disease can lead to problems for both mother and fetus. When IV antibiotics, fluids, and analgesics are not successful in treating the sequelae of acute cholecystistis, operative intervention is indicated. Percutaneous cholecystostomy may be used as a temporizing measure, but the second trimester patient is best managed with laparoscopic cholecystectomy. In the absence of other complications, there is no reason to sacrifice the pregnancy or to deliver the not yet viable fetus. Changing antibiotics is unlikely to be of significant benefit, and may delay definitive management.

34. C. *E. coli* is the most common bacterium cultured from gallbladder or common bile duct bile. Colonization with other gram-negative organisms and some gram-positive cocci (such as *S. faecalis* or *Enterococcus*) is also common. However, the virulence of the gram-positive cocci is low. The most common anaerobic bacterium is *C. perfringens*.

35. A. Obturator hernias are the most common type of pelvic floor hernia, though they are infrequently encountered. They occur almost exclusively in older, thin women who lack a protective layer of perperitoneal fat at the obturator canal. They are generally asymptomatic until strangulation develops. The clinical presentation is usually one of intestinal obstruction in a patient with no history of previous abdominal operation. Compression of the obturator nerve results in symptoms of pain in the ipsilateral hip, medial thigh, and knee that is exacerbated by extension and relieved by flexion of the thigh (Howship-Romberg sign). This is pathognomonic but is present in only 25%–50% of patients. Diagnosis is usually made by CT imaging or at laparotomy.

36. C. Although it was originally feared that early laparoscopic cholecystectomy in acute cholecystitis would lead to an increased complication rate, this has proven NOT to be the case. In addition, early intervention has been associated with DECREASED operative time, rate of conversion to open procedure, length of hospital stay, and operative blood loss. When it is not possible to perform the operation within 72 hours of onset of symptoms, these benefits may be diminished, in which case many surgeons may opt to delay surgery (for 6 weeks) to allow for a "cooling down" period. Interval cholecystectomy may then be performed at that time.

37. D. Botulinum toxin blocks acetylcholine (Ach) release from nerve terminals, and is fatal in large doses. When used therapeutically, it can treat conditions resulting from excessive or inappropriate muscle contraction. It has been used in conditions such as chronic anal fissure, achalasia, various tremors and tics, and (perhaps most famously) upper facial wrinkles. There is no role for Botox in the treatment of the other conditions listed.

38. E. A CT scan will help determine whether there is underlying infection (such as abscess) or fistula in relationship to the mesh. If so, then the patient will need to be started on intravenous antibiotics, have the fluid drained, and possibly have the mesh removed. TPN might be considered if there is evidence of fistula to or through the mesh. It makes no sense to partially excise or cover the mesh, as it will all be infected. In some cases, it may be possible to preserve the mesh with percutaneous drainage as needed and intravenous antibiotics. If open operative intervention is required, then the mesh will almost certainly need to be removed, and replaced with either absorbable mesh (which will leave a hernia) or with autologous tissue (which is not always technically feasible). There is no reason to divert the enteral stream at this time.

39. C. Although optimal hernia management in a patient with ascites would allow for medical control of the ascites, this is sometimes not possible. An incarcerated hernia with skin ulceration demands immediate operative repair. Unfortunately, umbilical hernia repair in the setting of uncontrolled ascites is associated with significantly higher morbidity and mortality rates than when ascites is absent. Worsening ascites and plans for TIPS are both reasons to delay operative intervention. Leaking ascites is an urgent problem that is best managed with hospitalization, aggressive medical management with diuresis and sodium restriction, and intravenous antibiotics. Ideally, these measures can sufficiently control the ascites for repair of the leaking hernia during the same admission. Hernia size should not be a criterion for timing of surgery.

40. F. Enteroclysis is an intubation infusion contrast study of the small bowel. It is the most sensitive study to predict the presence of obstruction, with a >98% sensitivity and a 90% specificity. In addition, it can show the level of the obstruction in 89% of cases. It is the definitive study when the diagnosis of low-grade intermittent small-bowel obstruction is clinically uncertain. Plain abdominal films and abdominal CT are quicker and easier to obtain, and so are unlikely to be replaced by enteroclysis as a first line study, particularly in the acutely presenting patient. Plain films are diagnostic in 50%–60% of patients and equivocal in 20%–30%. When diagnostic, these studies are usually not sufficient to identify the site of the obstruction.

Abdominal CT scan has a sensitivity of 80%–100% for high-grade and 45%–60% for low-grade obstruction. CT can reveal the cause of the obstruction in 73%–95% of cases.

41. B. Insulin is produced in the beta cells of the pancreatic islets of Langerhans. Patients with insulinoma suffer from an overproduction of insulin, which renders them hypoglycemic. Whipple's triad is the combination of low fasting glucose levels, symptom reproduction concurrent with the finding of low serum glucose, and symptom amelioration with the administration of dextrose. Insulinoma is treated by operative enucleation.

42. B. Patients in hypercalcemic crisis may have symptoms of anorexia, vomiting, constipation, dehydration, acute pancreatitis, shortened QT interval, polyuria, polysdipsia, nephrocalicnosis, apathy, drowsiness, coma, and, if untreated, death. It is usually caused by a progressive marked primary hyperparathyroidism, producing accelerated bone resorption and excessive elevation in serum and urinary levels of calcium. It is unclear what causes the sudden progression of hyperparathyroidism. Treatment is geared toward correcting dehydration, enhancing renal excretion of calcium, inhibiting accelerated bone resorption, and treating the underlying disorder. Initial treatment is with administration of large volumes of saline until normovolemia is achieved. This is followed by administration of a loop diuretic (i.e., furosemide), which inhibits calcium reabsorption in the ascending limb of the loop of Henle. Thiazide diuretics are contraindicated because they enhance distal tubular reabsorption of calcium. Bisphosphonates, gallium, and calcitonin inhibit osteoclast-mediated bone resorption. Oral phosphates and mithramycin may also be used as needed.

43. D. A solitary thyroid nodule in a child younger than 5 years of age (though rare) is much more commonly malignant than in an adult, with an incidence of thyroid cancer ranging from 18%–50%. If cancer is found on fine needle aspiration (FNA), then surgical excision is indicated. Benign solid lesions should be carefully followed, as the nearly 6% false negative rate seen for FNA may be quite significant when the incidence of malignancy approaches 50%. Serial examinations with ultrasound, thyroid scintigraphy, history, and physical examination may all be utilized. Benign cystic lesions may be aspirated for cure. There is some debate as to when children with a history of multiple endocrine neoplasia type 2A or 2B should be treated, with many recommending prophylactic thyroidectomy in childhood, due to the high penetrance of medullary thyroid cancer in those patients. Fewer children are being exposed to neck irradiation, with a concomitant decrease in the incidence of childhood thyroid cancer. Iodine deficiency is usually associated with diffuse goiter.

44. A. The thyroid is the only organ that accumulates iodine, which it uses to produce thyroid hormone. Thus, radioactive iodine (RAI) therapy is useful in well-differentiated thyroid cancers of papillary or follicular origin. It is NOT useful in medullary, anaplastic, or other cancers metastatic to the thyroid, as these cells do not uptake iodine. RAI is usually recommended in patients with well-differentiated tumors who are at increased risk for recurrence (primary tumor larger that 1–1.5 cm in diameter, invasive or locoregional metastases, age >45).

45. E. The standard, time-honored technique for removal of hyperplastic parathyroid glands is the (bilateral) 4-gland exploration. In this way, both sides of the neck are dissected, and all 4 glands are visualized. Because the diagnosis of parathyroid adenoma versus hyperplasia is dependent on the finding of enlarged as well as normal-sized glands (the histology is similar, so this is a clinical diagnosis), this approach is the surest way to confirm the diagnosis. The operation is typically done through a transverse collar incision that measures 6–10 cm in size. Though the cosmetic result is improved by careful placement of the incision, it still tends to leave a fairly noticeable scar because of its location.

More recently, the *focused*, or *directed* approach to parathyroidectomy has fallen into favor. This approach relies on preoperative imaging with sestamibi scanning and/or ultrasound, often in conjunction with intraoperative PTH (IOPTH) monitoring. In this way, a limited cervical incision (or set of incisions, if a laparoscopic approach is used) can be made directly over the tumor. This arguably leads to a more cosmetic incision (usually 2.5 to 4 cm in length). There is no reported difference in pain with this technique. It has been hypothesized that a higher rate of injury to the recurrent nerve would be seen because of the limited view, but this has not yet been reported. However, this potential effect may be balanced by the lack of risk to the contralateral side when only the involved side is explored. When preoperative studies are concordant (i.e., both ultrasound and nuclear imaging suggest the same location for the enlarged gland), the likelihood of the finding the involved gland at that location is >90%–95%. With the addition of a 50% decrease in IOPTH, the success rate is even higher. This is consistent with the historical >95% success rate seen in 4-gland approaches.

46. B. Normal expansion rates for AAA are estimated at 0.2 to 0.4 cm per year. The rate of rupture over 5 years for AAA of <5 cm is 2%, 5 to 7 cm 25% to 40%, and >7 cm □50%.

47. C. The overall survival benefits for breast conservation therapy as compared with modified radical mastectomy are equivalent. This has lead to an increased effort at preserving breast tissue in surgery for patients diagnosed with breast cancer.

48. C. As in women, the most common histology of breast cancer in men is *invasive ductal carcinoma*, accounting for about 90%. DCIS, Paget's disease, colloid, medullary, secretory, lobular, and inflammatory cancers have all been described. About 85% of male breast cancers are estrogen positive, a good prognostic feature. Principles of treatment are the same as in women, though it is more common to perform total mastectomy (as opposed to breast conservation therapy). Data for adjuvant therapy is derived from studies done in women.

49. E. In a large meta-analysis of 41 published reports, it was found that laparoscopic procedures involved a longer duration of operation (nearly 15 minutes, on average), a slight increase in visceral and vascular injuries (though low rates overall), no major difference in length of hospital stay, earlier return to usual activity, and less persistent postoperative pain. The use of mesh is associated with a reduction in the risk of hernia recurrence, such that a laparoscopic repair compared with an open nonmesh repair has a significantly lower recurrence rate. This advantage is lost if laparoscopic repair is compared against open mesh methods of hernia repair.

50. D. With the exception of the colon operation, multiple meta-analyses of the above-mentioned procedures have shown NO significant reduction in the rate of postoperative infections when routine administration of antibiotic prophylaxis is used. However, many surgeons continue to give preoperative antibiotics despite the paucity of evidence to support the practice. Some studies have suggested that good perioperative care, including adequate hydration, oxygenation, and warming may be equally effective.

51. A. Current recommendations hold that surgical margins of 5 mm are appropriate for melanoma in situ. Margins of 1 cm are recommended for melanomas up to 1 mm in depth (low-risk primaries). Randomized prospective studies show that 2-cm margins are appropriate for tumors of intermediate thickness (1–4 mm depth), although there is some evidence that 1-cm margins may be sufficient for tumors up to 2 mm thick. Margins of at least 2 cm are recommended for melanoma >4 mm thick. These considerations may have significant cosmetic implications, depending on the location of the tumor.

52. E. The diagnosis of osteomyelitis can generally be made in a patient with 2 of the 4 following criteria: (1) purulent material on aspiration of affected bone, (2) positive findings on bone or blood culture, (3) local classical findings of bony tenderness to palpation, with overlying soft tissue erythema/edema, and (4) positive imaging (x-ray or bone scan).

53. B. In the United States, estimates indicate that 1 in 10 men will develop prostate cancer in their lifetime. Findings of incidental prostate cancer (as in autopsy specimens) suggest rates that are considerably higher. The incidence of prostate cancer increases with age.

54. C. Splenic artery aneurysms account for nearly 60% of all visceral aneurysms. The risk of rupture and subsequent mortality is high if found in a pregnant woman. The indications for operation include symptoms, diameter >2 cm, woman of child-bearing age, and preoperative status for liver transplant. Most hepatic artery aneurysms occur in the common, extrahepatic segment. Most SMA aneurysms are mycotic and related to endocarditis. Both rupture and thrombosis are concerns.

55. A. TMA increases the energy of walking by 5%, while a BKA increases requirements by 9%–25%. In contrast, AKA requires a 50%–150% increase in energy expenditure for ambulation. Almost all AKAs will heal, compared to approximately 80% of BKAs.

56. D. A head CT is the first diagnostic test and should be performed immediately to rule out a hemorrhagic event. If there is no evidence of an intracranial hemorrhage, then catheter-directed or systemic thrombolysis may be initiated if appropriate (i.e., acute onset, no contraindications). Close neurologic monitoring is required for such therapy, as an ischemic stroke can be converted to a hemorrhagic stroke. If thrombolysis is not an option, a carotid duplex or CT angiogram may be performed and an emergent carotid endarterectomy considered if the appropriate anatomy is identified.

57. C. An infrarenal AAA should be considered for repair if diameter is >5.5 cm in men and >4.5 cm in women. Once an aneurysm grows to >4 cm, surveillance should be done biannually. The annual incidence of rupture for small aneurysms is <1%, compared to >20% for aneurysms >7cm.

58. B. Although all of the options are important in slowing the progression of atherosclerosis, smoking cessation is the single most effective intervention that can affect both disease progression and symptoms.

59. D. The ankle-brachial index is calculated by taking the highest systolic pressure measured at either the dorsalis pedis or posterior tibial artery and dividing it by the highest systolic brachial pressure. Both of these measurements should be taken by Doppler on each side. In addition to symptomatology, the ABI is a simple way of following patients and progression of disease over time. Claudication can occur with ABIs between 0.5 and 0.9, while tissue loss and gangrene generally does not occur until the ABI is <0.3. ABIs may be falsely elevated with severe vessel calcification, as occurs in diabetics and patients on chronic dialysis.

60. A. Nonocclusive mesenteric ischemia occurs in critically ill patients. Treatment is primarily supportive, with weaning of vasopressors as much as possible. In severe cases, infusion of a vasodilator directly into the SMA can be performed.

61. C. A retrospective cohort study of 780,000 patients who underwent major noncardiac surgery found a reduced risk of mortality in those receiving statins (Lindenauer, et al, JAMA 2004). Based on this study and others, it is recommended that statin therapy be continued up to and including the day of surgery. Most oral hypoglycemics should be held on the day of surgery, and insulin doses should generally be halved or held. There is no particular benefit to continuing the iron therapy through the NPO period. Coumadin should be discontinued 3–5 days before surgery.

62. C. Corrective surgical treatments for chronic atrial fibrillation include the Cox-Maze procedure, which consists of numerous incisions in the left and right side of the heart to block the signals coming from the atria and going to the ventricle. This may also be accomplished with radiofrequency and cryoablation techniques. Chronic atrial fibrillation is associated with mitral valve disease and other structural abnormalities, but valve replacement does not often fix the arrhythmia. Transplant is not indicated.

63. E. The mediastinum is typically divided into three parts (anterior, middle, and posterior), each extending from the thoracic inlet to the diaphragm. Knowing what structures reside in each of these areas will help with identification of aberrant masses. In the absence of other (previous) imaging studies, this understanding will be the most useful guide to further evaluation and workup. The anterior mediastinum is bounded by the sternum anteriorly and the anterior pericardium posteriorly. Structures found here include the thymus, fat, thyroid, and lymph nodes. Thus, the most common masses found here are sometimes recalled as the "terrible Ts" of the mediastinum: Thymoma, Thyroid (cancer, occasionally), Teratoma, and "Terrible" lymphoma. The middle mediastinum extends from the anterior pericardium to the anterior surface of the vertebral bodies; masses here are of the heart, great vessels, esophagus, nerves or lymph nodes. The posterior mediastinum extends posteriorly from the anterior vertebral bodies, encompassing the nerve roots and ganglion cells. A ganglioma would therefore be the most likely of the choices to be found in this region. See Table 2.

TABLE 2   Mediastinal Masses and their Expected Locations

Anterior (sternum to anterior pericardium)

Middle (anterior pericardium to anterior vertebral bodies)

Posterior (posterior to anterior surface of vertebral bodies) Contains

Thymus, fat, lymph nodes, thyroid if present

Heart, great vessels, trachea, esophagus, vagus, phrenic nerves, thoracic duct, most mediastinal lymph nodes

Sympathetic ganglia and paraganglionic cells, descending thoracic aorta, vertebral bodies

Masses

Thymoma

Teratoma/other germ cell tumors

Thyroid (substernal goiter, including tumor)

Lymphoma

Pericardial cyst

Lipoma

Diaphragm hernia (Morgagni hernia, a congenital defect)

Esophageal tumors

Tumors of the vagus or phrenic nerves

Aneurysm/angioma of the great vessels

Thoracic duct cyst

Foregut cyst

Lymphoma

Neurogenic tumors: ganglioma, paraganglioma, neuroblastoma, ganglioneuroblastoma

Descending thoracic aortic aneurysm

Meningocele

Tumors of the thoracic vertebra

64. A. Small cell lung cancer (SCLC) accounts for 15%–20% of all lung cancer cases, with cigarette smoking cited as a primary causative factor. Associated paraneoplastic syndromes are frequent, with the most common being the syndrome of inappropriate antidiuretic hormone (SIADH). Because SCLC is frequently extensive or metastatic at the time of diagnosis, operative therapy is rarely indicated. Treatment is with chemotherapy, and a complete response is seen in up to 80% of patients with limited disease. Still, overall survival remains dismal, with a median survival of 7–18 months, and a five-year survival of 2–25%, depending on the stage at diagnosis. The addition of radiation therapy may improve survival by 5%. Primary treatment for the other tumors listed is operative.

65. A. In this patient, the chest mass is cancer until proven otherwise. Although the most common site for distant metastasis from colon cancer is to the liver, isolated metastases to the lung are well described. Diagnosis can often be confirmed by percutaneous biopsy, though this is seldom necessary. Primary treatment is surgical, with reported survival rates for resection of isolated lung metastases similar to those for resection of isolated hepatic metastases. It is important to assess for other distant disease before proceeding with resection, as you would not want to subject the patient to metastatectomy for asymptomatic disease if not for curative intent. PET scanning can help to assess for foci of disease that may not be visible on other imaging. CEA levels are a good method for detecting (recurrent or) metastatic disease, but serum levels may not rise in all cases; therefore, a normal level does not exclude metastatic disease.

66. D. Treatment of malignant pleural effusion is focused on improving patient quality of life. Because persistent shortness of breath is quite distressing, management focuses on removing the fluid and preventing reaccumulation. Multiple thoracenteses or chest tube placement will remove fluid, but will not prevent reaccumulation. Pleurodesis causes the lung to adhere to the chest wall, eliminating the potential pleural space, and subsequent fluid accumulation. This can be accomplished by installation of bleomycin or talc into a chest tube, or via thoracoscopy. Thoracosopic approaches tend to be more effective, with long-term relief of symptoms exceeding 50%. There is no reason to drain the fluid via open thoracotomy.

67. C. Thymectomy is the surgical treatment for patients with myasthenia gravis. Complete remission occurs in 28%–42% of patients, and substantial improvement occurs in 58%–94%. The most reliable prognostic factor is amount of time between the onset of symptoms and thymectomy, with the shorter amount of time being the most favorable; the best chance for remission is seen if the operation is performed within 8 months of diagnosis. Complete remission is less common in patients over the age of 60. Men and women do equally well after thymectomy.

68. **D.** Renal calculi are often seen in patients who have undergone jejuno-ileal bypass for obesity, and calcium oxalate stones are most common. This is thought to be related to steatorrhea, which leads to increased calcium saponification, limiting the amount of free calcium available to bind with oxalate. Oxalate, an end product of metabolism, thus remains soluble, and can only be excreted in the urine. An increased concentration of oxalate in the urine is associated with urolithiasis.

69. **E.** There is no (immediate) indication for laparotomy in a patient with a renal laceration who is hemodynamically stable, has no peritoneal signs, and has no active extravasation of blood or urine on CT scan. Nonoperative management (bed rest, serial exams, and hematocrits) is successful in 85%–90% of cases. Renal artery embolization is not indicated when there is no active hemorrhage on CT scan, and/or when it is apparent that there is a significant amount of functioning renal parenchyma.

70. **A.** Although prostate cancer and benign prostatic hypertrophy (BPH) can occur simultaneously, there is no known causal relationship. It is the most common cancer in men in the United States and the second leading cause of cancer death. Serum prostate specific antigen (PSA) is specific for the prostate, but may be elevated in BPH, prostatitis, or prostate cancer. Prostate cancer incidence increases with age, and has been identified in more than 30% of men over the age of 50, and more than 75% of men older than 80, suggesting a gap between the microscopic presence and clinical significance of the disease. Prostate cancer usually metastasizes to locoregional lymph nodes, and commonly to bone.

71. **B.** Gastrointestinal stromal tumors (GIST) are rare, slow-growing mesenchymal tumors that probably arise from intestinal pacemaker cells (the interstitial cells of Cajal). These cells stain positive for the antigen CD-34 and for the proto-oncogene c-kit. The clinical behavior of these tumors is quite variable, but complete surgical resection offers the best chance for cure. Tumor size and number of mitoses per high powered field are the best predictors of malignant potential. Surgical resection for GIST may offer cure in up to 50% of patients, particularly if the tumors are small and localized. Disease-free survival of completely resected GIST ranges from 30%–60% at 5 years. These tumors do not generally involve the lymph nodes, but commonly recur in the peritoneal cavity and liver.

GISTs are NOT typically responsive to conventional chemotherapy or radiation. A relatively new agent, ST-571 (Gleevec), selectively inhibits the tyrosine kinase receptors of tumors that possess c-kit mutations. This has been the most effective adjuvant treatment for GIST, and is frequently offered to patients with c-kit positive tumors who recur.

72. D. The patient has a stage II rectal carcinoma (Table 3). Patients with stage II or III rectal cancer are at high risk for both local and distant disease recurrence. It is recommended that these patients undergo combined (radio-sensitization) chemo-radiotherapy, typically involving fluorouracil (5-FU). This treatment has reduced the rate of recurrence by 30%–40%. Neither therapy alone offers similar benefit. Preoperative (neoadjuvant) therapy remains somewhat controversial in patients with resectable disease.

TABLE 3   Staging for Rectal Cancer

Stage
Tumor (T)
Node status (N)
Distant metastases (M)
I
T1: invasion into submucosa
T2: invasion into muscularis propria
N0: no regional lymph node metastases
M0: no distant metastases
IIa
IIb
T3: invasion into subserosa
T4: invasion of adjacent structures or organs and/or perforation of visceral peritoneum
N0
M0
IIIa
IIIb
IIIc
T1-2
T3-4
N1: mets to 1–3 regional nodes
M0
Any T
N2: mets to e□ nodes
IV
Any T
Any N
M1: distant metastases: mets to ≥4 nodes
IV
Any T
Any N
M1: distant metastases

73. A. The marker for familial adenomatous polyposis (FAP) is the adenomatous polyposis coli (APC) tumor suppressor gene. The p53 tumor suppressor gene predicts whether Barrett's esophagus will progress to esophageal cancer. Programmed cell death (apoptosis) in breast cancer is affected by presence of the bcl-2 gene, probably in conjunction with p53. BRCA1 and -2 are genes that predispose to breast cancer, probably through enhanced oncogenesis. The RET proto-oncogene is associated with medullary thyroid cancer and the MEN syndrome.

74. E. Adenocarcinoma is the most common small bowel malignancy in industrialized countries. Peak age incidence is in the 60s, with a slight male predominance. There is an increased incidence in patients with familial adenomatous polyposis (FAP), Peutz-Jeghers syndrome, and Crohn's disease. Presenting symptoms include pain, weight loss, obstruction, anemia, and heme-positive stools. Tumors typically occur in the duodenum and proximal jejunum, and tend to appear as constricting "apple-core"–type lesions. This is in contrast to carcinoid tumors, which typically occur as small, submucosal nodules. Five-year survival for small bowel adenocarcinoma is 15%–20%. Neither chemotherapy nor radiation has been shown to effectively prolong survival.

75. C. Elevated 5-HIAA levels are seen in patients with carcinoid tumors, though relatively few (approximately 10%) will ever manifest a "carcinoid syndrome" (flushing, diarrhea, palpitations). 50% of all carcinoids occur in the appendix, and approximately 25% in the distal ileum; the rest occur throughout the GI tract.

76. A. Keloids extend beyond the original area of skin injury, whereas hypertrophic scar remains within the boundaries of the original wound. Hypertrophic scars tend to regress with time, while keloids remain elevated. Both scars are more commonly seen on the trunk and shoulders, and are typically seen in patients aged 10–30 years. Keloids may be treated with steroid injection into the wound, but recurrence is common.

77. B. Epidural anesthesia is delivered by way of a micro-catheter introduced into the epidural space. Symptom relief is achieved by continuous infusion of local anesthetics and opiates. Known complications include hypotension, bradycardia, mental status changes, respiratory depression, nausea, vomiting, and epidural hematoma. Several studies have shown that epidural anesthesia reduces the length of postoperative ileus, perhaps due to a decreased requirement for systemic opiates. Patients may be allowed to get out of bed and ambulate with an epidural in place.

78. D. Perioperative beta-adrenergic blockade has been shown to reduce both cardiac and all-cause mortality for up to 2 years following operation in patients who are at high-risk for perioperative cardiac events. Ideally, beta-blockade is started preoperatively, and is continued for up to 30 days postoperatively. The goal heart rate is 55–70 beats per minute. Neither calcium channel blockers nor nitroglycerine have been shown to similarly decrease the rate of postoperative cardiac events. Bradycardia, rather than hypotension, has been cited as an occasional problem, though treatment to correct it is rarely required.

79. C. Thoracic outlet syndrome (TOS) is defined as the symptomatic compression of the neurovascular bundle at the thoracic outlet. Patients may have symptoms related to compression of any of the components of the bundle—arterial, venous, or neural. This patient likely has venous TOS, and diagnosis can be made by duplex ultrasound to demonstrate an upper extremity deep venous thrombosis. A CXR may also be performed to identify an anomalous, or cervical, rib. Treatment consists of anticoagulation initially, although thrombolysis can be considered if symptoms are persistent or severe. Exploration, anterior scalenectomy, and first rib resection may be considered following thrombolysis.

80. E. Popliteal artery entrapment occurs when there is an anomalous anatomic relationship between the gastrocnemius muscle and the popliteal artery. Ninety percent of patients are men. The most common variation in this syndrome is with the artery running medial to the medial head of the gastrocnemius. This leads to compression of the artery with muscle contraction. Physical exam can suggest the diagnosis whether positional pulse changes are present, but MRI/MRA is the test of choice. Treatment requires popliteal exploration and release of the compressive musculotendinous bands.

81. D. Leg bypass with greater saphenous vein (GSV) has excellent long-term patency (>75% at 5 years); however, only 1/3 of patients will have a single, dominant vein. The lesser saphenous vein can also be used but obviously is of limited length. The cephalic vein is the longest vein in the arm and may be considered when the GSV has already been used for other procedures. Synthetic conduits, made of either PTFE or Dacron, have moderate long-term patency (40%–60% at 5 years) but may be necessary when no autogenous conduit is available. Cryopreserved cadaveric GSV is an option but has similar patency rates to synthetic grafts and is expensive.

82. A. SVC syndrome occurs when there is stenosis or occlusion of the SVC or its branches (subclavian, innominate, or jugular veins). Long-term dialysis catheters placed in the subclavian vein are now the most common cause of central venous stenosis/thrombosis. Therefore, the subclavian vein should not be used for dialysis catheter access unless absolutely necessary.

83. B. Primary vascular infections occur when septic emboli lodge in the wall of a native vessel. This is in contrast to secondary infections of prosthetic bypass grafts. The most common causes of primary infection are trauma, endocarditis, and contiguous seeding. The abdominal aorta is the most frequent location, followed by the femoral artery. Signs and symptoms include elevated white count, positive blood cultures, fever, localized pain, and palpable pulsatile mass.

84. D. Non-selective portosystemic shunts conduct all visceral venous outflow to the IVC and completely divert portal flow from the liver. In contrast, selective shunts maintain mesenteric venous blood flow to the liver. Both are effective in decompressing esophageal varices and preventing variceal bleeding, but nonselective shunts have a much higher incidence of encephalopathy and progressive hepatic failure.

85. D. The left iliac vein runs posterior to the right iliac artery on its way to join the right iliac vein and form the inferior vena cava.

86. B. Delayed primary closure should ideally be performed within 2–4 days, after granulation tissue has started to form but before wound contracture begins. Closure beyond 10 days postoperative is associated with higher rates of wound infection, so healing by secondary intention should be allowed at that point. DPC can be done with local anesthesia only using sutures or steristrips, or if sutures were placed at the time of surgery, no anesthesia may be needed.

87. C. The first stage of healing is inflammation, which involves the processes of hemostasis and cellular migration/recruitment. Initially, neutrophils accumulate, but by two to three days, monocytes predominate. Epithelialization is accomplished by the basal cells at the wound margins and is usually completed within 48 hours. This provides a barrier to bacteria, albeit a thin, relatively weak one. Fibroplasia marks the beginning of the proliferative phase of healing, where fibroblasts replace monocytes around day five as the primary cell type in the wound. Collagen production is maximized at day five and continues for more than six weeks. Maturation or remodeling completes the wound healing process and lasts for months to years. Wound tensile strength approximates 80% of normal at six weeks but never regains that of unwounded skin. Sun protective measures are recommended for at least the first six months to prevent hyperpigmentation of the scar.

88. A. Preoperative radiation is associated with slow healing, increased risk of infection, and reduced wound tensile strength. Moreover, risk of skin necrosis is higher due to the impaired vascularity in irradiated skin.

89. E. Fascial dehiscence occurs in 1% of abdominal operations, usually 4–14 days postoperatively. When accompanied by evisceration of abdominal contents, this is a surgical emergency. An incisional hernia is defined by fascial disruption with intact peritoneum, subcutaneous tissue and skin. Incisional tension is proportional to its length; therefore, longer incisions are at greater risk of dehiscence. Suture problems, such as suture breakage, knot failure, and excessive stitch interval, can be a factor. Fascial necrosis can also occur, leading to suture pulling through the fascia. Fascial necrosis may result from infection, or sutures placed too close to the fascial edge or drawn too tightly causing local tissue ischemia. A dehisced wound should be immediately covered with a moist dressing and binder and then explored in the operating room. All devitalized tissue should be debrided and the fascia reclosed with reinforcing retention sutures. The use of retention sutures at the initial operation should be considered in patients at high risk for dehiscence (i.e., obesity, radiation).

90. A. Esophageal atresia with or without TEF is a common congenital anomaly (1 in 4,500 live births). The most common (85%) is EA with distal TEF, where the esophageal gap is usually only 1–2 cm and the TEF joins the trachea at the carina. EA with proximal TEF is rare (1%), while pure EA is found in 8%–10% and is usually associated with a long esophageal gap. EA with both proximal and distal TEF accounts for 2%, while TEF without EA occurs in 4–5% (the TEF most commonly originates from the cervical esophagus). Repair is usually performed through a right posterolateral thoracotomy with extrapleural dissection. Complications include anastomotic leak, recurrent fistula, stricture, reflux, dysphagia, and tracheomalacia. >40% of patients with EA will have other congenital anomalies; the most well-known is the VACTERL syndrome (vertebral, anorectal, cardiac, tracheoesophageal, renal, and limb).

91. B. Omphalocele (1 in 5,000 live births) is a midline abdominal wall defect where a peritoneal/amniotic sac contains the abdominal viscera (often liver and nonrotated bowel). It is associated with other congenital anomalies in 30%–70%. Gastroschisis, in contrast, is twice as common, usually much smaller, occurs through a right paramedian abdominal wall defect, and has no sac. Other congenital anomalies are unusual. The herniated contents are nonrotated bowel but not liver, and amniotic peritonitis is ubiquitous. Repair is urgent, and postoperative ileus is often prolonged.

92. **B.** Operative repair of congenital diaphragmatic hernia (CDH) is deferred until the baby is stabilized and has no or minimal pulmonary hypertension. A sump gastric tube should be placed to minimize bowel distention, which could further compress the contralateral lung and heart. Peak inspiratory pressures should be kept <35 mmHg, if possible, and ECMO would be indicated in this case for inadequate oxygenation or ventilation despite maximal ventilatory support. A left-sided chest tube is not needed and would risk bowel injury. CDH affects 1 in 2,000 live births and, nowadays, is often diagnosed prenatally by ultrasound. Fetal intervention is a possibility in severe cases. CDH results from a failure of the components of the diaphragm to fuse, particularly posterolaterally (foramen of Bochdalek), and occurs on the left side in 90%. It is associated with other congenital anomalies in 20%. Pulmonary hypoplasia is not uncommon and is due to compression of the developing fetal lungs by abdominal contents.

93. **E.** The absence of parasympathetic ganglion cells in Hirschsprung's disease (congenital intestinal aganglionosis) begins just above the dentate line and extends proximally. There are no skipped regions, and the length of bowel involved varies. Most cases (75%) involve only the rectosigmoid colon, while 5% affect the whole colon and another 5% involve small bowel. The affected areas are unable to relax and therefore create a functional obstruction. Biopsies are taken of the mucosa and submucosa at least 1 cm proximal to the dentate line. Manometry and colonoscopy are not performed in neonates but can be done in older children who often present with chronic constipation. Treatment is surgical and involves resection of the affected bowel and a pull-through procedure to restore intestinal continuity.

94. **C.** All fluids given to a pediatric trauma patient should be warmed, as infants and children can lose body heat rapidly.

95. **C.** The patient gets 2 points for eye opening, 3 for verbal response, and 4 for motor response.

96. B. Zone I is the thoracic outlet, defined by the area of the neck below the cricoid cartilage and the sternal notch. Zone II extends from the cricoid to the angle of the mandible. Zone III is above the angle of the mandible to the base of the skull. Stable patients with stab wounds to Zones I and III should be evaluated with arteriography, as repair in these areas is difficult and requires careful planning. Injuries to Zone II have traditionally been managed with exploration in the operating room, although more recently initial evaluation of stable patients with neck CT has been reported. Zone II injuries that penetrate the platysma should have complete evaluation of the esophagus and trachea after surgical exploration (i.e., laryngoscopy, bronchoscopy, and esophagoscopy).

97. A. Primary spontaneous pneumothorax is most common in tall young men and is thought to be due to rupture of subpleural blebs. Smokers are more likely than nonsmokers to have spontaneous pneumothoraces. Chemical pleurodesis can be effective but is still associated with a 7%–25% recurrence rate. Video-assisted thoracoscopic resection of blebs is now the procedure of choice in treating spontaneous pneumothorax.

98. B. Hyperacute rejection occurs within the first minutes to hours of transplant and is caused by donor-specific antibodies (or significantly cross-reactive antibodies) already present in the recipient's serum. Prior sensitization is usually the result of previous transplant, pregnancy, or blood-product transfusion. It can ly be avoided by an adequate preoperative crossmatch and blood typing. A panel reactive antibody assay (PRA) can also be med; this screens recipients against random donor cells to an estimate of sensitization. Acute rejection is T-cell mediated occurs most often within the first six months of transplant specific inhibition is a standard part of post-transplant nd prevents acute rejection in 40%–70% of patients. jection does occur, prompt recognition and treatse the process in most cases. Monitoring for acute ticularly rigorous in the first year after transplant ires tissue biopsy. Chronic rejection occurs over and is characterized by the gradual replacement of ous tissue. It has no effective treatment.

nly used antiproliferative agents are azathioprine ophenolate mofetil (Cellcept). Calcinuerin inhibitors ine and tacrolimus. The antilymphocyte globulins re ATGAM and thymoglobulin; both are polyclonal ed from horse and rabbit, respectively. OKT3 is a murine monoclonal antibody targeting the CD3 signal transduction subunit on T-cells. Anti-IL-2 receptor drugs are the newest monoclonal preparations, which target CD25 on the IL-2 receptor of activated T-cells.

100. B. Carotid body tumors are located in the adventitia, are highly vascular, and may often be treated with embolization prior to resection. Needle biopsy is contraindicated due to bleeding risk. Tumors should be resected despite their typically benign histology, because the natural history is one of gradual growth and encasement of the carotid artery and surrounding cranial nerves. Cranial nerve injury is the most common complication of resection and occurs in up to 40%.

Index

Page numbers followed by *f* or *t* indicate figures or tables, respectively.

Pneumothorax (*Cont.*)
  diagnostic evaluation, 171–172,
    171*f*, 174
  etiology, 172, 173–174
  management, 170–171, 369
  spontaneous, 369, 400
Poikilothermia, 207
Poiseuille's law, 277
Popliteal artery entrapment, 365, 396
Portal hypertension, 80–81
Portosystemic shunts, 366, 397
Postoperative care
  fever, 270–272, 274
  hypoxia, 264–266
  pain management, 266
  respiratory symptoms, 321
Pregnancy
  cholecystitis in, 355, 382
  hepatic adenoma in, 110
Preoperative considerations
  anesthesia selection, 259–260
  beta blockade, 365, 396
  cardiac risk evaluation, 268, 268*t*
  medication schedule, 361, 388
  radiation therapy effects, 367, 398
Prilocaine, 262
Primary sclerosing cholangitis, 39
Prinzmetal's angina, 191–192
Procidentia. *See* Rectal prolapse
Prostate cancer
  diagnostic evaluation, 307
  grading, 308–309
  incidence, 359, 387, 392
  management, 307
  risk factors, 307, 392
  survival rates, 308–309
Prostate enlargement, 307
Prosthetic valves, 186
Proton pump inhibitors, 350, 377
Pseudo-obstruction, colonic, 351, 377
Pseudocyst, pancreatic, 28, 28*f*,
    354, 381
Psoas sign, 383
Pulmonary artery catheter, 323
Pulmonary embolism, 274–275
Pulse volume recording, 204
Pyloric stenosis
  clinical presentation, 102–103

diagnostic evaluation, 103
management, 104
pathophysiology, 105

Quincke sign, 185

Radiation therapy, preoperative,
    367, 398
Ranson's criteria, acute
    pancreatitis, 27, 27*t*
Rectal bleeding, 86–87
Rectal cancer, 363, 393, 394*t*. *See
    also* Colorectal cancer
Rectal prolapse, 98, 351, 377–388
Rectovaginal fistula, 38
Regional anesthesia, 260
Renal cell carcinoma
  clinical presentation, 160, 308–309
  diagnostic evaluation, 158
  management, 159–161
  metastatic spread, 160
  risk factors, 161
  screening, 161
Renal laceration, 363, 392
Renal mass
  clinical presentation, 156–157
  diagnostic evaluation, 157–158
  differential diagnosis, 157
Respiratory quotient, 280
Rest pain, 206
RET proto-oncogene, 395
Reynold's pentad, 12
Rinne test, 313–314
Rovsing's sign, 383

Saphenofemoral junction ligation,
    222
Scintigraphy
  technetium-labeled red blood cell,
    89, 109
  technetium-labeled sulfur
    colloid, 109
Sclerotherapy, 222
Scrotal varicocele, 156–159
Segmental pressures, 204
Seminoma
  clinical presentation, 152
  diagnostic evaluation, 153